Oxford Medical Publications

Geriatric consultation liaison psychiatry

Geriatric consultation liaison psychiatry

Edited by

Pamela S. Melding

Consultant in Psychiatry of Old Age
Waitemata District Health Board, North Shore Hospital, Takapuna, Auckland 10,
New Zealand

Honorary Senior Lecturer in Psychiatry of Old Age
Division of Psychiatry and Behavioural Science, Faculty of Medicine and Health Science,
University of Auckland, New Zealand

and

Brian Draper

Assistant Director and Senior Staff Specialist
Academic Department for Old Age Psychiatry, Prince of Wales Hospital, Randwick,
NSW 2031, Australia

Conjoint Senior Lecturer
School of Psychiatry and School of Community Medicine, University of New South
Wales, Sydney, Australia

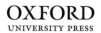
OXFORD
UNIVERSITY PRESS

OXFORD
UNIVERSITY PRESS

Great Clarendon Street, Oxford OX2 6DP

Oxford University Press is a department of the University of Oxford.
It furthers the University's objective of excellence in research, scholarship, and
education by publishing worldwide in

Oxford New York Athens Auckland Bangkok Bogotá Bombay Buenos Aires
Calcutta Cape Town Dar es Salaam Delhi Florence Hong Kong Istanbul Karachi
Kuala Lumpur Madrid Melbourne Mexico City Mumbai Nairobi Paris São Paulo
Shanghai Singapore Taipei Tokyo Toronto Warsaw
and associated companies in Berlin Ibadan

Oxford is a registered trade mark of Oxford University Press in the UK and in
certain other countries

Published in the United States
by Oxford University Press Inc., New York

© Oxford University Press, 2001

The moral rights of the authors have been asserted

Database right Oxford University Press (maker)

First published 2001

British Library Cataloguing in Publication Data

Data available

Library of Congress Cataloging in Publication Data

Geriatric consultation liaison psychiatry/edited by Pamela S. Melding and Brian Draper.
   p. ; cm. — (Oxford medical publications)
   Includes bibliographical references and index.
   1. Geriatric psychiatry. 2. Consultation-liaison psychiatry. I. Melding, Pamela S.
   II. Draper, Brian. III. Series.
   [DNLM: 1. Mental Disorders—therapy—Aged—Great Britain. 2. Geriatric Psychiatry—
Great Britain. 3. Psychiatric Department, Hospital—Aged—Great Britain.
4. Referral and Consultation—Aged—Great Britain. WM 400 G369 2001]
RC451.4.A5 G463 2001   618.97′689—dc21   2001032141

ISBN 0 19 263084 9 (Pbk)

10 9 8 7 6 5 4 3 2 1

Typeset by Phoenix Photosetting, Chatham, Kent
Printed in Great Britain
on acid-free paper by Biddles Ltd, Guildford & King's Lynn

To Debbie and to the memory of Alice

Foreword

The challenge and the thrill of old age psychiatry is its complexity—the interplay between multiple physical, psychological and social factors in the cause of mental disorders and in their treatment. Psychogeriatrics is not simply linear, where cause leads to disease from which follows treatment. The practice of psychiatry of old age requires the clinician to think in terms of interacting forces in many dimensions.

> An 86 year old man is for the first time in his life in tears, wishing he were dead and not coping. He has been experiencing severe arthritic pain limiting mobility and independence, change in family dynamics consequent to his wife's declining cognitive abilities, recently diagnosed hypertension requiring new medication and deteriorating financial circumstances.

This man has a myriad of reasons to be depressed and a single line of therapy, such as antidepressant medication, may be appropriate but in itself is hardly likely to be sufficient. Yet another lay of complexity is added when the man is admitted to hospital for his chest pain. He becomes fearful of death and preoccupied with concerns about the care of his wife. The nurses report that he is irritable and demanding, refuses to eat and is suspicious of what 'they are doing to (him)' and he is non-compliant with the doctors' recommendations.

This is the stuff of consultation liaison old age psychiatry. Extra dimensions of complexity have developed: the relationship of the elderly man to his doctors, his interaction with the nurses, their reaction to him – ambivalence, concern and resentment at his behaviour, and the need to ensure that the wife is safe at home.

Call in the CL psychogeriatrician. How can this man's predicament be best understood? Where should intervention be directed? Pharmacotherapy for his depression? Supportive therapy for, counselling or reassurance of the patient? Involvement of his extended family in the care of the patient and his wife? Discussion with and education of his nurses to help them develop ways of coping? Cardiac rehabilitation? Or inevitably, a combination of all? What if ECT is indicated? Is it safe given his recent cardiac history? And has he given informed consent? What if he states that he wishes to die? What are the ethics of intervention?

This excellent book concisely and practically provides a scholarly exposition of these and many other topics. It is timely to bring together the infant disciplines of CL and old age psychiatry. Older patients occupy almost half the bed days of general hospitals; and compared to their younger counterparts stay in hospital longer, have more complications, have more side effects from medications, exhibit more behavioural disturbances and pose more ethical dilemmas.

Specialties develop when there is sufficient new knowledge for a bud to break off from the main body or when there is evidence of inadequate standards of care by the mainstream medical practice. Medicine witnessed such a development in the second half of the 20th century as *Geriatrics* took its place on the clinical stage. Psychiatry has witnessed similar developments in its child and adolescent, forensic, consultation-liaison and now psychogeriatric branches. Should there be now a separate specialty of CL PG? Probably not, but there is an accumulating body of knowledge that will be useful to the CL psychiatrist attending older patients and for the psychogeriatrician. This book is relevant to clinicians caring for older people in general hospitals, nursing homes and other settings and for those practicing at the interface between psychiatry and old age medicine.

The pressure for the knowledge and skills described in this volume is set to intensify as the world population ages, as the proportion of the very old rises spectacularly, as life expectancy lengthens and as what was accepted as just old age becomes increasingly medicalised. Fancifully, we have reached midnight and this volume heralds the emergence of these two Cinderella subspecialties into adulthood if not quite a hybrid princess.

Professor Henry Brodaty
University of New South Wales   July 2001

Introduction

This book is a first. It was the only book on geriatric consultation liaison psychiatry retrieved by a recent literature search, and appropriately, it was listed as 'not yet available'. Whenever there is a first, in education and training, in medicine as well as in other disciplines, the question arises: Is it necessary? As always, I am reminded of a meeting half a century ago, when one of the most eminent leaders of United States medicine was asked to comment about the then newly emerging field of geriatric medicine. In his response, he stated, in no uncertain terms, that he could see no reason for fostering its development. After all, internists and internal medicine sub specialists already had the highest degree of expertise, since their practices consisted of a large proportion of older patients. Since that time, that proportion has continued to increase with the aging of the population and, as pointed out in the very first chapter of this volume, during the last 15 years, the proportion of elderly referrals to consultation liaison services in the United States increased from 20%–30% to over 50%.

These days, the need for special training in geriatric medicine is rarely questioned. Nevertheless, according to a recent count, just one of the 127 Medical Schools in the United States had an established department of geriatric medicine (Rowe,1997). By comparison, every Medical School in the United Kingdom has such a department. Since only about '100 physicians annually complete fellowships in geriatric medicine or geriatric psychiatry—3 percent of all physicians taking fellowship training in internal medicine' (Rowe,1997), the pool of physicians trained in geriatric medicine in the United States is unlikely to show rapid growth in the immediate future.

Geriatric psychiatry and consultation liaison psychiatry both developed during the second half of the 20th century in the United States. Old age psychiatry in the United Kingdom and the Commonwealth has had a much longer history. Those of us across the oceans have greatly benefited from their experience.

Geriatric consultation liaison psychiatry is still in an early stage of development, but considering the fact that in many countries up to half of inpatients are over the age of 65 years, the appearance of this volume is well timed. With increasing numbers of geriatric patients throughout the world straining health care resources, a book devoted to geriatric consultation liaison psychiatry, which brings together information from diverse sources into one readable volume meets a clear need.

In my opinion, this book fulfills an unmet need not only for consultation liaison psychiatrists, but also for trainees and practitioners in other specialties, especially geriatric medicine, internal medicine and its subspecialties, psychiatry, geriatric psychiatry and other medical specialties, and particularly for primary care physicians. In addition, it will be a most valuable reference also for members of other health professions who provide services for geriatric patients in general hospitals. Nursing, occupational and physical therapy, as well as social work are obvious examples.

The editors, Pamela Melding and Brian Draper, bringing together expertise from consultation liaison psychiatry and geriatric psychiatry, have organized the material into 3 sections and 16 chapters. The sections are: Issues in Assessment (Chapters 1–5), Important Disorders (Chapters 6–11) and Aspects of Treatment (Chapters 12–16).

The chapters provide information culled from research throughout the world. Many of the authors go beyond presenting the data to include critical evaluation of the findings. Nearly all chapters have extensive, up-to-date and carefully selected reference lists, and several chapters include informative tables, illustrations and case studies. The summaries are a welcome feature for the busy reader.

The book is as relevant for readers in the United States as it is for those dwelling in other parts of the English-speaking world. Actually, it is probably more relevant because of the exposure it provides to perspectives other than North American. Books widely used in consultation-liaison psychiatry often represent the national perspective with authors almost exclusively from the United States, and in one text-book predominantly from one area of that country (Cassem et al, 1997), with a few contributions from Canada (Stoudemire et al, 2000). Sometimes, as in Rundell et al., (1996) there is a chapter or so giving an international perspective.

None of the texts cited above has a chapter dealing with geriatric psychiatry, although one has a chapter on geriatric medicine authored by geriatric psychiatrists (Rundell et al,1996). In another book (Stoudemire et al, 2000), lack of emphasis on geriatric psychiatry stands in contrast to three chapters devoted to medically ill children and adolescents. Searching the indices of these books for entries to older patients tends to be relatively unrewarding. For example, in one book with over 600 pages (Cassem et al, 1997), I found only eight pages cited in the index . Another yielded 14 pages out of over 1200 for 'age, aging, elder, geriatric, old' (Stoudemire et al, 2000). So, an entire volume devoted to this age group is most welcome.

In the first chapter, co-editor Brian Draper gives a concise overview of geriatric consultation liaison psychiatry and provides an analysis of published data on service provision from which he concludes: 'Service provision by general CL psychiatry mainly occurs in North America', 'and by geriatric psychiatry in the UK and Europe'. His careful approach is illustrated by his tabular material. For example, table 1 contains information on CL Psychiatry Services reported from 28 studies over the 15-year period (1976–2000). They are compared by categories listing service type, sample size reported, age and gender of patients, sample features (e.g.

12-month retrospective), psychiatric history, referring service, reasons for referral, psychiatric diagnoses, and management recommendations. Of the 28 studies, ten are from the United States, seven from the United Kingdom, two each from Australia, Canada and Ireland, and one each from Hong Kong, Italy, the Netherlands, Sweden and Switzerland. This material constitutes a valuable resource. Among Draper's conclusions is the following: 'Formal service evaluation has found that the benefits of geriatric psychiatry CL services include reduction in lengths of hospital stay and costs, increase in depression recognition, improved physical functioning, fewer nursing home transfers and increased utilization of community services post-discharge.'

The second chapter, in contrast to the data-filled first chapter, takes the reader through a bird's eye view of the complex landscape encompassed by the title, 'The Effects of Ageing'. Even for someone like myself, who has a fair knowledge of the field, Pamela Melding's well-written chapter—objectively evaluating facts, theories and speculation—can provide valuable information about patients in the last decades of their lives. The third chapter, 'Coping with Illness in Late Life', which she co-authored with Andrew Cook, examines coping mechanisms as well as variables that enhance or compromise coping with illness. Three case studies illustrate different compromising factors. In Chapter 4, a geriatric medicine perspective is presented by Philip Wood. He uses two case studies to illustrate the importance of a team approach with input from both geriatricians and geriatric consultation liaison psychiatrists. Chapter 5, co-authored by Draper and Melding completes the first section with a thorough discussion of procedures for assessment (e.g. harm, medical and psychiatric conditions, ward environment, urgency of referral is laid out in table 1). Several case studies illustrate the authors' view that 'Assessment is the linchpin of quality service delivery in geriatric liaison psychiatry.' Potential barriers to com-munication with older patients range from the language difficulties of an immigrant, to the conviction of a physician-in-training that his 85-year-old demented patient had begun to hallucinate, until the psychiatrist arrived and actually saw the 'hallucina-tory' cockroaches crawling over the bed!

The six chapters in Section III are devoted to specific types of mental disorders seen in geriatric consultation liaison psychiatry, starting with Affective Disorders (Mavis Evans, chapter 6), Anxiety (Alastair Flint, chapter 7) and Somatoform Disorders in Late Life (Pamela Melding and Louise Armstrong, chapter 8). These are followed by Psychosis and Medical Illness (Osvaldo Almeida, chapter 9) with further discussion of Organic Mental Disorders (David Taylor and Ajit Shah, chapter 10) and ending with a most useful sampling of Specific Patients and Problems (Ajit Shah, chapter 11). Going through these six chapters, I believe, will offer every reader a fruitful experience. Some chapters emphasize facts and nosology, some concen-trate on diagnostic issues, some add literary spice, some devote much attention to treatment and care. There are useful cautions, for example, '... a diagnosis of pain disorder, which implies that the medical condition plays a lesser role than the psychological factors, is potentially an unsafe diagnosis.'(chapter 8). In addition, there is a warning to those managing psychotic patients on general medical wards, that the '... "plots" to get rid of patients do not only take place in their' (the patients') 'imagination–consultation requests are frequently used to persuade the psychiatrist to take responsibility for the care of psychiatric patients and move them to psychiatric wards.' (chapter 9) Or, the observation that in a 'meta-analysis of the naturalistic outcomes of depression in eight studies of elderly medical inpatients', '... the study that reported the best outcomes was one in which all depressed patients were treated and followed up by the investigator' (chapter 6). As most cases of late-onset generalized anxiety are associated with depression, it behooves us to remember that '... antidepressant medication, not a benzodiazepine, is the primary pharmacological treatment of generalized anxiety associated with depression.' (chapter 7). Not everyone may be familiar with the approach expressed in chapter 10 that, not only should the diagnosis, management plan and possible sequelae of delirium be provided to the relatives and the medical team, but during lucid periods, to the patients themselves. In the same chapter, we find the following observation on dementia: 'Although the issue of genetic counselling in the liaison context is un-common, well read or internet familiar patients and families are increasingly assertive in seeking information and advice on genetic risk to family members.' I can testify to the importance of this observation having heard from trainees unable to respond to such questions, that they turned to a supervisor for help only to find the latter less well informed than the patient! As a final comment, I want to point out that many authors evaluate evidence supporting clinical practices, and they generally agree that in the treatment of behavioral disturbances, the efficacy of various psycho-tropic drugs is unclear. For example, in chapter 11, there is the statement: 'It is not clear whether they (neuroleptics) reduce behaviour disturbance or simply sedate the patient.' There is also general consensus as to the clinical impression that non-pharmacological treatments of behavioral disturbances can be helpful, but that data for geriatric medical inpatients are notable for their absence.

Indeed, in this era of rapidly advancing knowledge in neuropsychopharma-cology—in the presence of extraordinary pressures to reduce health care expenditures, geriatric consultation liaison psychiatry, like geriatric psychiatry and liaison psychiatry, as well as mainstream psychiatry, rarely recommends non-pharmacological interventions as first-line treatment. Appropriately, an extensive discussion of Psychopharmacological Management of the Medically Ill Older Person (Alastair Flint, chapter 12) opens the third section, and is followed by ECT in Older Patients with Physical Illness (James Tew, Benoit Mulsant and Adele Towers, chapter 13). This chapter contains details of ECT administration and physiologic response, taking into account also the impact of cardiac, neurological and other disorders. In addition, the chapter contains recommendations for evaluations required before initiating ECT in an older patient with physical illness. The next chapter, which is the last chapter devoted to treatment approaches, examines Non-Biological Therapies (Julia Payne and Ken Wilson, chapter 14), and encompasses a wide range of them from psychotherapies to less structured psychosocial, supportive and other interventions. Although their examination of the state of the field is, as they put it, '... far from exhaustive and highly selective in the interventions and evidence examined', it does provide persuasive evidence that non-biological therapies have a place in '... non-psychiatric settings and work with physically ill, older people.'

The last two chapters are devoted to ethical and legal issues in geriatric consultation liaison psychiatry. Ethical Issues in Geriatric Psychiatry Liaison (Christine Perkins, chapter 15) examines in depth issues of particular relevance to geriatric consultation liaison psychiatry such as end of life decisions, the role of the family, and advocacy. Many questions are raised, not all have the answers we would like.

The final chapter, A Legal Perspective on Issues in Geriatric Liaison Psychiatry (Hanneke Bouchier, chapter 16) written by a lawyer and health law consultant in Auckland, New Zealand, concentrates on competency of patients with psychiatric disorders to consent to medical and surgical treatment and legal mental capacity. The author emphasizes that those '... involved with the medical care or treatment of geriatric psychiatric patients need to become familiar with the locally applicable laws and procedures. Medical practitioners need to be familiar with statutory provisions which apply in the country and place where they work.' She points out '... law is a matter for each sovereign state, and unlike medicine, sovereign laws have no universal application. Nevertheless, there is considerable uniformity in the substantive principles in the western world even where administrative processes differ.' After reading her chapter, I agree. I was surprised by the extent to which the opinions expressed by someone halfway around the world, could sound so familiar.

At the end, readers from outside the Commonwealth who have looked at all of the chapters will be impressed how similar to their own are the experiences described in this volume. Aging humans have much in common, especially when stricken by physical illness, and yet, at the same time there are great cultural as well as individual differences in their responses to the trauma—just as there are at any other age.

This volume is bound to become a useful resource to physicians and other health professionals from a wide variety of disciplines, regardless of their training, background and orientation, and no matter what their patients' socio-cultural milieu.

References

1. Rundell, J.R. and Wise, M.G. (1996). Textbook of Consultation Liaison Psychiatry, American Psychiatric Press, Washington,D.C.
2. Cassem, N.H., Stern, T.A., Rosenbaum, J.F., and Jellinek, M.S. (1997). Massachusetts General Hospital Handbook of General Hospital Psychiatry. Mosby, St.Louis.

3. Stoudemire, A., Fogel, B.S., and Greenberg, D. (2000). Psychiatric Care of the Medical Patient. Oxford University Press, New York.

4. Rowe, J.W. In Cassel, C.K., Cohen, H.J., Larson, E.B., Meier, D.E., Resnick, N.M., Rubinstein, L.Z., and Sorenson, L.B. (1997). Geriatric Medicine, pp.vii–ix. Springer-Verlag, New York.

Lissy Jarvik
Professor Emeritus
Department of Psychiatry and Biobehavioral Sciences
University of California, Los Angeles
and
Distinguished Physician Emeritus
US Department of Veterans Affairs   July 2001

Preface

Why have a book on geriatric consultation liaison psychiatry? There are plenty of excellent texts that cover old age psychiatry and more in the repertoire that cover consultation liaison (CL) psychiatry. However, when we started this project we could find no texts that married these two important aspects of psychiatry togethc Indeed, the idea for the book was suggested by students on an old age psychiatry training course who were frustrated at only finding scattered papers on the subject. They wanted a collection of pertinent CL psychiatry articles that would not only provide some theoretical background from the old age perspective, but also some practical guidance in dealing with the issues they confronted daily on hospital wards. That suggestion prompted this volume.

So, is CL psychiatry different in a geriatric population? Well, no and yes! The *principles* of geriatric CL psychiatry are no different. Irrespective of the age of the patient, the CL psychiatrist deals with patients who have mental disorders, in the context of an unfamiliar medical system, and aims to provide effective advice and treatment using non-psychiatric staff. However, the *problems* have a different intricacy in comparison to those of younger adults, with the added dimensions of the ageing process, increased vulnerability to degenerative diseases, together with relatively rapid and major changes leading to a need for major psychological adjustments in many aspects of living. The *practice* of Geriatric CL Psychiatry is also quite different. In the older age groups the emphasis is on care not cure. Not only are the patients assessed within a wider system, but their subsequent care needs to be undertaken by an extended group. Few patients would be treated outside a family or caregiving context. All this adds up to a complexity that Philip Wood, a geriatrician, describes in Chapter 4 as a 'Technicolor' representation of adult consultation liaison psychiatry.

All psychiatrists, but particularly those in old age or consultation liaison training schemes, need to develop expertise in geriatric consultation liaison psychiatry. As the world ages, so do hospital populations. Most physical illness affects people at the extremes of life, but especially in late life. In addition to people admitted to geriatric assessment, treatment, and rehabilitation units, a considerable number of the patients in general medical and surgical wards are over 65 years of age. With greater longevity the spectrum of disease is also changing, with the increasing emergence of degenerative diseases that can be associated with significant mental health or psychological adjustment problems. Addressing such problems in a comprehensive management plan shortens patient episodes of care and improves overall outcome. Yet, older people are less likely to be referred to liaison psychiatry services for a variety of reasons, ranging from subtle ageism to an inability to meet their needs. Not all general hospitals have specialist psychiatry services for older people. Hospital and medical units lacking specialist geriatric psychiatry services largely rely on adult psychiatry CL services for geriatric referrals. Accordingly, the generalist CL psychiatrist has to take over the role of a geriatric CL psychiatrist by default. Consultation and liaison psychiatric services to medical, surgical, and geriatric units have value not only for treating patients holistically, but also have the added value of forging productive and co-operative relationships with other medical disciplines.

Consultation and liaison psychiatry is complex. It requires sound medical knowledge as well as psychiatric ability, psychotherapeutic wisdom, an astute comprehension of human and organizational systems, and the resilience required of intrepid pioneers who venture into unknown and alien territory! Indeed, a few years ago a psychiatrist colleague (Dr Jeremy Anderson, of the University of Melbourne) used the metaphor of the Fool as depicted in the Tarot, as portraying the Consultation Liaison Psychiatrist. The 'fool', open, spontaneous, and fresh but standing in his own universe outside the mainstream 'pack', observes what others cannot see, embraces whatever problems come his way, but seems simultaneously oblivious of the abyss he is about to cross! In many ways this metaphor aptly captures the complex role of the consultation liaison psychiatrist.

This volume is intended to increase the confidence of those who dare to cross the geriatric medical 'abyss', by providing some theoretical and contextual background to the assessment of the medically ill older person and to providing some practical guidance for the treatment of older patients with psychiatric problems in medical, surgical, or geriatric wards. Case studies and adapted patient stories are used in many of the chapters to illustrate some of the issues. Hopefully, the reader should recognize and relate to many of these case studies as typical of patients they come across on medical wards, since they have mostly been adapted from our contributors' own clinical experiences.

The book is intended for geriatric psychiatrists and CL psychiatrists and those in training for these specialties. However, the book might also provide some insights into the psychiatric aspects of geriatrics for geriatricians, including those in training. General practitioners and others in primary care, particularly those who have practices in areas with high elderly populations or who consult to nursing homes, might also find the book useful. Some material may also be of interest to the nursing, physiotherapy, or occupational-therapy staff of psychiatric and medical wards.

The book is divided into five sections. The first section covers the context of a geriatric consultation liaison referral. We have included a theoretical discussion of the current status and effectiveness of geriatric consultation liaison psychiatry services by Brian Draper from Sydney. Next come two related chapters. The first covers the effects of ageing and the interface with disease by Pamela Melding from Auckland. For the second, Andrew Cook, a clinical psychologist from the University of Virginia, Charlottesville, joins Pamela Melding in a discussion on the psychological responses to late-life disease. As the geriatric ward is the most common setting for the patient and a geriatrician is the physician most commonly involved with the consultation-liaison psychiatrist, we have included a chapter from Philip Wood, a geriatrician who has taken a special interest in the interface between psychiatry and geriatrics. He presents his view of the geriatric perspective, indicates the important areas that precipitate referrals to psychiatry, and also discusses the complementary role of the geriatrician who consults to psychiatry.

The second section has only one chapter—Assessment. This chapter is a practical 'cook-book' guide to the geriatric consultation. Space precludes us from making it comprehensive. Indeed, an entire book could possibly be devoted to this aspect alone. Accordingly, we have kept the discussion brief and practical, in keeping with the 'brief and practical' nature of a real assessment. We have kept discussion of assessment practices or investigations to those that can be completed at the bedside and do not require the full resources of a psychiatric unit or clinical psychology department.

The third section deals with specific disorders encountered in the geriatric consultation liaison setting. Mavis Evans and Pat Mottram, from the University of Liverpool and well known for their work in geriatric consultation liaison psychiatry, have contributed a chapter on depression. Acknowledged as an international expert in the field, Alastair Flint from the University of Toronto provides a 'state of the art' analysis of anxiety disorders as they present within the medical setting. The complexity of the somatoform disorders and their relationship to the affective and anxiety disorders complements the trio of 'dysphoric' disorders. Osvaldo Almeida, from the University of Western Australia, Perth, has built on his previous work in the field and contributes a careful analysis of psychotic disorders, how and why they arise in a medical setting, and the possible relationships of psychotic symptoms with the organic mental disorders. One of the commonest referrals for a geriatric consultation liaison referral is to assess the patient who is dementing or for whom this diagnosis is being entertained. David Taylor and Ajit Shah, from London, clarify the important issues in the diagnosis and treatment of these disorders. Ajit Shah teams up with David Ames from Melbourne to conclude the section, with their interesting contribution on the stranger, unfamiliar, or simply problematic syndromes seen in older people, such as senile squalor syndrome, food refusal, or patients that staff find undesirable!

Of course, what referrers want from the consultation is for the patient 'to be fixed'. Thus, an important aim of the book is to provide guidelines for the appropriate treatment of psychiatric disorders when medical illness complicates the picture. The fourth section deals with these aspects, and both biological and non-biological treatments for mental illness are discussed. Alastair Flint contributes another chapter reviewing the important aspects of psychopharmacology to be considered in the medical patient. We have also included a chapter specifically devoted to ECT, contributed by James Tew, Ben Mulsant, and Adele Towers, from the University of Pittsburgh, also acknowledged experts in this area. Geriatric consultation liaison psychiatrists are commonly requested to see patients on medical wards who have failed to respond to medical treatment and whose severe depression has been missed until it becomes life-threatening. ECT may be the only option for such patients. The chapter provides a comprehensive overview of the safety and efficacy of ECT in a variety of medical disorders. Psychotherapy is not commonly thought of as an option for most consultation liaison patients as their setting is not generally conducive to more protracted non-biological therapies. Nevertheless, many patients can start therapy whilst in this setting, or even complete briefer therapies. Some very brief techniques or psychotherapeutic interventions can be highly effective even in a short-stay or very physically ill patient. Accordingly, Julia Payne and Ken Wilson, from the University of Liverpool, have addressed what possibilities might be considered in this context. The authors have discussed a range of options from cognitive–behavioural techniques to therapy pets. This is an area where space, sadly, has had to limit the discussion of such therapies, but it is hoped the reader will be inspired to further develop their knowledge in this area.

The final section deals with some ethical and medicolegal perspectives that might arise within the geriatric consultation liaison setting. Perhaps more than all other age groups combined, the treatment of the elderly medically ill continually raises ethical issues. Patient management often has to include consideration of the need for paternalism versus a patient's autonomy, beneficence of a treatment versus any potential harm or complication, and an assessment of a patient's competence to make treatment decisions. The consultation and liaison psychiatrist for older people needs to have a sound working knowledge of all these dilemmas. Christine Perkins, an old age psychiatrist with a medical ethics background, and Hanneke Bouchier, a lawyer who has specialized in medicolegal issues, both from Auckland, discuss these important aspects.

In any book such as this one, there will be omissions and exclusions. Some topics are worthy of whole volumes in their own right but have been only dealt with briefly. However, we hope that the reader will have enough material in this volume to enable them to increase their confidence in negotiating the CL 'abyss' and to make it more an interesting traverse than an unfathomable chasm.

Many people have helped us with this project. First, we would like to thank our international contributors from the United States, the United Kingdom, Canada, Australia, and New Zealand who have generously shared their knowledge and withstood our editing process with fortitude and good humour. Second, we would like to thank Oxford University Press, and particularly Richard Marley, for the support and encouragement in bringing this book to fruition. Third, we would like to thank our colleagues, trainees, and support staff who variously have peer-reviewed, proofread, checked references, or otherwise provided constructive criticism of the work whilst in progress. In particular, we would like to thank the following: Cheryl Ackoy,

Stephanie Allison, Lisa Blake, Chris Collins, Patrick Firkin, Rafael Fraser, Marie Israel, Bede McIvor, Alice Melding, Paul Merrick, and Felicity Roche. Finally, our gratitude goes to our older patients, who have provided not only the need but also the inspiration for this book and whose stories illustrate the text.

Auckland, New Zealand
Sydney, Australia
July 2001

P.S.M.
B.D.

Contents

Contributors

Osvaldo P. Almeida Department of Psychiatry and Behavioural Science of the University of Western Australia, Queen Elizabeth II Medical Centre, Nedlands, Perth, Australia.

David Ames University of Melbourne, Parkville, Australia.

Louise Armstrong Consultant in Liaison Psychiatry, Takapuna, Auckland 10, New Zealand.

Hanneke Bouchier Fortune Manning Ltd, Price Waterhouse Centre, 66 Wyndam Street, Auckland 1, New Zealand.

Henry Brodaty Professor of Psychogeriatrics, University of New South Wales and Director of the Academic Department for Old Age Psychiatry, Prince of Wales Hospital, Sydney, Australia.

Andrew Cook Department of Anesthesiology, Division of Pain Management, University of Virginia Health System, Charlottesville, Virginia, USA.

Brian Draper Assistant Director and Senior Staff Specialist Academic Department for Old Age Psychiatry, Prince of Wales Hospital, Randwick, NSW 2031, Australia; Conjoint Senior Lecturer School of Psychiatry and School of Community Medicine, University of New South Wales, Sydney, Australia.

Mavis Evans Clinical Director of Old Age Psychiatry, Clatterbridge Hospital, Wirral, Cheshire, UK.

Alastair J. Flint Associate Professor, Department of Psychiatry, University of Toronto; Head, Geriatric Psychiatry Program, University Health Network, Toronto, Canada; Toronto General Hospital, 200 Elizabeth St, 8, Eaton North, Room 238, Toronto, Ontario M5G 2C4, Canada.

Lissy Jarvik Professor (Emeritus), Department of Psychiatry and Biobehavioral Sciences, UCLA, CA, USA.

Pamela Melding Consultant in Psychiatry of Old Age, Waitemata District Health Board, Auckland, New Zealand; Honorary Senior Lecturer in Psychiatry of Old Age, Division of Psychiatry and Behavioural Science, Faculty of Medicine and Health Science, University of Auckland, New Zealand.

Patricia Mottram Department of Psychiatry, Section of Old Age, University of Liverpool, UK.

Benoit Mulsant Western Psychiatric Institute and Clinic, Department of Psychiatry, University of Pittsburgh School of Medicine, 3811 O'Hara St, Pittsburgh, PA 15213, USA.

Julia Payne Clinical Lecturer in Psychiatry of Old Age, University of Liverpool, UK.

Christine Perkins Consultant in Psychiatry of Old Age, 2A Dodson Ave, Milford, North Shore, Auckland 10, New Zealand.

Ajit Shah Honorary Senior Lecturer in Psychiatry of Old Age, Imperial College School of Medicine, London, UK.

David Taylor Consultant Psychiatrist, Ealing, John Connolly Wing, Hammersmith and Fulham Mental Health NHS Trust, Uxbridge Rd, Southall, Middlesex, UK.

James Tew Western Psychiatric Institute and Clinic, Department of Psychiatry, University of Pittsburgh School of Medicine, 3811 O'Hara St, Pittsburgh, PA 15213, USA.

Adele Towers Western Psychiatric Institute and Clinic, Department of Psychiatry, University of Pittsburgh School of Medicine, 3811 O'Hara St, Pittsburgh, PA 15213, USA.

Ken Wilson Professor in Psychiatry of Old Age, University of Liverpool, UK.

Philip Wood Consultant in Geriatric Medicine, Waitemata District Health Board, Private Bag, Takapuna, Auckland, New Zealand; Senior Lecturer, Geriatric Medicine, Faculty of Medicine and Health Science, University of Auckland, New Zealand.

Abbreviations

ACE	angiotensin-converting enzyme
AD	Alzheimer's disease
ADARDS	Alzheimer's Disease and Related Disorders Society
ADL	activities of daily living
ADR	adverse drug reactions
AMTS	Abbreviated Mental Test Scale
APA	American Psychiatric Association
Apo	apolipoprotein
APP	amyloid precursor protein
BPRS	brief psychiatric rating scale
BPSD	behavioural and psychological symptoms of dementia
BUN	blood urea nitrogen
CAM	Confusion Assessment Method
CBT	cognitive–behavioural therapy
CEI	cholinesterase inhibitor
CHF	congestive heart failure
CIDI	Composite International Diagnostic Instrument
CL	consultation liaison
COPD	chronic obstructive pulmonary disease
CPB	cardiopulmonary bypass
CT	computed tomography
CYP	cytochrome P family of enzymes
DAT	dementia of the Alzheimer's type
DBRS	Disruptive Behavior Rating Scale
DHEA	dehydroepiandrosterone
DLB	dementia with Lewy bodies
DVLA	Driver and Vehicle Licensing Agency (UK)
ECA	Epidemiological Catchment Area
ECG	electrocardiogram
ECT	electroconvulsive therapy
EEG	electroencephalogram
ELDRS	Evans Liverpool Depression Rating Scale
EPS	extrapyramidal symptoms

ER	emergency room
EXIT	Executive Interview
FBC	full blood count
FRS	first-rank symptoms
FTLD	frontotemporal lobar degeneration
GDS	Geriatric Depression Scale
GP	general practitioner
HDRS	Hamilton Depression Rating Scale
HPA	hypothalamo–pituitary–adrencortical
IADL	instrumental activities of daily living
INR	international normalized ratio
IPC	interpersonal counselling
IU	international unit
IV	intravenous
LOS	length of stay
MI	myocardial infarction
MMSE	Mini-Mental State Examination
MRI	magnetic resonance imaging
NOS	not otherwise specified
OCD	obsessive–compulsive disorder
OMD	organic mental disorders
OT	occupational therapist
PD	Parkinson's disease
PET	positron emission tomography
PrP	prion protein
PRT	progressive resistance training
PTSD	post-traumatic stress disorder
RCT	randomized clinical trial
REM	rapid eye movement
RO	reality-orientation therapy
SIADH	secretion [which is] inappropriate of antidiuretic hormone
sMMSE	standardized Mini-Mental State Examination
SPECT	single-photon emission computed tomography
SSRI	selective serotonin-reuptake inhibitor
TCA	tricyclic antidepressant
TIA	transient ischaemic attack
TSH	thyroid-stimulating hormone
TURP	transurethral resection of the prostate
UTI	urinary tract infection
VaD	vascular dementia

Section 1:
The context

1 Consultation liaison geriatric psychiatry

Brian Draper

Summary

Nearly 50% of general hospital inpatients are over 65 years of age and they comprise an increasing proportion of referrals to consultation liaison (CL) services. Between 27 and 95% of older patients in general hospitals have mental disorders, particularly organic disorders and depression. Service delivery models for CL geriatric psychiatry vary according to the type of service provider and the style of service delivery. A literature review of psychiatric service delivery to the elderly in general hospitals found that there were few differences in outcomes according to service type, though geriatric psychiatry is more likely than CL psychiatry to consider post-discharge issues. The liaison style has advantages, particularly when targeting high-risk groups (e.g. those with hip fractures). The most frequent reasons for the referral of older people are for assessment of depressive and confusional symptoms, mental state and competency assessments, and behavioural problems. Management recommendations most frequently include the use of psychotropic agents, further medical evaluation, and general advice. Formal service evaluation has found that the benefits of geriatric psychiatry CL services include shorter hospital stays and reduced costs, an increase in depression recognition, improved physical functioning, fewer nursing home transfers, and the increased utilization of community services postdischarge. Only modest effects on outcomes have been demonstrated for the treatment of depression and delirium. Geriatric psychiatry service delivery in emergency rooms, nursing homes, and primary care that utilize CL models are also briefly reviewed.

Introduction

Consultation liaison (CL) psychiatry is that aspect of psychiatry which involves non-psychiatric health workers in a variety of teaching and consultative roles (Lipowski

1983*a*). Despite such a broad definition, the focus of CL psychiatry has traditionally been in the general hospital setting.

In contrast, the patient's age rather than the setting defines geriatric psychiatry. However, 'the ability to work with other disciplines' is a basic principle for the delivery of geriatric psychiatry services, irrespective of the setting (Jolley and Arie 1978). Thus, it could be argued that geriatric psychiatry services are also CL services for a significant part of their work. In this chapter, although the focus will be on the general hospital setting, aspects of CL work in geriatric psychiatry will also be considered in other settings.

The development of CL psychiatry has been closely linked to the emergence of general hospital psychiatry units in North America during the early part of the twentieth century (Lipowski 1986). Theoretically, CL psychiatry has its roots in Meyerian psychobiology, which attempted to reintegrate the sciences of body and mind after the earlier separation of psychiatry from general medicine in the nineteenth century (Lipowski 1986; Clarke and Smith 1995). Engel's biopsycho-social model, as frequently utilized by CL psychiatry, captured this reintegration and has currency in geriatric psychiatry (Engel 1980). CL psychiatry service develop-ment over the last 40 years, however, has been essentially needs-driven due to the high rates of psychiatric disorders in patients in general hospitals (Lipowski 1983*a*; Clarke and Smith 1995).

The worldwide ageing of the population is mirrored in the general hospital setting where the proportion of elderly patients is increasing. In 1995, 40% of hospital discharges and 49% of bed days in the United States involved patients over 65 years of age (Duncker and Greenberg 1999). Similarly, in Australia, during 1997–98, the over-65 group made up 31% of hospital discharges and 46% of bed days (Australian Institute of Health and Welfare 1999). In this context, it is not surprising that there is an overlap of geriatric psychiatry and CL psychiatry, sufficient for Lipowski to call for the integration of the two disciplines (Lipowski 1983*b*).

Prevalence of mental disorders in older patients in general hospitals

There is a higher prevalence of mental disorders in hospitalized elderly people than in the general community. Between 27 and 95% of older patients in general hospitals have mental disorders (Bergmann and Eastham 1974; Cooper 1987; Ramsay *et al.* 1991; Rapp *et al.* 1991; Shamash *et al.* 1992; Evans 1993; Ames *et al.* 1994) compared with around 20–30% in the community (Gurland 1996).

A recent review has found that clinically significant depression occurs in 18–45% of older patients, major depression in 4–45%, and minor depression in 3–29% (Draper 2000*a*). Some 13% of patients in acute geriatric wards have been reported to express suicidal ideation, while a further 29% felt life was not worth living (Shah *et al.* 1998). Organic mental disorders (OMD) have been found in 20–68% of older patients (Bergmann and Eastham 1974; Ramsay *et al.* 1991; Shamash *et al.* 1992; Evans 1993; Ames *et al.* 1994). Delirium occurs in 10–61% (Millar 1981; Seymour and Pringle 1983; Francis *et al.* 1990; Gustafson *et al.* 1991; Inouye *et al.* 1993, 1999), and dementia in 14–61% (Gustafson *et al.* 1991; Ramsay *et al.* 1991; Shamash *et al.* 1992; Evans 1993). Comorbidity is common. For example, in a sample of 119 consecutive admissions with a median age of 83 years, 12% had dementia with depressive symptoms, 6% dementia and delirium, and a further 7% dementia, delirium, and depressive symptoms (Ramsay *et al.* 1991).

Service delivery

A psychiatrist treating the elderly in a general hospital setting requires a number of areas of expertise. These include an understanding of the stress of forced dependency, the impact of hospitalization and unfamiliar environments upon the older person, and the uncertainties of treatment (Goldberg 1989). Other areas include familiarity with diagnostic difficulties due to multiple physical morbidity, the ability to modify assessment techniques, and knowledge of the biological determinants of mental impairment. Furthermore, these areas of expertise need to be administered with a non-ageist attitude. It is also necessary to understand those laws that have a bearing on the elderly (for example, living wills, guardianship, elder abuse) (American Psychiatric Association 1993). To this can be added a knowledge of medical gerontology and the identification and utilization of appropriate community resources (Starkman and Hall 1979). Many of these issues also imply a good understanding of clinical ethics (Lederberg 1997).

Styles of service delivery

Although there are numerous styles of service delivery, these can be essentially categorized into: (1) the type of service provider; and (2) the model of service provision.

Geriatric psychiatry or CL service delivery

The service provider may be geriatric psychiatry, where CL is just one component of a comprehensive service, or general CL psychiatry, where the focus is the general hospital setting in which the elderly are not a specific target group. Service provision by general CL psychiatry mainly occurs in North America (see Table 1.1), and by geriatric psychiatry in the United Kingdom and Europe (see Table 1.2). The patient profiles, reasons for referral, diagnoses, and management are similar in both types of service provision, although it is difficult to generalize from uncontrolled descriptive studies. The only study to compare services found that the introduction of a specific

Table 1.1 CL psychiatry services (Part (i))

	Shevitz et al. (1976) USA	Krakowski (1979) USA	Rabins et al. (1983) USA	Popkin et al. (1984) USA	Folks and Ford (1985) USA	Pérez et al. (1985) Canada
Service type	Psychiatric consultation	CL service	CL service	CL service	CL service	Psychiatric consultation service
Sample size	255	113	139	266	195	66
Age (years)	60+	65+	60+	60+	60+	65+
Gender	64% female (all referrals)	52.3% female	Not available	Not available	68.2% female (> than age-matched controls)	Not available
Sample features	Retrospective 25.5% CL referrals (age 70+ = 9.7% referrals)	2-yr, prospective 30.4% CL referrals	12-mo, retrospect. 21% CL referrals (lower rate than those < 45 yr)	Prospective 25% CL referrals (lower referral rate than those < 60 yr)	Retrospective 19.5% CL referrals (lower proportion than control admissions)	12-mo retrospect. 26.2% CL referrals (no age differences in referral rate)
Psychiatric history	Not available	Not available	Not available	30% (lower than those < 60 years)	Not available	Elderly less frequent than < 65 years
Referring service	Not available specific. for age gp.	Medicine, 39% Family pract., 29% Surgery, 28% Neurology, 2% Other, 3%	Not available	Medicine, 50% Surgery, 22% Neurology, 14% Gynaecology, 7% Orthopaedics, 4%	Medicine/neurology, (75%) Surgery (19%) Gynaecology (3%)	Elderly more likely to be hospitalized for medical than surgical reasons compared to younger referrals
Reasons for referral	Not available specif. for age gp.	Not available	Mental state evaln, 38%	Not available	Not available	Elderly more likely than younger

	patients to be referred for: –behavioural disruption –refusal to follow treatment recommends. –conflict with health personnel	Management (inc. suicide + behav. problems), 25% Depression or stress, 22% Psychogenic cause, 11%				OMD, 44% Depression, 36% –dysthymia, 25% –major depression, 11% Adjustment disord., 8% Personality disorder, 3% Anxiety, 3% Schizophrenia, 2% Substance abuse, 2% No diagnosis, 3%
Diagnoses	Depression, 52% OMD, 33% Anxiety, 4% Schizophrenia, 1% Somatoform disorder, 1%	OMD, 66% –dementia, 52% –delirium, 14% Depression, 25% Personality disorder + neuroses, 6% Schizophrenia, 1% No diagnosis, 2%	OMD, 54% –dementia, 30% –delirium, 27% Depression, 27% Personality disorder, 5% Anxiety, 4% Schizophrenia, 1% No diagnosis, 4%	OMD, 46% Affective disorder, 23% Adjustment disord., 9% Substance abuse, 8% Personality disord., 3% Anx./somatoform, 2% No diagnosis, 8% Deferred, 5%	OMD, 42% –dementia, 23% –delirium, 18% Depression, 33% Somatoform disord., 6% Schizophr./paranoid, 5% Personality dis., 3% Substance abuse, 3% Bipolar–mania/mixed, 3% No diagnosis, 6%	
Management recommends.	Not available specif. for age gp.	Psychiatric transfer, 10%	Not available	Psychotropics, 42% (higher than < 60) Diagnostic action recommends., 48%	Not available	Elderly more likely than younger patients to be recommended for psychotropics. Elderly less likely than younger patients to be recommended for psychiatric ambulatory care

Table 1.1 CL psychiatry services (Part (ii))

	Mainprize and Rodin (1987) Canada	Small and Fawzy (1988) USA	Levitte and Thornby (1989) USA	Roulaux et al. (1993) Netherlands	Swanwick et al. (1994) Ireland	Leo et al. (1997) USA
Setting	University affiliated	University affiliated	VA medical centre	General hospital	General hospital	Tertiary hospital
Sample size	70	88	384	417	39	329
Age (years)	65+	> 60 (mean 75.2)	60+	65+ (mean 74.6)	65+ (mean 72)	65+
Gender	59% female	67% female	< 5% female	55% female	Not available	60% female
Sample features	Retrospective and prospective Non-emergency 29% CL referrals	All geriatric referrals, 55% CL referrals	1-yr retrospective 51% CL referrals 6.9% elderly admissions	10-yr retrospective, 26% CL referrals	6-month prospective	2-yr retrospective 5.6% Geriatric admissions,
Previous psychiatric contact	Not available	Psychiatric history 26%, hospitalization, 16% Psychotherapy, 8%	Not available	Psychiatric history. 20% Previous treatment, 9%	29%	Psychiatric history, 46%
Referring service	Medicine, 77% Surgery, 17% Gynaecology, 4% ICU, 1%	Medicine, 66% Surgery, 15% Neurology, 10%	Medicine, 60% Surgery, 17% Neurology, 11% Rehabilitation, 6%	Medicine, 61% Neurology, 20% Surgical, 14%	'Majority from medical wards' Surgical, 21%	'Majority from medical wards' Surgical, 8%
Reasons for referral	Depression, 37% Behaviour, 17% Confusion, 14% Competency/certification, 12% Psychosis/paranoia, 4%	Depression, 47% MSE, 34% Psychiatric follow-up, 16% Behaviour problems, 10% Suicide assessment,	Competency assessment, 26% Depression, 26% Agitation, 16% Anxiety, 8% Poor compliance, 7% Psychosis, 6%	Not available	Depressive symptoms, 39% Behavioural disturbance, 23% Other, 38%	Depression, 23% Behavioural, 21% Psychosis, 14% Confusion, 11% Dementia, 8% Capacity, 7% Suicidal, 7%

Reasons for referral	Diagnosis, suicide assessment, psychotropics, discharge advice, alcohol, functional cause (each 3%)	9%	Suicide assessment, 6% Medication management, 5%				Anxiety, 4% Medication rev., 3% Psychiatry transfer, 2% Placement, 1%
Diagnoses	OMD, 51% Affective disorder, 17% Adjustment disorder, 17% Personality disorders, 14% Substance use, 6% Somatoform disorders, 4% Schizophr./paranoid states, 1% No diagnosis, 11%	Affective disorder, 55% OMD, 47% Adjustment disorder, 22% Psychotic disorder, 16% Alcohol abuse, 7% Anxiety/somatoform disorder, 5% Personality disorder, 5% No diagnosis, 7%	OMD, 55% –dementia, 26% –delirium, 11% Depression, 25% Anxiety, 8% Alcoholism, 8% Personality disorder, 8% Schizophr/paranoid states, 5% No diagnosis, 2%	OMD, 31% –dementia, 10% –delirium, 8% Depression, 28% Adjustment, 2% Schizophrenia/ paranoid states, 2% Substance use, 8% Anxiety, 1% Uncertain, 17% No diagnosis, 16%	OMD, 31% Mood disorder, 28% Adjustment, 8% Anxiety, 8% Schizophr., 5% Personality, 5% Substance abuse, 3% No diagnosis, 13%	OMD, 34% Mood disorder, 28% Substance abuse, 7% Anxiety, 5% Personality, 5% Adjustment, 4% Schizophrenia, 4% No diagnosis, 15%	OMD, 42% Mood disorder, 17% Psychotic disorders, 15% Adjustment, 7% Substance use, 6% Bereavement, 3% Anxiety, 2% Other, 3% No diagnosis, 6%
Management recommends:	Psychotropics, 43% Discharge planning, 30% Medical work-up, 29% Psychotherapy, 13% Ward management, 13% Psychiatry admission, 9% Neuropsychology, 7% Certification, 7%	Psychotropics, 42% Psychotherapy, 32% Diagnostic recommendations, 25%: –neuroimaging, 10% Medical review, 23% Psychiatry admission, 13%	Psychotropics, 46% Competency assessment, 26% Medical work-up, 18%	Not available	Treatment: –advice, 46% –pharmacother./ ECT, 44% –psychotherapy, 10% Follow-up: –psychiatric, 33% –Med./surg., 46% –GP, 21%	Treatment: –advice, 41% –pharmacother./ ECT, 55% –psychotherapy, 4% Follow-up: –psychiatric, 26% –Med./surg., 59% –GP, 15%	Medication, 41%: –prescribed, 27% –adjusted, 13% Investigations, 20% Med. review, 14% Placement, 6% Staff education, 5% Psychotherapy, 5% Psychiatry admiss., 3% Other, 6%

Abbreviations: CL, consultation liaison; OMD, organic mental disorders; VA, Veterans Administration; ICU, intensive-care unit; MSE, Mental State Evaluation; GP, general practitioner (primary-care physician).

Table 1.2 Geriatric psychiatry CL services (Part (i))

	Ruskin (1985) USA	Pauser et al. (1987) Sweden	Benbow (1987) UK	Poynton (1988) UK	Scott et al. (1988) UK	
Setting	Univ.-affil. general hospital	Univ.-affil. hospital	Univ.-affil. hospital	Univ.-affil. hospital	Univ.-affil. hospital	
Service type	Consultation	Consultation	Consultation	Consultation	Consultation, years 1 and 2	CL—year 3
Sample size	67	294	112	79	98	119
Age (years)	60+	70+ (mean 78)	65+	65+	65+ (median 79.5)	
Gender	64% female	63% female	68% female	57% female	62% female	
Sample features	Retrospective CL referrals, 16.5% Geriatric admiss., 2.7%	Retrospective CL referrals, 54% Geriatric admiss., 2.5%	12-mo. retrospective	16-mo. retrospective less than < 65 years	14-mo. retrospective lower rate than < 65 years	All referrals from geriatric unit with sufficient information, 94%
Psychiatric history	Not available	53% contact	Not available	33%	33%	Not available
Referring service	Medicine, 34% Neurology, 16% Surgery, 15% Orthopaedics, 10%	Medicine, 52% Geriatric, 19% Surgery, 8% Neurology, 8% Other, 13%	Geriatrics, 58%	Medicine, 73%	Medicine, 58% General surgery, 9% Orthopaedics, 21% Other, 11%	Medicine, 70% Surgery, 6% Orthopaedics, 18% Other, 6%
Reasons for referral	Competency, 19% Psychosis, 12% Depression, 10% Behaviour, 10%	Diagn./assess., 84% Psychotropic use, 27% Transfer to	Depressed, 36% Psychotic, 13% Psychiatric FU, 11% Behaviour, 9%	Depression, 30% Confusion, 26% Dementia, 3%	Confusion, 32% Failure to cope/ discharge advice, 21%	Depression, 31% Confusion, 20% Behaviour, 11% Diagnosis/advice, 21%

Reasons for referral	Cognition, 9% Somatization, 7% Psychotropic use, 7% Suicide attempt, 7% Confusion, 6%	psychiatric care, 19% Discharge advice, 17%	Confusion, 8% Suicidal, 8% Placement, 7% No cause for symptoms, 4%			Depression, 18% Behaviour, 16% Psychosis, 6% Diagnosis/treatment advice, 4% Suicide attempt/ personality, 3%	11% Failure to cope/ discharge, 9% Diagnosis/treatmentPsychosis, 8% Suicide attempt/ personality, 6%
Diagnoses	OMD, 54%: –dementia, 39% –delirium, 22% Depression, 36% Schizophrenia, 19% Personality, 15% Alcohol abuse, 13% Somatoform, 6%	OMD, 49%: –dementia, 38% –delirium, 11% Depression, 22% Neurosis, 5% Paranoid states, 2% Uncertain, 8% No diagnosis, 9%	OMD, 38%: –dementia, 32% –delirium, 6% Depression, 27% Neurosis, 8% Personality, 3% Paranoid states, 2% Alcohol, 1% No diagnosis, 21%	OMD, 36%: –dementia, 17% –delirium, 19% Depression, 27% No diagnosis, 10%	OMD, 38%: –dementia, 18% –delirium, 20% Depression, 22% No diagnosis, 15%	OMD, 53%: –chronic, 29% –acute, 24% Depression, 12% Anxiety/adjust., 5% Personality, 4% Funct. psychos., 2% Alcohol abuse, 2% No diagnosis, 14%	OMD, 41%: –chronic, 19% –acute, 22% Depression, 28% Anxiety/adjust., 8% Personality, 5% Alcohol, 5% Funct. psychos., 3% No diagnosis, 7%
Management recommends.	Psychotropics, 61% Medical review, 36% Psychotherapy, 28% Competency assess., 25% Discharge plan, 24% Behaviour manage., 13% Psychiatr. admiss., 12% Neuropsychology, 4%	Psychotropics, 45% Psychiatric admiss., 22% Transfer to long-term care, 22% Medical rev., 22% Geriatric psychiatry community review, 7%	Psychiatric FU, 43% –community, 19% –admission, 13% –outpatient, 8% Psychotropics, 38% Placement, 23% Social, 13% No change, 11% Medical rev., 10% Psychotherapy, 8% Behaviour management + OT (each 6%)	Not available	Not available	Not available	Not available

Abbreviations: CL, consultation liaison; OMD, organic mental disorders; FU, follow-up; CPN, community psychiatric nurse.

Table 1.2 Geriatric psychiatry CL services (Part (ii))

	De Leo *et al.* (1989) Italy	Grossberg *et al.* (1990) USA	Anderson and Philpott (1991) UK	Wrigley and Loane (1991) Ireland
Setting	University-affiliated geriatric hospital	University-affiliated general hospital	University-affiliated hospital	General hospital
Service type	Consultation—years 1–6 CL—years 6–7	Geriatric psychiatry consultation	Geriatric psychiatry consultation	Geriatric psychiatry CL
Sample size	245	147	811	107
Age (years)	Mean age, 72.3	60+ (> 70 years, 72%)	65+ (mean 78 years)	65+ (mean 79 years)
Gender	66% female	Approx 2:1 female	64% female	68% female
Sample features	All traceable referrals from geriatric unit, 50% Geriatric admiss., 2.0%	All referrals from geriatric unit Geriatric admiss., 4.7%	2-year retrospective of all referrals	8-year retrospective Referral rate increased from 0.7% to 1.3% over study period	18-month retrospective
Psychiatric history	Not available	Not available	Not available	Not available
Referring service	All from geriatric service Neurological conditions, 9%	All from geriatric service Neurological conditions, 9%	Internal medicine, 71% Surgery/orthopaedics, 18% Neurology, 6% Gynaecology, 4% Emergency room, 1%	Not available	General hospital, 82% Psychiatric hospital, 18%
Reasons for referral	Affective disorders, 57% Anxiety disorders, 17% Organic mental disorders, 12%	Depression, 48% Confusion/dementia, 22% Behavioural problems, 7% Competency evaluation, 7%	Not available	Placement, 47% Psychological problem, 33% Behavioural problem,

Reasons for referral	Somatoform disorders, 4% Weight loss, 4% Schizophrenia, 3% Hypochondria, 1% Alcohol, 1%	Anxiety, 6% Medication, 2% Suicide evaluation, 2% Psychosis, 1%			11% Forgetfulness, 6% Alcohol abuse, 2%
Diagnoses	Depression, 69% Anxiety disorders, 9% OMD 9%—dementia, 4% Schizophrenia/paranoid disorders, 3% Personality disorder, 3% Somatoform disorders, 1% Alcohol abuse, 1% No diagnosis, 6%	OMD 36%: –dementia, 22% –delirium, 14% Affective disorder, 28% Adjustment disorders, 26% Anxiety, 3% Schizophrenia, 2% Personality disorder, 1% No diagnosis, 2%	OMD 49%: –dementia, 40% –delirium, 9% Depression, 30% Other, 11% No psychiatric diagnosis, 10%		OMD 54%: –dementia, 44% –drelirium, 10% Depression, 11% Functional disorder, 14% Alcohol abuse, 2% No psychiatric diagnosis, 19%
Management recommends.	Psychotropics, 96% Referral to mental health centre, 12% Neurological consultation, 11% Psychological treatment, 7% Psychiatric admiss., 1%	Psychotropics, 87% Psychological treatment, 47% Referral to social workers, 10% Neurological consultation, 7% Referral to mental health centre, 5% Psychiatric admiss., 1%	Psychotropics, 73% FU plan, 12%: –placement, 7% –social service, 4% –rehabilitation, 1% Medical review, 21% Ward management, 12% Psychotherapy, 13% Psychiatric transfer, 5% FU, 32%	Not available	Advice, 62% Medication, 28% CPN, 5% Psychiatric admission, 5% Psychiatric extended care, 3% Community services, 2% Day hospital, 2% Other, 12%

Table 1.2 Geriatric psychiatry CL services (Part (iii))

	Camus et al. (1994) Switzerland	Chiu and Leung (1995) Hong Kong	Collinson and Benbow (1998) UK	Loane and Jefferys (1998) UK
Setting	Univ-affiliated general hospital	Univ-affiliated hospital	General hospital	General hospital
Service type	Geriatric psychiatry consult.	Geriatric psychiatry consult.	Geriatric psychiatry CL	Geriatric psychiatry CL
Sample size	126	97	71	20
Age (years)	65+ (mean 77.5 years)	65+	65+	60+ (mean 80.8 years)
Gender	57% female	52% female	Not available	68% female
Sample features	12-month retrospective < 3% elderly admissions	12-month prospective 0.9% geriatric patients, 80.4% of referral rate of under 65s	12-month prospective 19% referrals to old age psychiatry service, proportion increased with a liaison nursing service	Retrospective All general hospital inpatient referrals to geriatric psychiatry service
Psychiatric history	Psychiatric history, 26%	Not available	Not available	35% contact with geriatric psychiatry service in past year, 6% current contact with CPN
Referring service	Medicine and neurology, 44% Emergency room, 25% Surgery, 14% Rehabilitation, 10%	Medicine, 64% Orthopaedics, 13%	Not available	Not available

Reasons for referral	Not available	Suicide attempt/idea, 22% Confusion, 17% Depression, 15% Past psychiatric history 15% Refusing food, 5% Psychosis, 5% Psychological factors, 5% Violent behaviour, 3%	Not available	Psychological symptoms, 51% Forgetfulness, 23% Behavioural problem, 14% Placement advice, 11%
Diagnoses	OMD, 44%: –dementia, 30% –delirium, 27% Affective disorder, 16% Adjustment disorder, 12% Anxiety, 6% Psychoses, 5% Substance use, 4% Personality disorder, 1% No diagnosis, 3% (deferred 8%)	OMD, 28%: –dementia, 15% –delirium, 13% Depression, 25% Substance use, 5% No psychiatric diagnosis, 19%	OMD, 55%: –dementia, 45% –delirium, 10% Affective disorder, 28% Adjustment disorder, 6% Personality disorder, 3% Substance use, 3% Schizophrenia, 2%	OMD, 58%: –chronic, 45% –acute, 13% Functional disorder, 38% Alcohol misuse, 1% No diagnosis, 3%
Management recommends,	Geriatric psychiatry admission, 17% Transfer to nursing home, 15% Outpatient clinic, 3% Day hospital, 3%	Medication advice, 44% Psychiatric follow-up, 36% Psychiatric advice, 28% Psychiatric admission, 6%	Not available	Community psychiatric FU, 59% Psychotropics. 42% Psychiatric advice, 30% Transfer to residential care, 21% Diagnostic invest., 6% Psychiatric admission, 6% Refer to social services, 62%

Table 1.2 Geriatric psychiatry CL services (Part (iv))

	Kitching (1999) Australia	Baheerathan and Shah (1999) UK	Kisely and Axten (2000) Australia
Setting	Univ-affil. general hospital	General hospital	Univ-affil. general hospital
Service type	Geriatric psychiatry consultation	Geriatric psychiatry consultation	Geriatric psychiatry consultation integrated with CL service
Sample size	169	227	151
Age (years)	Mean age 77.5	Median age 84 (range 65–98)	65+
Gender	53% female	66% female	Not available
Sample features	Retrospective. All general hospital inpatient referrals to geriatric psychiatry service	Retrospective, 30 months. All referrals from geriatric medicine	Retrospective. All catchment area referrals
Psychiatric history	Not available	Not available	Not available
Referring service	Geriatric medicine, 62% Medical specialties, 15% Palliative care, 9% Surgery, 9% General psychiatry, 5%	Geriatric medicine, 100%	Not available

Reasons for referral	Not available	Dementia management, 46% Depressive symptoms, 36% Delirium management, 14% Competency, 14% Psychosis management, 10% Aggressive behaviour, 10% Placement, 4%	Not available
Diagnoses	OMD, 44%: –dementia, 26% –delirium, 18% Depression, 31% Schizophrenia/psychosis, 9% Substance abuse, 5% Anxiety, 2% Factitious, 2% Personality disorder, 2% No diagnosis, 4%	OMD, 71%: –dementia, 51% –delirium, 20% Depression, 19% Schizophrenia, 3% Anxiety, 1% Other diagnosis, 6%	Major depression, 42% OMD, 37%
Management recommends.	Psychotropics, 41% Psychotropics ceased, 5%	Diagnostic investigations, 71% Social-work referral, 58% Psychotropic medication, 52% Occupational therapy referral, 46% Correction of sensory deficits, 35% Placement advice, 31% CPN follow-up, 18% Psychiatric outpatients, 13% Medical review, 13% Social-care package, 11% Competency advice, 11% Neuroimaging, 6% Psychiatric admission, 5% Psychologist, 4%	Not available

geriatric psychiatry service resulted in few changes apart from a higher referral rate (Poynton 1988).

One possible difference noted in Tables 1.1 and 1.2 is that discharge advice is requested in around 20% of referrals to geriatric psychiatry services, particularly about placement, an issue infrequently mentioned by general CL psychiatry service evaluations. Furthermore, geriatric psychiatry services are more likely to arrange community psychiatric follow-up. This extended-care approach has been found to be the most effective style of service delivery for the elderly (Cole 1991) and is consistent with a comprehensive geriatric psychiatry service. It also points to the fundamental limitation of institutionally based general CL psychiatry. There may be too much emphasis on the patient in the hospital setting and insufficient recognition of community issues including discharge planning (Huyse *et al.* 1990). This has been recognized as a particular challenge to all CL psychiatry practitioners in an era where hospital stays are becoming shorter (Wright *et al.* 1996).

Loane and Jefferys (1998) found that 35% of CL referrals had been seen by the geriatric psychiatry service in the previous year and 6% were in current contact. Thus, it is likely that many patients are already known to the geriatric psychiatry service from other settings. Such knowledge often simplifies the assessment through awareness of the patient's premorbid functioning, previous treatment response, and social circumstances.

Consultation or liaison models

Greenhill (1979) reviewed mental health services in medical settings and described several service delivery models. The consultation model, in which the physician refers the patient for psychiatric assessment, forms the basis of other models. A variant of this includes the biological psychiatry model in which there is a predominant emphasis on neurosciences and psychopharmacology, with less emphasis on psychodynamics and social factors. A second variant is the integral model in which any member of the healthcare team may request a consultation, with a particular focus on primary prevention by the early identification of patients at high risk for mental disorder.

The liaison model involves the consulting psychiatric service working with patients and physicians in specific units. A variant of this, the milieu model, encompasses the social psychology of patient care, with the psychiatric consultant becoming an 'insider' by attending ward rounds and having greater collaboration with ward staff (Mohl 1981). This model requires the CL psychiatrist to have a good understanding of systems theory.

Several authorities have proposed hybrid models. For example, collaboration between CL psychiatry and geriatric psychiatry services (Small and Fawzy 1988; Kisely and Axten 2000) and medical psychiatric units where old age psychiatrists work together with geriatricians on joint patient care (Arie and Dunn 1973; Pitt and Silver 1980; Fogel 1985). These may take the form of joint departments where the geriatric medical and geriatric psychiatry wards are in close proximity to each other (Arie and Jolley 1982). While it could be suggested that educational models are another variant, it is probably more reasonable to regard education as a component of each model.

There have been four comparisons of liaison and consultation models in the elderly (Scott et al. 1988; De Leo et al. 1989; Swanwick et al. 1994; Baheerathan and Shah 1999). While findings have been inconsistent, liaison models appear to have some advantages. Liaison models had a higher referral rate in some (Scott et al. 1988; De Leo et al. 1989), but not all studies (Baheerathan and Shah 1999). Other reported advantages include more referrals for depression (Scott et al. 1988), a higher degree of diagnostic accuracy by referring doctors (Swanwick et al. 1994), increased reviews by the psychiatric consultant (De Leo et al. 1989), and improved compliance with psychotropic recommendations (De Leo et al. 1989).

Over the last 20 years, CL psychiatry services in the United States have tended to move from liaison to consultation models, with programmes that focus on high-risk groups, e.g. hip fractures in the elderly (Sharpe and Hawton 1990; Strain et al. 1991). This change is due to shorter hospital stays, the lack of data on cost-effectiveness, understaffing, and reimbursement mechanisms that do not compensate for liaison services (Sharpe and Hawton 1990; Cavanaugh and Milne 1995; Unützer and Small 1996). Furthermore, the increased number of referrals of elderly people has resulted in the recommendation that CL psychiatrists should have specific training in geriatric psychiatry (Lipowski 1983b). In the UK, a shortage of geriatric psychiatry consultants has also restricted service provision; one service has described the employment of a nurse in a CL role to supplement psychiatric consultations (Baldwin 1998; Collinson and Benbow 1998).

Referral patterns of older patients

In the US over the last 15 years, the proportion of elderly referrals to CL services increased from around 20–30% to over 50%. In the UK, 15–20% of referrals to geriatric psychiatry services come from a general hospital ward (Wattis 1997, cited in Baldwin 1998). Between 0.9 and 5.5% of older patients admitted to a general hospital are referred for consultation (see Tables 1.1 and 1.2). The majority of referrals are from general medical, geriatric, and neurological services, while most surgical referrals are from orthopaedic services (e.g. patients who have received hip replacement). Some studies have reported that referrals occur late in the course of admission (Pérez et al. 1985; Roulaux et al. 1993), which may be due to the increased risk of psychological decompensation found in longer admissions (Incalzi et al. 1991).

Many studies report lower referral rates in the elderly (Rabins et al. 1983; Popkin et al. 1984; Folks and Ford 1985; Poynton 1988; Chiu and Leung 1995), although there are some exceptions (Pérez et al. 1985; Levitte and Thornby 1989). Postulated reasons for lower referral rates mainly relate to the attitudes of physicians. These include a greater concern with acute medical problems and the beliefs that cognitive dysfunction is part of normal ageing, or that it is a medical rather than a psychiatric problem. Patient refusal, discomfort in treating psychiatric problems, concern about psychiatric stigma, or beliefs that treatment is ineffective are additional reasons (Popkin *et al.* 1984; Unützer and Small 1996). Racial characteristics may also influence referral, with Caucasians having higher referral rates than African–Americans in the US (Leo *et al.* 1997).

Under-utilization of psychiatric consultation is a common problem. Less than 25% of older patients meeting a high-risk profile, involving four or more risk factors, were referred for consultation at one centre (Swigar *et al.* 1992). The majority of depressed older patients are either undiagnosed or misdiagnosed, and are infrequently referred for psychiatric advice (Folks and Ford 1985; Koenig *et al.* 1992, 1997*a*; Shah and De 1998). Use of screening instruments, such as the Geriatric Depression Scale, by non-psychiatric health workers improves the recognition of depression and increases psychiatric referrals (Shah and De 1998). Furthermore, the educational influence of geriatric psychiatry consultations over a period of years may improve the rate of appropriate referrals (Anderson and Philpott 1991).

Reasons for referral

From the studies listed in Tables 1.1 and 1.2, the most frequently mentioned reason for consultation is the assessment of depressive symptoms ($n = 14$, range 10–57%, median 31%). Other common referral reasons mentioned include 'confusion, dementia' ($n = 12$, range 6–46%, median 19.5%), discharge advice and placement ($n = 10$, range 1–47%, median 17%), 'mental state evaluation/competency' assessment ($n = 10$, range 7–84%, median 15%), and behavioural problems ($n = 14$, range 7–35%, median 14.5%). Suicide evaluation ($n = 9$, range = 2–22%, median = 6.5%) and psychosis ($n = 10$, range 1–14%, median = 6%) are also regularly mentioned. Between 20 and 53% of patients have a previous psychiatric history.

Referral reasons for older and younger patients differ. Older patients are more frequently referred for evaluation of depression (Pérez *et al.* 1985; Small and Fawzy 1988), mental state evaluation/competency assessment (Rabins *et al.* 1983; Small and Fawzy 1988; Levitte and Thornby 1989), behavioural problems (Pérez *et al.* 1985; Levitte and Thornby 1989), and psychosis (Pérez *et al.* 1985). They are less frequently referred for assessment of suicide risk (Pérez *et al.* 1985; Levitte and Thornby 1989) and psychogenic causes of physical symptoms than younger patients (Rabins *et al.* 1983).

There are often overt and covert reasons for the referral. For example, while the overt request to see a dementing patient with a behavioural disturbance may be for management advice, often the covert reason is to facilitate a psychiatric transfer. The prevalence of covert reasons for referral in the elderly is unknown, although across the age range it has been reported to occur in about 13% of cases (Bustamente and Ford 1981).

Lipowski (1986) described three types of consultations—patient-oriented, consultee-oriented, and situation-oriented. While most of the reasons for referral listed in the studies reviewed are overtly patient-oriented, covertly many are likely to have been situation- and consultee-oriented; that is to say, the referral is really requesting advice on behavioural problems, competency assessments, or discharge/placement. Situation-oriented referrals require a systems approach to assessment and management, with an understanding of the ward system, its interface with other parts of the hospital, other health services, community services, and long-term care providers. The referral of any patient with 'behavioural problems' should immediately alert the consultant to the fact that the situational aspects might require attention.

Possibly, the staff has contributed to the patient's behaviour by their management approach. Staff conflicts over behaviour management often lead to inconsistent responses to the patient's needs that serve to exacerbate the problem. Sometimes the staff conflicts over the patient mirror more fundamental problems with staff morale. Other systems factors such as complaints by other patients, poor ward design, and pressure from administration to reduce costs may also contribute.

Consultee-oriented referrals are influenced by the attitudes, beliefs, and motivations of the consultee. The referral may reflect the consultee's lack of gerontological knowledge, ageist attitudes, or discomfort with addressing issues of conflict with elders. Older patients are more likely to be in conflict with health personnel and to refuse to follow advice from their treating physician than younger patients (Pérez et al. 1985). Request for a competency assessment may be the overt reason for referral that masks such conflicts. An educational approach is often required as part of the consultation.

Diagnostic profile

The referral pattern for older patients is similar to the prevalence rates described earlier, with the majority of cases being organic mental disorders (OMD) or depression. OMDs are the most prevalent psychiatric diagnoses reported (see Tables 1.1 and 1.2), occurring in 9–71% of cases ($n = 27$, median = 44%). Dementia accounts for 4–52% ($n = 20$, median 29.5%) and delirium for 6–27% ($n = 19$, median 14%) of cases. The higher prevalence of OMD in the elderly, particularly dementia, distinguishes them from younger CL referrals (Shevitz et al. 1976; Rabins et al. 1983; Pérez et al. 1985; Small and Fawzy 1988; Levitte and Thornby 1989; Smith et al. 1997). In many cases, the referral has been precipitated by a behavioural disturbance or competency assessment (Levitte and Thornby 1989; Smith et al. 1997).

Depression is found in 11–69% of referrals ($n = 26$, median = 27%). Although the type of depression has been infrequently specified, major depression is reported in 4–26%, dysthymia in 4–41%, and adjustment disorder with depressed mood in 3–9% of referrals (Folks and Ford 1985; Pérez et al. 1985; De Leo et al. 1989; Chiu and Leung 1995; Kitching 1999).

Other diagnoses are less common. Anxiety, adjustment, and somatoform disorders occur in 1–29% of referrals ($n = 21$, median = 8%), substance abuse in 1–13% ($n = 19$, median = 5%), personality disorders in 1–15% ($n = 17$, median = 4%), and schizophrenia/paranoid disorders in 1–19% ($n = 21$, median = 3%). In comparison with younger CL referrals, fewer older patients are diagnosed with substance abuse, anxiety, somatoform, and personality disorders (Shevitz *et al.* 1976; Rabins *et al.* 1983; Small and Fawzy 1988; Levitte and Thornby 1989). No psychiatric diagnoses are made in 0–21% ($n = 24$, median 7%) of referrals, which is less frequent than in younger patients (Shevitz *et al.* 1976; Rabins *et al.* 1983; Small and Fawzy 1988; Levitte and Thornby 1989).

The majority of older patients have multiple medical diagnoses, with cardiac, cerebrovascular, neurological, endocrine, gastrointestinal, and neoplastic disorders prominent (Popkin *et al.* 1984; Pauser *et al.* 1987; Scott *et al.* 1988; Small and Fawzy 1988; De Leo *et al.* 1989; Wrigley and Loane 1991; Roulaux *et al.* 1993; Camus *et al.* 1994; Kisely and Axten 2000). Only 5–16% of cases have no medical diagnoses, further emphasizing the relatively infrequent diagnosis of somatoform disorder in the older clinical population (Popkin *et al.* 1984; Pauser *et al.* 1987; Wrigley and Loane 1991; Roulaux *et al.* 1993).

Management recommendations

The appropriateness and effectiveness of any management recommendation depends on whether the consultant has identified and answered the right questions, namely both the overt and covert reasons for referral. This process is enhanced if the consultant has established a working relationship with the consultee (Unützer and Small 1996).

Consistent with the high rates of somatic comorbidity, between 6–71% of referrals need further medical review or investigations (see Tables 1.1 and 1.2). This is more frequent than in younger referrals (Levitte and Thornby 1989). The differences between psychiatric and somatic symptoms in the elderly may be subtle. Many referrals with depressive symptoms do not meet the diagnostic criteria for clinical depression (Grossberg *et al.* 1990). Depressive symptoms such as apathy, anorexia, and fatigue are excluded from some diagnostic systems in the physically ill due to their lack of specificity, and this may result in under-diagnosis (Koenig *et al.* 1997b). Further review of symptoms and clinical investigations are a feature of the diagnostic approach for OMDs.

The most frequent management recommendation is for psychotropic medication ($n = 15$, range 28–96%, median = 44%). Antipsychotic drugs, prescribed in 20–26% of referrals, are mainly used to treat OMD, particularly behavioural problems and psychosis (Smith *et al.* 1997). Antidepressants are prescribed in 8–26% of referrals and minor tranquillizers in 4–24%. Several studies have reported higher rates of psychotropic recommendations for the elderly (Popkin *et al.* 1984; Pérez *et al.* 1985;

Levitte and Thornby 1989), but this is not a consistent finding (Small and Fawzy 1988).

The use of psychotherapy is variable, ranging from 4 to 47% of referrals ($n = 8$, median = 11.5%). The nature of the therapy is infrequently mentioned, but has been variously described as 'focal', 'supportive', 'cognitive', or 'psychoanalytical' (Krakowski 1979; Ruskin 1985; De Leo et al. 1989). 'Ward management and advice' is mentioned for 5 to 62% of referrals ($n = 10$, median = 20.5%). Studies with the elderly have provided no details of what these recommendations involve. However, they are likely to include advice about behaviour management, staff–patient and staff–family interactions, psychological support of the patient, education, and the use of restraints (Huyse et al. 1990).

As mentioned earlier, one of the major distinguishing features of service provision by CL and geriatric psychiatry is the increased likelihood that the latter will make recommendations about discharge planning, placement, and psychiatric follow-up. For geriatric psychiatry services this occurs in up to 62% of cases. Psychiatric transfer occurs in 1–22% of referrals ($n = 14$, median = 6%).

The effectiveness of CL services

Evaluations of CL services for the elderly are limited. One randomized clinical trial (RCT) evaluated the effectiveness of geriatric psychiatry consultation in reducing the severity of confusion, anxiety, depression, abnormal behaviour, and functional disability in older patients over a period of 8 weeks (Cole et al. 1991). Only modest results were obtained. Patients with delirium and depression improved most often, but overall the differences, when compared with controls, were not statistically significant. An RCT of the treatment of depression with fluoxetine in elderly, physically ill, medical inpatients, while not strictly a CL intervention, also found a non-significant trend towards improvement in the treatment group (Evans et al. 1997).

A more focused, experimental, multi-site controlled study of psychiatric CL intervention in elderly patients with hip fractures produced a significant reduction in the length of stay (LOS) and hospital costs (Strain et al. 1991). While there were no overall significant improvements on mental health parameters, one site demonstrated a significant improvement in cognitive function and another a significant reduction in depressive symptoms. An earlier controlled study of elderly patients with hip fractures also demonstrated a reduction in LOS and a higher rate of home discharges, although the study had a number of flaws (Levitan and Kornfeld 1981).

The detection of depression and cognitive dysfunction was the focus of a randomized trial of consultation and intervention by a geriatric liaison multidisciplinary team led by a geriatrician who also had training in geriatric psychiatry (Slaets et al. 1997). Although this intervention resulted in improved physical functioning, shorter lengths of stay, and fewer nursing home transfers for the patients, unfortunately no mental health outcomes were reported.

Few service audits have included outcome data. An Italian study described the effects of establishing a formal psychogeriatric unit upon psychiatric consultations in a geriatric hospital (De Leo *et al.* 1989). Consultation rates, frequency of contact with each consultation, use of psychological interventions, and implementation of psychiatric prescriptions by referring agents all increased, while length of stay reduced after the unit's establishment. The presence of a formal, geriatric psychiatry liaison service may also increase the recognition of depression by referring agents (Scott *et al.* 1988). A 3-month follow-up of a CL intervention showed an increased utilization of community services and community nursing, while 54% of patients had further psychiatric contact and 14% a psychiatric admission (Loane and Jefferys 1998).

In summary, the benefits of geriatric psychiatry CL services include shortened hospital stays and reduced costs, increased recognition of depression, improved physical functioning, fewer nursing home transfers, and increased utilization of community services post-discharge. However, only modest effects on outcomes have been demonstrated for the treatment of depression and delirium. A recent review of the effectiveness of geriatric psychiatry CL services concluded that, on a four-level evidence hierarchy, the overall quality of evidence for their effectiveness was only level 3 (Draper 2000*b*). There is no evidence of a difference in treatment outcomes between CL services and geriatric psychiatry services.

CL services for the elderly in other settings

It is impossible within the scope of this chapter to provide an in-depth discussion of CL services in emergency rooms, nursing homes, and general practice (primary care). In view of the importance of these other areas, however, a brief overview is provided.

Emergency rooms

A general hospital may have an emergency room (ER) serviced by the CL psychiatry unit or have a distinct psychiatric ER administered by the mental health service. In general, psychiatric referrals to the ER occur less often in the elderly (Pérez and Blouin 1986; Thienhaus *et al.* 1988; Puryear *et al.* 1991; Shulman *et al.* 1996). The reasons for attending the ER have not been well characterized, although 69% of referrals in one study were behaviourally disturbed, particularly in public settings (Puryear *et al.* 1991). One Canadian study found a high rate of referrals from primary-care physicians (Pérez and Blouin 1986), but this was not the case in the US (Puryear *et al.* 1991). It has been suggested that a lack of community geriatric psychiatry services may contribute to referrals (Herst 1983; Pérez and Blouin 1986; Shulman *et al.* 1996).

Most elderly patients in ER have been symptomatic for more than a month (Pérez and Blouin 1986; Puryear *et al*. 1991). Furthermore, a higher rate of previous psychiatric morbidity is evident in patients attending ER than CL referrals in the general hospital: between 51–75% of patients have a past psychiatric history, 36–57% have previous psychiatric hospitalizations, and 18–30% are in current treatment (Pérez and Blouin 1986; Thienhaus *et al*. 1988; Puryear *et al*. 1991; Shulman *et al*. 1996). In comparison with younger patients attending ER, the elderly are more likely to be diagnosed with OMD or major depression and have medical comorbidity (Pérez and Blouin 1986; Thienhaus *et al*. 1988; Shulman *et al*. 1996). Psychological factors affecting medical conditions are also common, and the ER may be the site where patients are 'shunted back and forth' between medical and psychiatric services (Bassuk *et al*. 1983; Pérez and Blouin 1986). They are less likely to have a diagnosis of schizophrenia or personality disorder (Pérez and Blouin 1986; Thienhaus *et al*. 1988; Shulman *et al*. 1996). Older patients are also less likely to attend due to parasuicidal behaviour (Pérez and Blouin 1986).

Approximately 20–50% of older patients are formally admitted, which is more than younger attendees (Pérez and Blouin 1986; Thienhaus *et al*. 1988; Shulman *et al*. 1996). Predictors of admission include delusions, aggression, major affective disorder, and referral for being a 'public nuisance' (Thienhaus *et al*. 1988; Puryear *et al*. 1991). Psychiatric follow-up is arranged for around 33–35% of patients (Pérez and Blouin 1986; Shulman *et al*. 1996). These data suggest that emergency rooms have an important function in service delivery, especially when there are gaps in specialized, geriatric psychiatry service provision.

Nursing homes

Nursing home residents have considerable unmet needs (Reichman *et al*. 1998). Over 20% have depressive disorders, 60–70% have dementia, severe behavioural problems have been identified in 14–20%, and psychosis in around 15% (Zimmer *et al*. 1984; Ames 1993; Rosewarne *et al*. 1997). Few have received formal diagnoses or specialist mental health interventions (Zimmer *et al*. 1984; Snowdon *et al*. 1995).

Psychiatric service provision to nursing homes is similar to CL in the general hospital, though the referrals tend to be older and are more likely to have dementia (Lippert *et al*. 1990). Over 80% of referrals are for behavioural problems such as aggression, agitation, and vocal disruption (Draper *et al*. 1998). The CL service is more likely to interface with primary-care physicians and may be the site of a broader, community geriatric psychiatry service (Oxman 1996).

Provision of psychiatric input on a regular basis may impact upon diagnosis, management, identification of medication side-effects, and better staff tolerance of behaviours (Goldman and Klugman 1990). Psychogeriatric nursing consultations to nursing homes have been shown to decrease hospital admissions and improve communication (Fuller and Lillquist 1995; Joseph *et al*. 1995). An uncontrolled study demonstrated a significant improvement in the behavioural disturbances of nursing-home and hostel residents treated by a community team. Some 87% of referring agents and 80% of caregivers rated the service as being 'helpful' or 'very helpful' (Seidel *et al*. 1992).

Tourigny-Rivard and Drury (1987) reported that monthly visits by an old age psychiatrist increased the nursing home staff's understanding and acceptance of emotional problems, and also increased the frequency of therapeutic programmes offered. An educational approach for the nursing staff was the key to this achievement. Rovner *et al*. (1996) further demonstrated the importance of this educational liaison model in a randomized trial of a dementia care programme consisting of activities, guidelines for psychotropic medications, and educational rounds. The prevalence of behaviour disorders, use of antipsychotic medication, and restraints all reduced. Such liaison programmes rely heavily on high levels of human resources, but reimbursement issues may constrain the wider applicability of this approach.

General practice (primary care)

General practitioners (GPs) may lack expertise in managing depression and dementia in the community, without additional training and support. A survey of GPs in Sydney found that dementia and depression were two of the conditions they had least confidence in diagnosing and managing in the elderly (Shah and Harris 1997). In dementia care, it is widely accepted that GPs have a central role, yet they often have insufficient information and training to fulfil it (Brodaty *et al*. 1994). Whilst an estimated 80% of older people with moderate to severe depression consult their family doctor with symptoms, GPs only detect about 25% of cases (Cole and Yaffe 1996).

The interface between geriatric psychiatry and primary care is best conceptualized in a CL framework. A survey of old age psychiatrists in the UK during 1991 revealed that 71% of psychogeriatric teams had a community psychiatric nurse regularly working in GPs surgeries, and that 23% of old age psychiatrists had clinics there. Most reported that there were more advantages than disadvantages to the arrangements, and these included improved management, decreased crisis referrals, reduced need for admission, and better GP education (Banerjee *et al*. 1993). There is evidence that collaborations between geriatric psychiatry services and GPs can improve the detection of depression and the treatment strategies employed (MacDonald 1986; Callahan *et al*. 1994), although good outcome data are lacking. The style of collaboration is important. Pure consultative models are ineffective (Ames 1990); however, 'shared care', where there is greater educational and supervisory interaction between the specialist service and the GP, may have a better outcome (Llewellyn-Jones *et al*. 1999).

Collaboration between GPs, other primary-care providers, and geriatric psychiatry services could effectively facilitate continuing education, improve identification of problems, and enhance the treatment of patients at the primary-care level. Further research examining the effectiveness of shared-care models should be encouraged.

References

American Psychiatric Association (1993). *Selected models of practice in geriatric psychiatry: a task force report of the American Psychiatric Association.* American Psychiatric Association, Washington DC.

Ames, D. (1990). Depression among elderly residents of local-authority residential homes: its nature and the efficacy of intervention. *British Journal of Psychiatry*, **156**, 667–75.

Ames, D. (1993). Depressive disorders among elderly people in long term care. *Australian and New Zealand Journal of Psychiatry*, **27**, 379–91.

Ames, D., Flynn, E., and Harrigan, S. (1994). Prevalence of psychiatric disorders among inpatients of an acute geriatric hospital. *Australian Journal on Ageing*, **13**, 8–11.

Anderson, D.N. and Philpott, R.M. (1991). The changing pattern of referrals for psychogeriatric consultation in the general hospital: an eight-year study. *International Journal of Geriatric Psychiatry*, **6**, 801–7.

Arie, T. and Dunn, T. (1973). A 'do-it-yourself' psychiatric–geriatric joint patient unit. *Lancet*, **ii**, 1313–16.

Arie, T. and Jolley, D. (1982). Making services work: organization and style of psychogeriatric services. In *The psychiatry of late life* (ed. R. Levy and F. Post), pp. 222–5. Blackwell, Oxford.

Australian Institute of Health and Welfare (1999). *Australian Hospital Statistics, 1997–98.* AIHW Catalogue No. HSE-6, Canberra.

Baheerathan, M. and Shah, A. (1999). The impact of two changes in service delivery on a geriatric psychiatry liaison service. *International Journal of Geriatric Psychiatry*, **14**, 767–75.

Baldwin, R.C. (1998). Re: Geriatric consultation and liaison service. *International Journal of Geriatric Psychiatry*, **13**, 820–1.

Banerjee, S., Lindesay, J., and Murphy, E., (1993). Psychogeriatricians and general practitioners: a national survey. *Psychiatric Bulletin*, **17**, 592–4.

Bassuk, E., Minden, S., and Apsler, R. (1983). Geriatric emergencies: psychiatric or medical? *American Journal of Psychiatry*, **140**, 539–42.

Benbow, S.M. (1987). Liaison referrals to a department of psychiatry for the elderly 1984–5. *International Journal of Geriatric Psychiatry*, **2**, 235–40.

Bergmann, K. and Eastham, E. (1974). Psychogeriatrics ascertainment and assessment for treatment in acute medical ward setting. *Age and Ageing*, **3**, 174–88.

Brodaty, H., Howarth, G.C., Mant, A., and Kurrle, S.E. (1994). General practice and dementia. *The Medical Journal of Australia*, **160**, 10–14.

Bustamente, J.P. and Ford, C.V. (1981). Characteristics of general hospital patients referred for psychiatric consultation. *Journal of Clinical Psychiatry*, **42**, 338–41.

Callahan, C.M., Hendrie, H.C., Dittus, R.S., Brater, D.C., Hui, S.L., and Tierney, W.M. (1994). Improving treatment of late-life depression in primary care: a randomised clinical trial. *Journal of the American Geriatrics Society*, **42**, 839–46.

Camus, V., De Mendonca Lima, C.A., Simeone, I., and Wertheimer, J. (1994). Geriatric psychiatry liaison-consultation: the need for specific units in general hospitals. *International Journal of Geriatric Psychiatry*, **9**, 933–5.

Cavanaugh, S. and Milne, J. (1995). Recent changes in consultation-liaison psychiatry. A blueprint for the future. *Psychosomatics*, **36**, 95–102.

Chiu, H.F.K. and Leung, C.M. (1995). Hong Kong psychogeriatric consultations. *Clinical Gerontologist*, **15**, 55–8.

Clarke, D.M. and Smith, G.C. (1995). Consultation-liaison psychiatry in general medical units. *Australian and New Zealand Journal of Psychiatry*, **29**, 424–32.

Cole, M.G. (1991). Effectiveness of three types of geriatric medical services: lessons for geriatric psychiatric services. *Canadian Medical Association Journal*, **144**, 1229–40.

Cole, M.G. and Yaffe, M.J. (1996). Pathway to psychiatric care of the elderly with depression. *International Journal of Geriatric Psychiatry*, **11**, 157–61.

Cole, M.G., Fenton, F.R., Engelsmann, F., and Mansouri, I. (1991). Effectiveness of geriatric psychiatry consultation in an acute care hospital: a randomized clinical trial. *Journal of the American Geriatrics Society*, **39**, 1183–8.

Collinson, Y. and Benbow, S.M. (1998) The role of a geriatric psychiatry consultation liaison nurse. *International Journal of Geriatric Psychiatry*, **13**, 159–63.

Cooper, B. (1987). Psychiatric disorders among elderly patients admitted to hospital medical wards. *Journal of the Royal Society of Medicine*, **80**, 13–16.

De Leo, D., Baiocchi, A., Cipollone, B., Pavan, L., and Beltrame, P. (1989). Psychogeriatric consultation within a geriatric hospital: a six-year experience. *International Journal of Geriatric Psychiatry*, **4**, 135–41.

Draper, B. (2000*a*). The effectiveness of the treatment of depression in the physically ill elderly. *Aging and Mental Health*, **4**, 9–20.

Draper, B. (2000*b*). The effectiveness of old age psychiatry services. *International Journal of Geriatric Psychiatry*, **15**, 687–703.

Draper, B., Meares, S., and McIntosh, H. (1998). A psychogeriatric outreach service to nursing homes in Sydney. *Australasian Journal on Ageing*, **17**, 184–6.

Duncker, A. and Greenberg, S. (1999). A profile of older Americans: 1998. *Online statistical data on aging*. Program Resources Department, American Association of Retired Persons and Administration on Aging, US Department of Health and Human Resources www.aoa.gov/aoa/stats/statpage.html.

Engel, G.L. (1980). The clinical application of the biopsychosocial model. *American Journal of Psychiatry*, **137**, 535–44.

Evans, M.E. (1993). Depression in elderly physically ill inpatients: a 12-month prospective study. *International Journal of Geriatric Psychiatry*, **8**, 587–92.

Evans, M., Hammond, M., Wilson, K., Lye, M., and Copeland, J. (1997). Placebo-controlled treatment trial of depression in elderly physically ill patients. *International Journal of Geriatric Psychiatry*, **12**, 817–24.

Fogel, B.S. (1985). A psychiatric unit becomes a psychiatric-medical unit: administration and clinical implications. *General Hospital Psychiatry*, **7**, 26–35.

Folks, D.G. and Ford, C.V. (1985). Psychiatric disorders in geriatric medical/surgical patients. Part 1: Report of 195 consecutive consultations. *Southern Medical Journal*, **78**, 239–41.

Francis, J., Martin, D., and Kapoor, W.N. (1990). A prospective study of delirium in hospitalized elderly. *Journal of the American Medical Association*, **263**, 1097–101.

Fuller, K. and Lillquist, D. (1995). Geropsychiatric public sector nursing: placement challenges. *Journal of Psychosocial Nursing*, **33**, 20–2.

Goldberg, R.L. (1989). Geriatric consultation/liaison psychiatry (Issues in geriatric psychiatry). *Advances in Psychosomatic Medicine*, **19**, 138–50.

Goldman, L.S. and Klugman, A. (1990). Psychiatric consultation in a teaching nursing home. *Psychosomatics*, **31**, 277–81.

Greenhill, M.H. (1979). Models of liaison programs that address age and cultural differences in reaction to illness. *Bibliothecha Psychiatrica*, **159**, 77–81.

Grossberg, G.T., Zimny, G.H., and Nakra, B.R.S. (1990). Geriatric psychiatry consultations in a university hospital. *International Psychogeriatrics*, **2**, 161–8.

Gurland, B. (1996). Epidemiology of psychiatric disorders. In *Comprehensive review of geriatric psychiatry–II* (2nd edn) (ed. J. Sadavoy, L.W. Lazarus, L.F. Jarvik, and G.T. Grossberg), pp. 3–41. American Psychiatric Press Inc., Washington DC.

Gustafson, Y., Brännström, B., Berggren, D., Ragnarsson, J.I., Sigaard, J., Bucht, G., *et al.* (1991). A geriatric-anesthesiologic program to reduce acute confusional states in elderly patients treated for femoral neck fractures. *Journal of the American Geriatrics Society*, **39**, 655–62.

Herst, L. (1983). Emergency psychiatry for the elderly. *Psychiatric Clinics of North America*, **6**, 271.

Huyse, F.J., Strain, J.J., and Hammer, J.S. (1990). Interventions in consultation/liaison psychiatry. Part 1: Patterns of recommendations. *General Hospital Psychiatry*, **12**, 213–20.

Incalzi, R.A., Gemma, A., Capparella, O., Muzzolon, R., Antico, L., and Carbonin, P.U. (1991). Effects of hospitalization on affective status of elderly patients. *International Psychogeriatrics*, **3**, 67–74.

Inouye, S.K., Viscoli, C.M., Horwitz, R.I., Hurst, L.D., and Tinetti, M.E. (1993). A predictive model for delirium in hospitalized elderly medical patients based on admission characteristics. *Annals of Internal Medicine*, **119**, 474–81.

Inouye, S.K., Bogardus, S.T. Jr, Charpentier, P., Leo-Summers, L., Acampora, D., Holford, T.R., *et al.* (1999). A multicomponent intervention to prevent delirium in hospitalized older patients. *New England Journal of Medicine*, **340**, 669–676.

Jolley, D. and Arie, T. (1978). Organization of psychogeriatric services. *British Journal of Psychiatry*, **132**, 1–11.

Joseph, C., Goldsmith, S., Rooney, A., McWhorter, K., and Ganzini, L. (1995). An interdisciplinary mental health consultation team in a nursing home. *Gerontologist*, **35**, 836–9.

Kisely, S. and Axten, C. (2000). Collaboration between general and old age psychiatrists in the provision of a consultation-liaison service. *The Royal Australian and New Zealand College of Psychiatrists 35th Annual Congress*. Adelaide, South Australia, 27–30 April 2000.

Kitching, D. (1999). The consultation-liaison psychogeriatrician—current experience in a general hospital. *Faculty of Psychiatry of Old Age (Royal Australian and New Zealand College of Psychiatrists), 1st Annual Clinical Meeting*, Sydney, Australia, 30 November, 1999.

Koenig, H.G., Goli, V., Shelp, F., Kudler, H.S., Cohen, H.J., and Blazer, D.G. (1992). Major depression in hospitalized medically ill older men: documentation, management, and outcome. *International Journal of Geriatric Psychiatry*, **7**, 25–34.

Koenig, H.G., George, L.K., and Meador, K.G. (1997*a*). Use of antidepressants by nonpsychiatrists in the treatment of medically ill hospitalized depressed elderly patients. *American Journal of Psychiatry*, **154**, 1369–75.

Koenig, H.G., George, L.K., Peterson, B.L., and Pieper, C.F. (1997*b*). Depression in medically ill hospitalized older adults: prevalence, characteristics, and course of symptoms according to six diagnostic schemes. *American Journal of Psychiatry*, **154**, 1376–83.

Krakowski, A.J. (1979). Psychiatric consultation for the geriatric population in the general hospital. *Bibliothecha Psychiatrica*, **159**, 163–85.

Lederberg, M.S. (1997). Making a situational diagnosis. Psychiatrists at the interface of psychiatry and ethics in the consultation-liaison setting. *Psychosomatics*, **38**, 327–38.

Leo, R.J., Narayan, D.A., Sherry, C., Michalek, C., and Pollock, D. (1997). Geropsychiatric consultation for African-American and Caucasian patients. *General Hospital Psychiatry*, **19**, 216–22.

Levitan, S. and Kornfeld, D. (1981). Clinical and cost benefits of liaison psychiatry. *American Journal of Psychiatry*, **138**, 790–3.

Levitte, S.S. and Thornby, J.I. (1989). Geriatric and nongeriatric consultation. A comparative study. *General Hospital Psychiatry*, **11**, 339–44.

Lipowski, Z.J. (1983*a*). Current trends in consultation-liaison psychiatry. *Canadian Journal of Psychiatry*, **28**, 329–37.

Lipowski, Z.J. (1983*b*). The need to integrate liaison psychiatry and geropsychiatry. *American Journal of Psychiatry*, **140**, 1003–5.

Lipowski, Z.J. (1986). Consultation-liaison psychiatry: the first half century. *General Hospital Psychiatry*, **8**, 305–15.

Lippert, G.P., Conn, D., Schogt, B., and Ickowicz A. (1990). Psychogeriatric consultation: general hospital versus home for the aged. *General Hospital Psychiatry*, **12**, 313–18.

Llewellyn-Jones, R.H., Baikie, K.A., Smithers, H., Cohen, J., Snowdon J., and Tennant, C.C. (1999). Multifaceted shared care intervention for late life depression in residential care: randomised controlled trial. *British Medical Journal*, 319, 676–82.

Loane, R. and Jefferys, P. (1998). Consultation-liaison in a geriatric psychiatry service. *Psychiatric Bulletin*, **22**, 217–20.

Macdonald, A. (1986). Do general practitioners miss depression in elderly patients? *British Medical Journal*, **292**, 1365–7.

Mainprize, E. and Rodin, G. (1987). Geriatric referrals to a psychiatric consultation-liaison service. *Canadian Journal of Psychiatry*, **32**, 5–9.

Millar, H.R. (1981). Psychiatric morbidity in elderly surgical patients. *British Journal of Psychiatry*, **138**, 17–20.

Mohl, P. (1981). A review of systems approaches to consultation-liaison psychiatry. *General Hospital Psychiatry*, **3**, 103–10.

Oxman, T.E. (1996). Geriatric psychiatry at the interface of consultation-liaison psychiatry and primary care. *International Journal of Psychiatry in Medicine*, **26**, 145–53.

Pauser, H., Bergström, B., and Wålinder, J. (1987). Evaluation of 294 psychiatric consultations involving in-patients above 70 years of age in somatic departments in a university hospital. *Acta Psychiatrica Scandinavica*, **76**, 152–7.

Pérez, E.L. and Blouin, J. (1986). Psychiatric emergency consultations to elderly patients in a Canadian general hospital. *Journal of the American Geriatrics Society*, **34**, 91–4.

Pérez, E.L, Silverman, M., and Blouin, J. (1985). Psychiatric consultation to elderly medical and surgical inpatients in a general hospital. *Psychiatric Quarterly*, **57**, 18–22.

Pitt, B. and Silver, C.P. (1980). The combined approach to geriatrics and psychiatry: evaluation of a joint unit in a teaching hospital district. *Age and Ageing*, **9**, 33–7.

Popkin, M.K., Mackenzie, T.B., and Callies, A.L. (1984). Psychiatric consultation to geriatric medically ill inpatients in a university hospital. *Archives of General Psychiatry*, **41**, 703–7.

Poynton, A.M. (1988). Psychiatric liaison referrals of elderly in-patients in a teaching hospital. *British Journal of Psychiatry*, **152**, 45–7.

Puryear, D.A., Lovitt, R., and Miller, D.A. (1991). Characteristics of elderly persons seen in an urban psychiatric emergency room. *Hospital and Community Psychiatry*, **42**, 802–7.

Rabins, P., Lucas, M.J., Teitelbaum, M., Mark, S.R., and Folstein, M. (1983). Utilization of psychiatric consultation for elderly patients. *Journal of the American Geriatrics Society*, **31**, 581–5.

Ramsay, R., Wright, P., Katz, A., Bielawska, C., and Katona, C. (1991). The detection of psychiatric morbidity and its effects on outcome in acute elderly medical admissions. *International Journal of Geriatric Psychiatry*, **6**, 861–6.

Rapp, S.R., Parisi, S.A. and Wallace, C.E. (1991). Comorbid psychiatric disorders in elderly medical patients: a 1-year prospective study. *The Journal of the American Geriatrics Society*, **39**, 124–31.

Reichman, W.E., Coyne, A.C., Borson, S., Negrón, A.E., Rovner, B.W., Pelchat, R.J., *et al*. (1998). Psychiatric consultation in the nursing home. *American Journal of Geriatric Psychiatry*, **6**, 320–7.

Rosewarne, R., Opie, J., Bruce, A., Ward, S., Doyle, C., and Sach, J. (1997). Care needs of people with dementia and challenging behaviours living in residential facilities. Main Report. *Aged and Community Care Service Development and Evaluation Reports*, Number 30. Australian Government Printing Service, Canberra, Australia.

Roulaux, T.A.H., Oei, T.T., and Jansen op de Haar, M.M.B.B. (1993). A decade of psychiatric consultation with elderly patients in a Dutch general hospital. *International Psychogeriatrics*, **5**, 103–8.

Rovner, B.W., Steele, C.D., Shmuely, Y., and Folstein, M.F. (1996). A randomized trial of dementia care in nursing homes. *Journal of the American Geriatrics Society*, **44**, 7–13.

Ruskin, P.E. (1985). Geropsychiatric consultation in a university hospital: a report on 67 referrals. *American Journal of Psychiatry*, **142**, 333–6.

Scott, J., Fairbairn, A., and Woodhouse, K. (1988). Referrals to a psychogeriatric consultation-liaison service. *International Journal of Geriatric Psychiatry*, **3**, 131–5.

Seidel, G., Smith, C., Hafner, R.J., and Holme, G. (1992). A psychogeriatric community outreach service: description and evaluation. *International Journal of Geriatric Psychiatry*, **7**, 347–50.

Seymour, D.G. and Pringle, R. (1983). Post-operative complications in the elderly surgical patient. *Gerontology*, **29**, 262–70.

Shah, A. and De, T. (1998). Documented evidence of depression in medical and nursing case-notes and its implications in acutely ill geriatric inpatients. *International Psychogeriatrics*, **10**, 163–72.

Shah, A., Dighe-Deo, D., Chapman, C., Phongsathorn, V., George, C., Bielawski, C., *et al*. (1998). Suicidal ideation amongst acutely medically ill and continuing care geriatric inpatients. *Aging and Mental Health*, **2**, 300–5.

Shah, S. and Harris, M. (1997). A survey of general practitioners' confidence in their management of elderly patients. *Australian Family Physician*, **26** (Suppl. 1), S12–S17.

Shamash, K., O'Connell, K., Lowy, M., and Katona, C.L.E. (1992). Psychiatric morbidity and outcome in elderly patients undergoing emergency hip surgery: a one-year follow-up study. *International Journal of Geriatric Psychiatry*, **7**, 505–9.

Sharpe, M.E. and Hawton, K.E. (1990). Liaison psychiatry and psychological sequelae of physical disorders. *Current Opinion in Psychiatry*, **3**, 199–203.

Shevitz, S.A., Silberfarb, P.M., and Lipowski, Z.J. (1976). Psychiatric consultations in a general hospital. A report on 1,000 referrals. *Diseases of the Nervous System*, **37**, 295–300.

Shulman, R.W., Marton, P., Fisher, A., and Cohen, C. (1996). Characteristics of psychogeriatric patient visits to a general hospital emergency room. *Canadian Journal of Psychiatry*, **41**, 175–80.

Slaets, J.P.J., Kauffmann, R.H., Duivenvoorden, H.J., Pelemans, W., and Schudel, W.J. (1997). A randomized trial of geriatric liaison intervention in elderly medical inpatients. *Psychosomatic Medicine*, **59**, 585–91.

Small, G.W. and Fawzy, F.I. (1988). Psychiatric consultation for the medically ill elderly in the general hospital: Need for a collaborative model of care. *Psychosomatics*, **29**, 94–103.

Smith, G.C., Strain, J.J., Hammer, J.S., Wallack, J.J., Bialer, P.A., Schleifer, S.S., *et al.* (1997). Organic mental disorders in the consultation-liaison setting. *Psychosomatics*, **38**, 363–73.

Snowdon, J., Vaughan, R., and Miller, R. (1995). Mental health services in Sydney nursing homes. *Australian Journal of Public Health*, **19**, 403–6.

Starkman, M.N. and Hall, G.G. (1979). Teaching medical gerontology: utilization of a psychiatry consultation program. *Journal of Medical Education*, **54**, 643–8.

Strain, J.J., Lyons, J.S., Hammer, J.S., Fahs, M., Lebovits, A., Paddison, P.L., *et al.* (1991). Cost offset from a psychiatric consultation-liaison intervention with elderly hip fracture patients. *American Journal of Psychiatry*, **148**, 1044–9.

Swanwick, G.R.J., Lee, H., Clare, A.W., and Lawlor, B.A. (1994). Consultation-liaison psychiatry: a comparison of two service models for geriatric patients. *International Journal of Geriatric Psychiatry*, **9**, 495–9.

Swigar, M.E., Sanguineti, V.R., and Piscatelli, R.L. (1992). A retrospective study on the perceived need for and actual use of psychiatric consultations in older medical patients. *International Journal of Psychiatry in Medicine*, **22**, 239–49.

Thienhaus, O.J., Rowe, C., Woellert, P., and Hillard, J.R. (1988). Geropsychiatric emergency services: utilization and outcome predictors. *Hospital and Community Psychiatry*, **39**, 1301–5.

Tourigny-Rivard, M-F. and Drury, M. (1987). The effects of monthly psychiatric consultation in a nursing home. *Gerontologist*, **27**, 363–6.

Unützer, J. and Small, G.W. (1996). Geriatric consultation-liaison psychiatry. In *Comprehensive review of geriatric psychiatry–II* (2nd edn) (ed. J. Sadavoy, L.W. Lazarus, L.F. Jarvik, and G.T. Grossberg), pp. 937–72. American Psychiatric Press, Washington DC.

Wright, M., Samuels, A., and Streimer, J. (1996). Clinical practice issues in consultation-liaison psychiatry. *Australian and New Zealand Journal of Psychiatry*, **30**, 238–45.

Wrigley, M. and Loane, R. (1991). Consultation-liaison referrals to the north Dublin geriatric psychiatry service. *Irish Medical Journal*, **84**, 89–91.

Zimmer, J.G., Watson, N., and Treat, A. (1984). Behavioural problems among patients in skilled nursing facilities. *American Journal of Public Health*, **74**, 1118–21.

2 The effects of ageing

Pamela Melding

> There is no perfect definition of ageing. But, as with love or beauty, most of us know
> it when we experience or see it.
> (Hayflick, L. (1994). *How and why we age*, p. 12.)

From prehistory to modern times, life expectancy has increased by about 32 years. Before the Common Era, the human lifespan averaged 22 years, by the turn of the twentieth century it averaged 50 years. The twentieth century saw an increase in life expectancy almost equivalent to the previous two millennia. Some people did live to great ages, but they were the exception rather than the norm. Cultures that traditionally venerated old people perhaps did so because they were rare, and considered the person who lived to 'three score and ten' to have survival strengths worthy of special reverence (Hayflick 1994).

Today, there are 580 million people aged over 60 years, with 171 million of them in the developing world (World Health Organization 1999). This worldwide 'elder boom' is very much a phenomenon of the modern times. Advances in public, antenatal, postnatal, child, and other healthcare have improved both the number of surviving young expected to grow old and also human longevity, that is, the expected length of life at birth. Population ageing is particularly rapid in the developing world (WHO 1999) with a projected nine times increase in the over-60 population by 2050. Worldwide, the over-80 age groups are the most rapidly expanding sector of the older population. The human lifespan may not yet have reached its limit and the potential may be as much as 115–120 years (Hayflick 1994; Finch and Pike 1996).

Lifespan potential is different from life expectancy, as disease tempers the latter. At the turn of the century, infectious diseases were the major causes of death, but as these have been eradicated or controlled, chronic degenerative diseases have gained prominence. Individuals remain free from disease for longer and morbidity is increasingly compressed into the seventh decade and beyond. Currently, in the developed world, women outlive men by 7 or more years (WHO 1999). It is difficult to ascertain the cause of this phenomenon. Possible factors include: (1) the cohort effect of a particular generation affected by one or more major wars; (2) increased health-risk behaviours in males; (3) male propensity to cardiovascular diseases; or possibly (4) a true gender-based biological advantage. Whatever the reason, there are approximately 15% more elderly women than men, the majority of whom are widows who have outlived their men-folk. Unfortunately, women do not benefit greatly from their extra longevity, as they are more prone to disabling diseases such as arthritis, Alzheimer's disease, and hearing and visual impairments. Women can expect about 2 years of disablement more than their male counterparts (Verbrugge 1989) and are more likely to require hospitalization.

What is ageing?

Ageing is a progressive accumulation of changes over time that causes the systems and structures of the organism to lose function, decline, and eventually die. No single measure accurately quantifies ageing changes. *Chronological age* is widely used in most societies as a social discriminator to determine who should or should not be eligible for various social benefits or services. Leonard Hayflick (1994), a prominent researcher and writer in the field of human ageing, ironically notes (page 108) 'much of what we think about human ageing is centered around the concept that the number sixty-five is somehow significant—there is still a widely held belief that at age sixty-five some mysterious biological event occurs that makes humans old at the stroke of midnight!'. People actually age at rates that have no relationship to the number of their birthdays.

Biological age is an alternative, as indicated by the phrase 'appears older' or 'appears younger' than the stated years commonly seen in health records. Some 80-year-olds may be as physiologically fit as 50-year-olds and vice versa. However, as ageing takes place in different human cells at different rates in different people, 'biological age' also has its limitations as a measure of ageing.

Social age refers to a society's expectation of older people's roles and norms. In New Zealand Maori culture, the tribal leaders are the elders, or *Kaumatua*, and great age is revered for bringing *mana* or great wisdom. This tribal leadership role starts at an age when many Europeans retire. Unfortunately, vulnerability to morbid diseases and premature death has left many Maori communities without elderly people to take on the role of tribal elders. This leaves a void in the social structure and consequently a *kaumatua* designee sometimes has to start this leadership role at a younger age than is usual. Quite often in this situation an interesting phenomenon occurs, with the youngish 'elder' starting to look and behave as one much older, in keeping with the community's expectation of eldership (Maaka 1993).

Other measures of age are *psychological age* or the degree to which the person has developmentally matured. Older people themselves have a self-perceived age. The age they inwardly feel is often decades younger than their chronological age. Commonly, many 80-year-olds perceive themselves to be 'too young' to go into a geriatric unit.

What causes ageing?

The precise process that makes a human age is unknown. Theories vary from determinist genetic to conjectural environmental hypotheses. There is much interest in, and some evidence for, a genetic basis to ageing. Before the 1960s, scientists considered that human diploid cells in laboratory culture would divide and replicate indefinitely. Hayflick and Moorhead (1961) conclusively demonstrated that, *in vitro*, human diploid fibroblast cells appeared to have a finite number of subcultivations (the 'Hayflick limit') specifically programmed into a cell strain. As the cell culture reaches this limit, growth slows, the cells shows signs of distress, and they die.

Further evidence for programmed ageing has come from *in vitro* cell-fusion experiments between defined-lifespan diploid cells (capable of senescence) and potentially immortal, transformed heteroploid cells (tumour cells without ageing potential) (Pereira-Smith and Smith 1983). This work indicates that the phenotype for senescence is dominant. So, how is the number of pre-programmed replications controlled? Engelhardt and Martens (1998) hypothesize that chromosomes have expendable ends called telomeres that act as biological clocks for the ageing process. These structures function to protect chromosomes from degradation, fusion, and recombination and are important regulators in cell division. Each cell replication shortens the telomere sequences until eventually the cell is no longer capable of division and it dies (Fossel 1998). Further evidence comes from the discovery of genes that command the expression or suppression of the enzyme telomerase, (a ribonucleoprotein reverse transcriptase), in somatic cells. Telomerase, when genetically 'switched on', maintains the base pair sequences of the chromosome ends thus preventing the shortening process. In some animal experiments (Engelhardt and Martens 1998) this process is linked to the onset of cancer (which consists of cells that replicate indefinitely and whose telomeres do not shorten i.e. are non-ageing). Whilst conceptually appealing, these phenomena have so far only been observed in the laboratory but the field is advancing rapidly. An implication of this work is that it might be possible to insert a gene for telomerase into ageing cells and delay or stop the ageing process. The challenge for science is to manage this without inducing malignant change.

Programmed ageing and telomere theory does not explain all the variance in ageing. Other genetic theories include instability and mutations of chromosomes, epigenetic error theories, and codon restriction theory. The reader is referred to Bittles (1997), who has reviewed the major theories and their limitations.

There are several non-genetic hypotheses. Of particular interest are the cross-linking, free-radical, and melatonin theories. With increasing age, macromolecules develop cross-links thus changing the properties of the molecules. Examples are the cross-linkage that occurs with collagen and elastin molecules which increase stiffness and brittleness. Consequently, skin and blood vessels lose elasticity (Kohn 1985).

Free radicals are produced by cell mitochondria during metabolism, but they may also be formed as the result of ionizing radiation. They are highly reactive oxidative molecules with an unpaired electron in the outer orbital shell that attacks neighbouring compounds autocatalytically. Free-radical theory (Harman 1992) conjectures that these reactive molecules are responsible for the progressive accumulation of ageing changes in cells over time. Terminally differentiated cells such as those in the brain, heart, and muscle seem to be the most severely affected, possibly because replication of these cells is slow, allowing the oxidative damage to accumulate (Miquel 1991). There is some evidence that some people's tissues may be more prone to free-radical attack than others because of a genetic susceptibility, expressed under environmental influences (Bittles 1997). Harman (1985) suggested that the greater longevity of females may be partly due to genetic resistance to free-radical attack. At least one of the key enzymes necessary to the inhibition of these reactions in body cells, is located on the X chromosome. The free-radical theory has gained wide attention and has been commercially successful for health-food retailers in the sale of antioxidants, which may protect against free-radical damage. Whilst animal experiments indicate that longevity is increased by the addition of these compounds to the diet, benefit to humans has yet to be proven (Bittles 1997).

Much interest has been expressed in the general and professional press on the possible role the pineal hormone melatonin might play in the ageing process. This hormone regulates the seasonal and circadian fluctuations of other hormones and synchronizes the biological light–dark and sleep–wake cycles. In addition, melatonin is one of the most powerful free-hydroxyl scavengers known (Reiter 1995) and may also have an immunoenhancing function (Zhang *et al.* 1997). Thus, melatonin features as a link in at least three ageing theories: that is, free-radical theory, lowered immunological function, and decline of hormone cycles. However, the evidence linking melatonin with the ageing process remains speculative but inconclusive. Zeiter *et al.* (1999) compared plasma concentrations of melatonin in young (under 30 years of age) and elderly (over 65) patients and did not detect a significant difference. Kennaway *et al.* (1999) analysed the excretion of a melatonin metabolite in 253 patients aged between 21 and 80 and found an age-associated reduction, but noted that this actually occurred around 20–30 years of age. It seems that ageing is associated with loss of the circadian melatonin rhythm rather than with the plasma melatonin level, and that this change destabilizes other circadian rhythms contributing to ageing and age-related diseases.

Other ageing theories are summarized in Table 2.1. Most are conjectural theories based on observations of changes associated with ageing in various organ systems. With our current knowledge, it is impossible to determine whether the changes are the cause or the result of ageing at the cellular level.

No theory explains all, and many theories overlap with others. Ageing probably depends upon genetic programming, which is influenced by favourable or detrimental environmental circumstances, and is modified by lifestyle factors such as caloric intake, nutrition, sun exposure, smoking, alcohol, exercise, and health behaviours.

Table 2.1 Theories of ageing

	Theory	Evidence for	Evidence against
System-based	Wear and tear	Vascular stiffness limiting blood circulation to vital organs	Ageing is observable in animal species that lack blood vessels
	Immune	T-cell loss related to characteristic changes of ageing	Difficult to isolate immune system from neuroendocrine systems. Ageing seen in animals without an immune system
	Neuroendocrine	Age-related changes could be ascribed to neuroendocrine loss, e.g. adrenal, thyroid, and gonadal hormones	Lacks universal application
	Melatonin	Melatonin important in neuroendocrine cycles. Potent free-radical scavenger. Melatonin immunoenhancer	Plasma melatonin does not decline after 20–30 years of age
Genetic	Programmed ageing in human cells	Hayflick limit; telomeres as programmable 'clock'	Generalizable to human ageing? Some animal models of ageing do not show telomere shortening
	Twin studies	Greater similarity in lifespans with monozygotic twins	HLA studies suggest monozygotic twins inherit susceptibilities to diseases that is the lifespan limiting factor
Phenomenological	Rate of living	Inverse relationship between basal metabolic rate and longevity	Research has not identified a salient factor controlling this relationship
	Accumulation of waste products	Accumulation of lipofuscin in cells with advancing age	Build-up does not affect cell function significantly and may be a secondary effect
	Oxygen-radical tissue damage (free-radical theory)	Mitochondrial DNA and cell organelles susceptible to oxidative damage by free radicals produced by metabolism	In *in vitro* cell cultures mitochondria still have potential function, despite free-radical attack at point of death

How does ageing interface with age-related disease?

Ageing changes the homeostasis of the organism and increases vulnerability to disease. Dynamically juxtaposed are the individuals' psychological responses to these events as they occur. Although changes occur at a cellular and organ level they eventually reach a threshold at which the individual person recognizes, responds, and has to adapt (Whitbourne 1996). Several human, longitudinal research studies of ageing cohorts, such as the Baltimore Aging Study (Shock *et al.* 1984) and the Duke Longitudinal Study (Busse and Maddox 1985), have provided a wealth of data on the effects of ageing alone and in conjunction with disease, as well as people's responses to both.

These studies indicate that:

◆ Some losses are the inevitable consequences of the ageing process and unrelated to disease. These tend to be very slow losses over time.

◆ Some slow losses can be the result of diseases such as arthritis and Alzheimer's disease.

◆ Sudden losses are the result of diseases rather than ageing.

◆ Primary changes lead to secondary changes. As losses occur, the body tries to compensate and this can cause further losses or change.

◆ Lifestyle factors can influence the occurrence or progression of age-related diseases (Hayflick 1994).

The interface between ageing, disease, and mental health

Appearance

Changes to the epidermis of the skin, reduction in sweat- and oil-producing glands, and loss and structural change in connective tissue collagen and elastin give the characteristic wrinkles and sagging skin of ageing (Kohn 1985). Sweat and sebaceous glands become less active (Kurban and Bhawan 1990). These changes accelerate with sun exposure and cigarette smoking. The physical changes increase the risk of skin diseases such as dermatitis, pruritus and skin cancer, particularly for those with previous sun damage. Depletion of hair follicles leads to hair loss, and reduction in melanin pigment gives the characteristic greying of the hair (Whitbourne 1998). Teeth lose enamel and periodontal disease may result in total loss of dentition. The bones lose mineral content, strength, and become osteoporotic. Men lose about 3 cm and women 5 cm in their height from the age of 30 to 70 years (Sorkin *et al.* 1999). Bone and muscle mass is lost but fat stores increase (O'Connor *et al.* 1998), giving midriff obesity or 'middle aged spread'.

It is often the outward, unmistakable signs of ageing that cause the person to acknowledge that they are growing older. Depending on an individual's attitudes and personality, such a self-admission may be tolerable or threatening. Some wear wrinkles proudly as a testament to a well-lived life, while others view ageing changes as an affront to their personal self-image.

Bone demineralization can result in painful fractures and collapse of vertebrae. Wear and tear losses to joint articular cartilage causes osteoarthritic changes that restrict movement, induce muscle wasting, and give discomfort (Ralphs and Benjamin 1994). The outcome is often stooped posture, loss of height, decreased mobility, and chronic skeletal pain. Reduced muscle strength, painful joints, and reduced mobility interfere with activities of daily living, decrease independence, lower a sense of well-being, and contribute to a fear of falling. A hip fracture may devastate an older person and, if they are poorly rehabilitated, lead to severe loss of confidence, long-term disability, and dependency (Roberto 1992)

Sensory system

Hearing

Many older people experience hearing difficulties in social conversational situations where there is background noise, for example in busy, noisy hospital wards.

The Baltimore Longitudinal Study found marked gender differences; men had a greater loss of hearing sensitivity with an earlier age of decline than women (Pearson et al. 1995). These subjects were controlled for otological disease and noise-induced hearing loss. Age-related decreases in hearing particularly affect the higher frequencies (presbycusis) and the hearing of consonant sounds. This may be accompanied by tinnitus and a loss of ability to hear loud sounds.

Deafness, even if mild, has psychological effects. Tinnitus reduces hearing further, may cause insomnia, and be extremely irritating. Tinnitus may be misinterpreted as other stimuli. Patients may complain of hearing noises from power cables or water pipes, and tinnitus can be the focus of delusions. Older people are often highly embarrassed if they miss parts of conversations and may confabulate or attempt to cover up for the deficits. On occasions, the misinterpretation may be severe enough to appear as if the person is cognitively impaired. The psychological consequences of deafness include persecutory ideation often due to misinterpretation, depression, social deprivation, and loneliness. Profound deafness does not preclude auditory hallucinations.

Balance

Age-related changes in the vestibular system produce dizziness and vertigo. These unpleasant sensations may lead to falls, nausea, and vomiting. Some medications, cardiovascular disease, or other debilitating physical illness may make matters worse (Anderson et al. 1995). Slopes, stairs, escalators, and an uneven floor surface can upset the person's balance and increase a fear of falling (Myers et al. 1996).

Older people can be trapped at the top of stairs or escalators or have panic attacks trying to negotiate them. The individual with balance problems often becomes very anxious or embarrassed and fears appearing intoxicated or mentally confused. Agoraphobia and social isolation may result.

Vision

Ageing affects the retina, lens, and vitreous humor of the eye. There is a loss of accommodation (presbyopia) due to the lens fibres becoming hard and less elastic. The accumulation of yellow pigment in the lens reduces an individual's ability to discriminate the green, blue, violet spectrum. Cataract formation severely reduces eyesight. The retina undergoes ganglion-cell degeneration, degeneration of the macula, thinning of the central retina, and a decrease in foveal cone density. Visual acuity decreases, particularly for distance vision, and the older person has more difficulty tracking moving objects, particularly in low-light situations (Whitbourne 1998). Older people become, realistically, nervous when driving at night.

Presbyopia, poor dark adaptation, and a decrease in depth perception increase people's vulnerability to falls (McMurdo and Gaskell 1991). If the visual losses are uncorrectable, then partial or total blindness severely limits independence and activities of daily living. Leisure pursuits such as reading, watching television, and movie or theatre going are lost. Low vision can cause visual misinterpretations. Social isolation, loneliness, and depression are often consequences of poor vision.

Taste and smell

Odour detection variably diminishes with age, with women performing better than men in such tests (Hayflick 1994; Ship et al. 1996). Olfactory decline, which starts in the twenties, is accelerated by smoking tobacco. Loss of the sense of smell can be dangerous if an older person cannot detect leaking gas or smoke.

The number of taste buds does not reduce with age, but some degeneration takes place within the cells of the buds themselves so that taste sensation declines slightly with age. Diseases or side-effects of medication, such as anticholinergic effects, may cause marked deficits.

Smell and taste sensations are important for nutrition. Loss of pleasure in eating can lead to poor nourishment. Debility and malnutrition may facilitate depressive illness that will further reduce taste sensation and appetite. Older people who suddenly develop increased sensitivity to smells may have an underlying medical problem or psychiatric disturbance.

Vital organs

Normally active, healthy older people show little change in cardiac output with age (Shock et al. 1984). However, Fleg et al. (1995), using data from the Baltimore

Longitudinal Aging Study, found gender differences in that ageing produced little change in the resting heart rate and systemic vascular resistance in healthy older men, but there was some decrease in older women. During exercise, the older men (but not the women) increased their stroke volume rather than their resting heart rate to maintain cardiac output, in contrast to younger people.

Even in normotensive people, age-associated increases in arterial stiffness occur (Vaitkevicius *et al.* 1993). At a microscopic level, the elastin and intima of blood vessel walls becomes thickened and rigid. These changes predispose the individual to atherosclerosis, a disease process that may actually start in early adult life. One of the first descriptions of the disease was by Leonardo da Vinci (1425–1519) who considered the consequent reduction in blood supply to be the cause of ageing (Hayflick 1994, p. 151). Atherosclerosis increases resistance and impedance to blood flow and circulation. It reduces blood supply to organ systems and increases vulnerability to cardiac disease. Genetic factors such as familial hypercholestero-laemia and lifestyle factors such as smoking, little exercise, dietary factors, and hypertension facilitate these changes. Interestingly, atherosclerosis appears to be a human disease as it rarely occurs naturally in old animals (Hayflick 1994, p. 152). Cardiac disease is the commonest cause of death for older people in the developed world, with autopsy studies indicating that 65–75% of men and 60–65% women have significant coronary stenosis. Approximately half of these are clinically silent (Rodeheffer and Gerstenblith 1985).

Cardiovascular function is essential to life and, at a psychological level, heart disease is perceived as a serious threat by the individual. Depression, anxiety, and fear of dying can be the reaction to a diagnosis of cardiac disease. Lowered cardiac output can have deleterious effects on mood, well-being, and functioning. Mitral incompetence is associated with panic and hyperventilation disorders, both of which can mimic angina pain.

Respiratory system

Lung function reduces by approximately 0.75% per annum after the age of 30 years (Smith 1985). As in other organ systems, lung alveoli walls lose elasticity and the pulmonary vasculature shows intimal thickening. Decreased vital capacity and forced expiratory volume lower the quality of gas exchange in ageing respiratory systems, particularly under exercise conditions. Bronchial mucous glands increase with age. Over time, pollution, smoking, and respiratory infections destroy cilia, the mechanical barrier to infections, in nasal passage, bronchi, and small airways (Smith 1985), making the older person more susceptible to respiratory tract infections.

In chronic, obstructive airways disease the airways become hypersensitive and close prematurely, entrapping air and mucus. The alveoli walls distend, disrupt, and eventually break down to form bullae. The total alveolar closing volumes increase. The major breathing difficulty is during expiration due to air trapping in closed alveoli. The effect of these is to limit ventilation capability, giving a sensation of shortage of breath. These together, assisted by ventilation perfusion mismatches, lead to hypoxia and carbon dioxide retention. Cardiorespiratory failure is usually the outcome.

The sensation of shortage of breath is usually alarming. Struggling for air is exhausting and fatigue is common. The person may lie awake fearful to sleep lest they stop breathing. Paradoxically, the sensation of shortage of breath often leads to hyperventilation that further reduces gas exchange. Hypoxia and hypercapnia may also cause delirium. Both may cause psychomotor retardation with or without accompanying depression. Drugs, particularly the injudicious use of opiate or benzodiazepine sedatives, in older people in end-stage respiratory disease can depress respiration. Steroids given for chronic, obstructive airways disease or severe asthma may give rise to depression, mania, or frank psychosis.

Regulatory organs

Renal function

Structural changes in nephrons diminish renal function, as measured by creatinine clearance, by about 0.75 ml/min per year from the age 20 years (Shock *et al.* 1984; Lindeman 1990). The kidney's ability to concentrate urine also diminishes with age. Age-related changes in the bladder cause it to lose expandability, resulting in a greater residual volume after voiding. Recumbent posture, as in sleep, increases the blood flow to the kidney, with the result that older people often have to wake in the night to void, thus disturbing sleep maintenance.

Urinary incontinence may cause great distress and embarrassment for older people. Women in particular suffer from stress incontinence (voiding whilst coughing or straining) and both genders may experience urgency incontinence (precipitate voiding). A patient may lie awake all night rather than face the embarrassment of wetting the bed. Altered kidney function can interfere with the excretion of drugs, as there is less renal reserve this renders older people more vulnerable to the nephrotoxic effects of drugs such as lithium.

Immune system

The functional decline of the immune system with age possibly accelerates secondary ageing changes, which, because of feedback mechanisms, further compromise the system. Many components of the extremely complex immune system lose effectiveness with age, for example, antigen-destroying T cells. Involution of the thymus gland, the major organ of the immune system, has been implicated in this ageing process as, by 50 years of age, only 5–10% of the original gland remains. Other ageing changes include a decline in the ability to produce antibodies to foreign substances, resulting in a greater chance of producing antibodies to self-proteins thus contributing to autoimmune diseases (Makinodan and Hirokawa 1985). Free radicals, produced by neutrophils and macrophages, may also compromise the effectiveness of the immune system (De la Fuente, *et al.* 1993). Diminished immune system function increases susceptibility to cancer, infection, and autoimmune diseases such as arthritis and diabetes. These diseases have secondary effects on bodily systems causing increased pain and debility, which may have detrimental psychological effects by precipitating depression or anxiety. Psychoimmunological studies have shown that older people with high levels of life- or illness-stress have lowered T-cell functioning. Conversely, good social support has a positive effect on T-cell functioning in older people (Thomas *et al.* 1985).

Neuroendocrine system

Since the hypothalamus–pituitary–axis action on target endocrine glands affects every cell in the body, many age-related changes start to emerge as endocrine function declines. The hypothalamus influences the sleep–wake cycle, menstruation, oestrus, and thermoregulation. These rhythms change with increasing age (Timaras 1985). Blood sugar rises with age due to decreased insulin efficiency (Davidson 1979). Dehydroepiandrosterone (DHEA) (a gonadal hormone precursor), oestrogen, testosterone, and growth hormone levels all decline with age.

Ageing has little effect on the thyroid gland itself, but thyroxine levels (T_4) decline slightly (Rowe and Devons 1996, p. 32) and there is, possibly, some loss in the ability of target receptor cells to respond to the hormone (Hayflick 1994). Ageing does produce an increase in autoimmune problems as discussed earlier, and thus the prevalence of anti-thyroid antibodies increases with age. It is more likely that this factor is responsible for the increased thyroid disease seen in older people rather than an age-related decline of the thyroid gland itself (Rosenthal *et al.* 1987). Hypothyroidism may present with a variety of mental symptoms including depression, memory loss, stupor, weakness, and constipation. This disorder may be confused with dementia. Hyperthyroidism can present in atypical ways in older people, for example with apathy and depression rather than nervousness.

A differential decrease in the neurotransmitters noradrenaline, dopamine, acetylcholine, and, possibly, serotonin, occurs with ageing. These deficiencies may result in cerebral neurotransmitter imbalances contributing to several psychiatric syndromes, including depression, anxiety, and psychosis.

Several mechanisms affect thermoregulation. Reduced sweat glands in the skin impair responses to heat, any decline in thyroid activity decreases the basal metabolic rate, and the reduction of monoamines in the autonomic nervous system inhibits the vasoconstriction response. The loss of sweat glands in the skin and poor vasodilator/vasoconstrictor responses can cause overheating in hot weather and hypothermia in cold.

The sleep–wake cycle changes in late life. Sleep latency is longer and sleep maintenance may be impaired. Older people seem to need more rest periods but less time asleep. Other ageing changes such as 'heartburn', urinary frequency, or sleep apnoea also disturb sleep. EEG studies show an age-related rise in stage-1 sleep and a large decrease in stage-4 sleep. By the late sixties and seventies, rapid eye movement (REM) sleep starts to diminish (Whitbourne 1998). Older people can get very upset about changes in their sleep pattern and believe that less than 8 hours sleep is abnormal. This is often a reason for them to seek night sedatives. Of course, sleep disturbance is a feature of several psychiatric disorders such as depression, anxiety, dementia, and delirium.

Central nervous system

Ageing changes occur at the cellular level, with cytoplasmic accumulation of lipofuscin, loss of neurons, and the formation of neuritic plaques and neurofibrillary tangles. These are seen in the normal ageing brain, but in Alzheimer's disease the numbers increase markedly. Macroscopically, the brain shows some shrinkage and ventricular enlargement with increased sulci. The brain at 90 years of age weighs 10% less than it did at 20 years. For most, these losses do not result in clinically significant problems as the brain has a vast surplus of neurons. In addition, neurons have some degree of plasticity and some can sprout new connections to compensate for broken circuits. It is only if the neuronal losses are in cells whose functions can not be assumed by other cells that significant deficits become manifest, or if the loss of cells is greater than the reserve (Hayflick 1994).

The EEG of a healthy elderly person shows a well-organized, dominant resting background rhythm centred in the alpha (12–18 Hz) frequency band. There is a shift in the dominant spontaneous rhythm, decreasing in frequency at about 0.5 Hz per decade between the ages of 60 and 90 years but remaining stable thereafter. There is an increase in diffuse slow-wave delta (0.5–4 Hz) and theta (4–8 Hz) activity, with increased focal slow-wave delta and theta activity in the left temporal area. A generalized increase in fast-wave beta (18–30 Hz) activity occurs up to 80 years of age, decreasing thereafter. Clinical activation procedures result in a general lowered responsiveness (Keller *et al.* 1985). Neurodegenerative diseases usually show changes in the EEG pattern late in the disease when there is considerable neuronal loss.

Cognitive function

The functional changes that occur with cognition and ageing are multiple and complex. Cognition is the effective, dynamic processing of information at any point in time, or 'fluid intelligence', and is also the accumulation of all the products and knowledge of previous cognitive processing or 'crystallized intelligence' (Horn 1982). 'Crystallized intelligence' does not decline in normal ageing—because it incorporates the full range of affective, analytical, emotional, conceptual, and intellectual processing, it often increases with maturity and wisdom. 'Fluid intelligence' does decline with ageing, with hierarchically superior mental operations giving way to more concrete cognition (Labouvie-Vief 1985). One major research difficulty is in determining the effect of age, culture, and educational level on a person's ability to perform cognitive tests of fluid processing. In general, short-term memory declines with age and new learning becomes more difficult. Older people often have particular difficulty with retrieving names, which is often socially very embarrassing. The ability to solve novel problems also declines. Processing response time slows; however, some individuals become more careful, resulting in a speed–accuracy trade-off (Salthouse 1996).

Age-related cognitive decline

When does age-related cognitive decline become pathological? Despite considerable debate, some agreement exists (Salthouse 1998) as summarized below.

1. Pathological cognitive decline occurs over a short time, months or a few years. Normal age-related decline takes place over decades.

2. The person's functional performance has declined relative to that person's peers (two standard deviations below the peer group). A demonstrable fall from a previous level of functioning means that pathological decline is likely.

3. Normal activities or level of functioning has declined *and* the person is unable to adapt or accommodate the change to maintain functioning in normal life. Thus, one might be worried about a former university professor who can no longer do a simple word game when he used to devise the newspaper's cryptic crossword, but not about his colleague who has taken to reading pulp fiction and thrillers instead of serious literature.

The central nervous system is vulnerable to age-related diseases such as Alzheimer's disease and related dementing disorders, cerebrovascular disease, tumours, and the neurodegenerative disorders such as Parkinson's disease.

Which older people are most at risk?

The literature generally supports the contention that problems of ageing, complications of disease, and poor psychological adaptation increase the risk for mental health problems (Lindesay 1990; Phillips and Murrell 1994; Garfein and Herzog 1995). The British Medical Research Council longitudinal study of adjustment in later life (Taylor 1994) assessed risk in 10 groups of older people, identifying 19 variables covering physical and psychological health, confidence, activity support, and material resources. The groups clustered into three main categories of risk. Those individuals recently discharged from hospital were clearly at more risk for

Table 2.2 The interface between ageing changes, disease, and psychiatric disorder

System	Ageing changes	Potential diseases	Common psychiatric problems
Cardiovascular	Structure of collagen and elastin in vessels and ventricles	Atherosclerosis Myocardial infarction Mitral valve prolapse Heart failure	Dementia Depressive episode Anxiety disorders Panic disorder Delirium
Respiratory	Reduced ventilation exchange	Pneumonia Late-onset asthma and obstructive respiratory disease Cancer	Anxiety disorders Panic disorder Depression Delirium Organic mood disorders
Immune	Decline in T-cell function Autoimmune antibodies	Infections Cancer Autoimmune disease Thyroid disease Rheumatoid arthritis Systemic lupus erythematosis	Depressive episode Anxiety disorders Delirium Psychotic disorder Organic mood disorders
Neuroendocrine	Altered thyroid function Decreased insulin efficiency Decreased neurotransmitters altering pituitary–hypothalamic function Diminished melatonin secretion	Hypothyroidism Hyperthyroidism Diabetes mellitus Pituitary failure	Sleep disorders Depressive episode Anxiety disorders Psychotic disorder Organic mood disorders Dementia Sleep disorders
Musculoskeletal	Demineralization Loss of muscle tone	Osteoporosis Mobility Fractures	Depressive episode Anxiety disorders Adjustment disorders

Skin	Loss of collagen and hair pigmentation	Dermatitis Pruritus Malignancies	Depressive episode Anxiety disorders Adjustment disorders
Genitourinary	Urinary frequency Prostatic hypertrophy	Incontinence Infection Cancer of prostate Urinary retention Loss of sexual function	Delirium Depressive episode Anxiety disorders Sleep disorder
Metabolic		Hyponatraemia Weight gain	Depressive episode Dysphoria Delirium
Brain		Dementia Cognitive impairment Cerebrovascular disease Cerebrovascular accidents Tumours	Psychotic disorder Depressive episode Delirium Dementia Organic mood disorder Mood disorder secondary to medical condition Personality change
Hearing	Loss of high-tone frequencies Vestibular stiffening	Deafness Balance problems	Paranoid disorders Depressive episode Agoraphobia Anxiety disorders
Vision	Macular degeneration Presbyopia	Blindness Distorted vision Glaucoma Cataracts	Depressive episode Anxiety disorders Adjustment disorders

physical and psychological ill health. The recently widowed, those living alone, the poor, and the socially disadvantaged were next most at risk. The childless and the never married showed a no greater risk than the sample as a whole.

Social contact and good social networks are beneficial for older people and may have the added advantage of enhancing immune function, thus decreasing their vulnerability to some diseases. Older people's social networks can break down because of high demands and dependency needs (Wenger 1997). Family-dependent networks consist of close family members who are committed to looking after their aged relative with high-dependency needs due to physical or mental frailty. These networks are vulnerable to caregiver stress and burnout. The independently minded, eccentric, or isolated individuals or couples may form restricted networks, with social isolation, absence of kin, and avoidance of neighbours or friends. There is a higher incidence of mental health difficulties in these social networks (Wenger 1997), which are often unmet as the patients usually refuse all offers of help. By the time of presentation, the mental health problems are usually florid and entrenched.

How is old age perceived?

Almost everyone has an opinion about old age, especially as old age is something to which most people aspire. Yet paradoxically, many people invest considerable physical and mental energy into denying that old age will ever affect them! Ubiquitous, cultural gerontophobia fuels a veritable gestalt of anti-ageing remedies and potions, lifestyle advice, and media standards of desired youthfulness. One possible, positive benefit is that fear of ageing may influence younger people to adopt positive lifestyle factors that will assist their personal ageing process.

The physical effects of ageing and diseases lead to myths and stereotypes about old people. Pejorative terms, such as 'wrinklies' or 'oldies' are widespread. Myths include beliefs that men and women age in the same way; older people are asexual (or at least should be); older people are frail and riddled with disease; older people are an economic and social burden; older people have no value to society; older people are querulous or complaining; older people are unable to think or cope by themselves; and that older people have a low resilience for stress (WHO 1999). Few people are actually consciously aware of the covert nature of the omnipresent gerontophobic and ageist tendencies that can affect not only their personal attitudes to ageing but also their attitudes to patients.

What is ageism?

Ageism is defined as any subjective, negative biases or prejudicial attitudes that discredit individuals based on chronological age. It includes stereotyping, patronizing superiority of younger over older, and social exclusion or avoidance of the aged (Palmore 1972). Ageism is externalized in discrimination, such as activities, institutionalized policies and practices that use the arbitrary discriminator of chronological age as a means of excluding older people from needed services or social groups (Butler 1980).

Fears and prejudicial attitudes against ageing are often concealed and have an automatic and unconscious psychological component. Unfortunately, doctors, nurses, and health professionals are as subject to pervasive ageist attitudes as any other member of the community. Perdue and Gurtman (1990) showed that negative-trait descriptors encoded with either old or young person references were recalled more often when primed with 'old person' and that for these, decisions concerning negative traits were made more quickly. The reverse was true for the positive traits and for the 'young 'category. Hospital doctors, particularly younger colleagues and medical students, have been shown to hold relatively negative attitudes and beliefs about older people. Younger psychiatrists (Draper *et al*. 1999), nurses (Stevens and Herbert 1997), and health visitors (Pursey and Luker 1995) are not immune from negative preconceptions. General practice physicians miss depression in older people because physical illness takes precedence over psychological symptoms (Tylee *et al*. 1993). Alternatively, symptoms are incorrectly attributed to ageing, or loneliness. Treatment nihilism can occur, and biases against treating mentally ill people with concomitant physical illness has been reported with New Zealand general practitioners (McIvor 1996), British general practitioners (Tylee *et al*. 1993). and US clinical psychologists (Haley 1995). Low exposure to the mental health problems of ageing in many undergraduate, medical school curriculae contributes to the low levels of diagnostic detection, which combined with treatment nihilism, leads to the undertreatment of reversible disorders such as depression.

Gender biases add further complications. For those unfortunate elders of either gender, who also have psychological or psychiatric problems, prejudice against the mentally ill can add yet another dimension. Several authors have demonstrated that this is one of the more pervasive prejudices in community (Williams and Taylor 1995) and general hospital services, and that personnel are just as vulnerable as other community institutions (Collings and Myers 1992).

These undesirable influences may cause older people at risk for psychological complications of illness to be under-referred to the appropriate services or to find the experience of hospitalization difficult or prolonged. Improving attitudes towards elderly people with physical illness requires awareness that health services and professionals are susceptible to inherent biases. It is important to dispel some of the more pervasive myths and stereotypes about older people. The liaison psychiatrist must develop a positive outlook on both the ageing process and to the disabilities associated with ageing.

References

Anderson, D.C., Yolton, R.L., Reinke, A.R., and Kohl, P. (1995). The dizzy patient: a review of etiology, differential diagnosis and management. *Journal of the American Optometric Association*, **66**, 545–58.

Bittles, A.H. (1997). Biological aspects of human ageing. In *Psychiatry in the elderly* (2nd edn) (ed. R. Jacoby and C. Oppenheimer), pp. 3–23. Oxford University Press, Oxford.

Busse, E.W. and Maddox, G.L. (1985). *The Duke longitudinal studies of normal ageing 1955–1980. An overview of history, design and findings.* Springer, New York.

Butler, R.N. (1980). Ageism: a foreword. *Journal of Social Issues*, **36**, 8–11.

Collings, S.C. and Myers, S. (1992). Psychiatric patients and their medical care. *Psychological Bulletin*, **16**, 88–90.

Davidson, M.B. (1979). The effects of ageing on carbohydrate metabolism: a review of the English literature and a practical approach to the diagnosis of diabetes mellitus in the elderly. *Metabolism*, **28**, 688–705.

De la Fuente, M., Ferrández, D., Muñoz, F., De Juan, E., and Miquel, J. (1993). Stimulation of the antioxidant thiopoline on the lymphocytic functions of old mice. *Mechanisms of Ageing and Development*, **68**, 27–36.

Draper, B., Gething, L., Fethney, J., and Winfield, S. (1999). The Senior Psychiatrist Survey III: attitudes towards personal ageing, life experiences and psychiatric practice. *Australian and New Zealand Journal of Psychiatry*, **33**, 717–22.

Engelhardt, M. and Martens, U.M. (1998). The implications of telomerase activity and telomere stability for replicative ageing and cellular immortality. *Oncology Reports*, **5**, 1043–52.

Finch, C.E. and Pike, M.C. (1996). Maximum life span predictions from the Gompertz mortality model. *Journals of Gerontology. Series A, Biological Sciences and Medical Sciences*, **5**, B183–94.

Fleg, J.L., O'Connor, F., Gerstenblith, G., Becker, L.C., Clulow, J., Schulman, S.P., *et al.* (1995). Impact of age on the cardiovascular response to dynamic upright exercise in healthy men and women. *Journal of Applied Physiology*, **78**, 890–900.

Fossel, M. (1998). Telomerase and the ageing cell: implications for human health. *Journal of the American Medical Association*, **279**, 1732–5.

Garfein, A.J. and Herzog, A.R. (1995). Robust ageing among the young-old, old-old, and oldest-old. *Journal of Gerontology: Social Sciences*, **50B**, S77–S87.

Haley, W.E. (1995). Age and health bias in practicing clinical psychologists. *Psychology and Ageing*, **10**, 610–16.

Harman, D. (1985). Role of free radicals in ageing and disease In *Relations between normal ageing and disease, Ageing series* 28 (ed. H.J. Johnson), pp. 45–84. Raven Press, New York.

Harman, D. (1992). Free radical theory of ageing. *Mutation Research*, **275**, 257–66.

Hayflick, L. (1994). *How and why we age*. Ballentine Books, New York.

Hayflick, L. and Moorhead, P.S. (1961). The serial cultivation of human diploid cell strains. *Experimental Cell Research*, **25**, 585–621.

Horn, J.L. (1982). The theory of fluid and crystallised intelligence in relation to concepts of cognitive psychology and ageing in adulthood. In *Ageing and cognitive processes* (ed. F.L.M Craik and S. Trehub), pp. 237–78. Plenum Press, New York.

Keller, W.J., Largen, J.W., Burch, N.R., and Maulsby, R.L. (1985). Physiology of the ageing brain: normal and abnormal states. In *Relations between normal ageing and disease. Ageing series* 28 (ed.. H.A. Johnson), pp. 165–90. Raven Press, New York.

Kennaway, D.J., Lushington, K., Dawson, D., Lack, L., van der Heuvel, C., and Rogers, N. (1999). Urinary 6-sulfatoxylmelatonin excretion and aging: new results and a critical review of the literature. *Journal of Pineal Research*, **27**, 210–20.

Kohn, R.R. (1985). Ageing and age related diseases: normal process. In *Relations between normal ageing and disease, Ageing Series 28* (ed. H.A. Johnson), pp. 1–44. Raven Press, New York.

Kurban, R.S. and Bhawan, J. (1990). Histologic changes in skin associated with ageing. *Journal of Dermatology and Surgical Oncology*, **16**, 908–14.

Labouvie-Vief, G. (1985). Intelligence and cognition. In *Handbook of the psychology of ageing* (ed.. J.E. Birren and K.W. Schaie), pp. 500–30. Van Nostrand Reihold, New York.

Lindeman, R.D. (1990). Overview: renal physiology and pathophysiology of aging. *American Journal of Kidney Diseases*, **16**, 275–82.

Lindesay, J. (1990). The Guys' Age Concern survey: physical health and psychiatric disorder in an urban elderly community. *International Journal of Geriatric Psychiatry*, **5**, 171–8.

Maaka, R. (1993). Te ao o te pakeketanga. In *New Zealand's Ageing Society: the implications* (ed. P.G. Koopman-Boyden), pp. 213–29. Daphne Brasbell Associates Press, Wellington, New Zealand.

McIvor, B.T. (1996). *Barriers to the diagnosis and treatment of depression in the elderly in primary care*. Unpublished dissertation. Australian and New Zealand College of Psychiatrists.

McMurdo, M.E. and Gaskell, A. (1991). Dark adaptation and falls in the elderly. *Gerontology*, **37**, 221–4.

Makinodan, T. and Hirokawa, K. (1985). Normal ageing of the immune system. In *Relations between normal ageing and disease, Ageing Series* Vol. 28 (ed. H.J. Johnson), pp. 117–32. Raven Press, New York.

Miquel, J. (1991). An integrated theory of ageing as the result of mitochondrial DNA mutation in differentiated cells. *Archives of Gerontology and Geriatrics*, **12**, 99–117.

Myers, A.M., Powell, L.E., Maki, B.E., Holliday, P.J., Brawley, L.R., and Sherk, W. (1996). Psychological indicators of balance confidence: relationship to actual and perceived abilities. *Journal of Gerontology: Medical Sciences*, **51**, 37–43.

O'Connor, K.G. Tobin, J.D., Harman, S.M., Plato, C.C., Roy, T.A., Sherman, S.S., *et al.* (1998). Serum levels of insulin-like growth factor-I are related to age and not to body composition in healthy women and men. *Journals of Gerontology. Series A, Biological Sciences and Medical Sciences*, **53**, M176–82.

Palmore, E. (1972). Gerontophobia versus ageism. *The Gerontologist*, **12**, 213.

Pearson, J.D., Morrell, C.H., Gordon-Salant, S., Brant, L.J., Metter, E.J., Klein, L.L., *et al.* (1995). Gender differences in a longitudinal study of age-associated hearing loss. *Journal of the Acoustical Society of America*, **97**, 1196–205.

Perdue, C.W. and Gurtman, M.B. (1990). Evidence for the automaticity of ageism. *Journal of Experimental Social Psychology*, **26**, 199–216.

Pereira-Smith, O.M. and Smith, J.R. (1983). Evidence for the recessive nature of cellular immortality. *Science*, **221**, 964–6.

Phillips, M.A. and Murrell, P. (1994). Impact of psychological and physical health: stressful events and social support on subsequent mental health help seeking among older adults. *Journal of Consulting and Clinical Psychology*, **62**, 270–5.

Pursey, A. and Luker, K. (1995). Attitudes and stereotypes: nurses work with older people. *Journal of Advanced Nursing*, **22**, 547–55.

Ralphs, J.R. and Benjamin, M. (1994). The joint capsule: structure composition ageing and disease. *Journal of Anatomy*, **184**, 503–9.

Reiter, R.J. (1995). The pineal gland and melatonin in relation to aging: a summary of the theories and of the data. *Experimental Gerontology*, **30**, 199–212.

Roberto, K. (1992). Coping strategies of older women with hip fractures: resources and outcomes. *Journal of Gerontology—Psychological Sciences*, **47**, 21–6.

Rodeheffer, R.J. and Gerstenblith, G. (1985). Effect of age on cardiovascular function. In *Relations between normal ageing and disease* (ed. H.A. Johnson), pp. 85–99. Raven Press, New York.

Rosenthal, M.J., Hunt, W.C., Garry, P.J., and Goodwin, J.S. (1987). Thyroid failure in the elderly: microsomal antibodies as a discriminant for therapy. *Journal of the American Medical Association,* **258**, 209–13.

Rowe, J.W. and Devons, C.A.J. (1996). Physiological and clinical considerations of the geriatric patient. In *Textbook of geriatric psychiatry* (2nd edn) (ed. E.W. Busse and D.G. Blazer), pp. 25–47. American Psychiatric Press, Washington DC.

Salthouse, T.A. (1996). The processing speed theory of adult age differences in cognition. *Psychological Review*, **103**, 403–28.

Salthouse, T.A. (1998). Cognitive and information processing perspectives on ageing. In *Clinical geropsychology* (ed. (ed. I.H. Nordhus, G.R. VanderBos, S. Berg, and P. Fromholt), pp. 49–59. American Psychological Association, Washington DC.

Ship, J.A., Pearson, J.D., Cruise, L.J., Brant, L.J., and Metter, E.J. (1996). Longitudinal changes in smell identification. *Journals of Gerontology. Series A, Biological Sciences and Medical Sciences*, **51**, M86–91.

Shock, N.W., Greulich, R.C., Andres, R., Arenberg, D., Costa, P.T., Lakatta, E.G., *et al.* (1984). *Normal human ageing: the Baltimore longitudinal study of ageing*, NIH publication 84–2450. US Government Printing Office, Washington DC.

Smith, I. M. (1985). Pneumonia and the ageing lung. In *Relations between normal ageing and disease, Ageing Series* 28 (ed. H.A. Johnson), pp. 101–15. Raven Press, New York.

Sorkin, J.D., Muller, D.C., and Andres, R. (1999). Longitudinal change in height of men and women: implications for interpretation of the body mass index: the Baltimore Longitudinal Study of Aging. *American Journal of Epidemiology*, **150**, 969–77.

Stevens, J. and Herbert, J. (1997). Ageism and nursing practice in Australia. *Nursing Review*, **17–18**, 23–4.

Taylor, R.C. (1994). Elderly persons at risk. In *Principles and practice of geriatric psychiatry* (ed. J.R.M. Copeland, M.T. Abou-Saleh, and D.G Blazer), pp. 116–22. Wiley, Chichester.

Thomas, P.D., Goodwin, J.M., and Goodwin, J.W. (1985). Effect of social support and stress related changes in cholesterol, uric acid level and immune function in an elderly sample. *American Journal of Psychiatry*, **142**, 735–7.

Timaras, P.S. (1985). Physiological ageing: brain and hormones set the pace of life. In *Relations between normal ageing and disease*, *Ageing series*, 28 (ed. H.A. Johnson), pp. 151–6. Raven Press, New York.

Tylee, A.T., Freeling, P., and Kerry, S. (1993). Why do general practitioners recognize major depression in one woman patient yet miss it in another? *British Journal of General Practice*, **43**, 327–30.

Vaitkevicius, P.V., Fleg, J.L., Engel, J.H., O'Connor, F.C., Wright, J.G., Lakatta, L.E., *et al.* (1993). Effects of age and aerobic capacity on arterial stiffness in healthy adults. *Circulation*, **88**, 1456–62.

Verbrugge, L. (1989). Gender ageing and health. In *Ageing and health perspectives on gender race ethnicity and class* (ed. K. Markides), pp. 23–78. Park Sage, Newbury.

Wenger, G.C. (1997). Social networks and the prediction of elderly people at risk. *Aging and Mental Health*, **1**, 311–20.

Whitbourne, S.K. (1996). *The ageing individual; physical and psychological perspectives*. Springer, New York.

Whitbourne, S.K. (1998). Physical changes. In *Clinical geropsychology* (ed. I.H. Nordhus, G.R. VanderBos, S. Berg, and P. Fromholt), pp. 79–108. American Psychological Association, Washington DC.

Williams, M. and Taylor, J. (1995). Mental illness: media perpetuation of stigma. *Contemporary Nurse*, **4**, 41–6.

World Health Organization (1999). *World population prospects: the 1998 revision.* United Nations Population Division, *http://www.popin.org/pop1998/8.htm.*

Zeiter, J.M., Daniels, J.E., Duffy, J.F., Klerman, E.B., Shanahan, T.L., Dijk, D.J., *et al.* (1999). Do plasma melatonin concentrations decline with age? *American Journal of Medicine*, **107**, 432–6.

Zhang, Z., Inserra, P.F., Liang, B., Ardestani, S.K., Elliott, K.K., Molitor, M., *et al.* (1997). Melatonin, immune modulation and aging. *Autoimmunity*, **26**, 43–53.

3 Coping with illness in late life

Pamela Melding and Andrew J. Cook

Summary

Of all life events, physical illnesses are the most common occurrences that signifi-cantly affect older people and represent the most significant losses in late life. Understanding how an older person perceives the personal significance of the illness is essential to the liaison clinician's own appraisal of the patient's problems. The chapter discusses not only how an illness may influence the individual, but also how the person's response may affect an illness. For the patient, the important aspects of primary appraisal include acuity and timing of events, their impact on social roles, the person's perception of illness, their emotional and physical health status, perceived social support, personality traits, sense of personal control, and perception of any stigma attached to the illness. The ageing person's primary appraisal of their illness influences the secondary appraisal process that assesses their ability to cope with the stressor. Aspects of coping discussed in this chapter are self-efficacy, outcome expectancy, focus for coping, and strategies employed.

Introduction

Sickness is different for older people, and hospitalization may be a great ordeal. What may be an inconvenience for a younger adult, may prove to be a highly significant stressor for an older person, due to their worry of having an illness, its potentially greater impact on daily functioning, and uncertainty about the possible outcomes. An older person's response and adjustment to illness stresses may be more problematic than that of a younger person, bringing added complications and possibly modifying outcomes. Consequently, liaison clinicians working with older people should understand the interaction between the person and their illness: not only how an illness may influence the individual, but also how the person's response may affect an illness.

Life events and health

We are all very aware of the relationship between stressful life events and deterioration in mental health. Whilst it is commonly thought that bereavements of spouses, friends, or peers and social losses are more likely to occur in late life, they are not particularly predominant. Krause (1994) interviewed over 1000 older people and found a surprising low incidence of such significant events. Similarly, Murrell *et al.* (1984) found that less than 3% of older people living in the community had experienced significant bereavements in the previous year, but over a quarter had experienced an illness of some sort. Half the people surveyed in this study had experienced a recent hospitalization, either of themselves or a close family relative. Of all life events, physical illnesses are the most common occurrences that significantly affect older people (Davies 1996). Further evidence from longitudinal ageing studies (Shock *et al.* 1984; Busse and Maddox 1985) indicates that the most significant losses in late life result from increasing physical debility.

Physical ageing can lead to deterioration in health status, often with resulting psychosocial ripple-effects that limit independence, reduce self-determination, and induce a loss of self-esteem. The response to illness stresses is as much a part of the total clinical picture as physical ageing, disease status, and pathology.

Disease versus illness

The impact of a medical disease is far greater than just the physiological upset. Certainly, physical debility may result from an acute change in health status and appetite, nutrition, and bodily rhythms may all be adversely affected. In addition, the disease may have secondary effects such as dehydration, metabolic or electrolyte upsets, severe pain, or constipation. A disease process may have a cascade effect, with one dysfunctional system putting additional strain on other marginal organ systems. Treatment may compound the patient's problem by sedation or drug inter-actions (Gurland *et al.* 1988).

Although a disease is a definable pathological state that can induce all the afore-mentioned adverse effects, an illness is a state of being (Eisenberg 1977). A person may be diseased but not feel ill, or they may feel ill but not have a disease. Similarly, a patient may have a delineated defect or impairment resulting from a disease process, but if this influences a person's ability to function either physically or socially, then disability is the result (Wolcott 1981). Several authors have identified chronic disability as a prominent correlate of psychological distress, depression, prolonged hospitalization, and suicide in older people (Aneshensel *et al.* 1984; Arling 1987; Catell 1988; Turner and Noh 1988; Kennedy *et al.* 1989; Lindesay 1990).

The older person's subjective experience of a medical illness

When confronted with objective evidence of lowered health status, the first reaction of an older person is often a state of disbelief. This may give way to anger and 'why me' questioning, expressions of a grief reaction to the loss of health or function. Lazarus, from his perspective as a life-long researcher of adaptation to stress through the adult lifespan (a viewpoint that is now enriched by insights from his personal ageing process), states that (Lazarus 1998, p. 113): 'appraisal is the central construct of cognitive mediation'. What the person thinks is happening is crucial to the subsequent response.

In the primary appraisal stage, the patient considers the personal significance of the stressor, and in the secondary appraisal stage assesses the options for changing the situation (Folkman *et al.* 1987).

Aspects of primary appraisal

Understanding how an older person perceives the personal significance of the illness is essential to the liaison clinician's own appraisal of the patient's problems. Multiple aspects impinge upon the primary appraisal process and all are inter-connected, rather like a jigsaw puzzle (Table 3.1).

Table 3.1 ASPECTS of primary appraisal of illness events

Anticipation and acuity
Social roles and issues
Personal beliefs
Emotional and physical health status
Control
Temperament and personality factors
Stigma of illness

Anticipation and acuity

Response to late-life stressful events can be influenced by both perceived normative-ness and timing. Late-life events can be normative 'on-time' events or non-normative 'off-time' events (Brim and Ryff 1980; Davies 1996). Many events in the older person's life are anticipated 'on-time' events such as retirement, loss of income, deaths of peers and spouses. The classic examples of 'off-time' events in late life are the loss of an adult child, a natural disaster, an accident, or a physical attack against the person. As there is often a discrepancy between chronological and self-perceived age, older people may accept intellectually that illness is likely as a normative 'on time' event in late life, yet view their own personal experience of an acute illness event as definitely occurring 'off-time'. Actual or self-perceived 'off-time' events have an immediate impact and the person often has a sense of unfairness about them. Similarly, an suddenly acute illness, such as a stroke, or one that is chronic but suddenly deteriorates, may have a more negative impact than might be predicted from the disease status (Young 1994; Davies 1996).

Social roles

Illness in older people, especially if accompanied by significant chronicity, pain, or disablement, has a major impact on the person's social roles and relationships. Krause (1994) postulated that the adverse effect of life events is more severe when the event threatens an aspect of self-image that identifies the person's concept of a salient social role, such as that of spouse, parent, grandparent, friend, or community contributor. A stressor that compromises a highly valued role will have a greater impact than one that affects a less salient domain. For older people, illness and disability changes many social relationships and roles to a greater degree than for younger people. A major insult to self-identity can occur when a person is no longer able to self-care and becomes reliant on adult offspring or other caregivers. The 'life and soul of the party' may lose social confidence or suffer agoraphobia following a serious fall. Physical or cognitive handicap can force an elderly car enthusiast to stop driving. These events have profound psychosocial effects that affect the person far beyond the physiological impact of the medical problems.

Illness stress may be moderated in older people if they feel cared for and esteemed by their social networks (Penninx *et al.* 1997; Cavanaugh 1998; Lang, *et al.* 1998; Roberto 1992; Burke and Flaherty 1993). Murphy's (1982) classic study found that older people with confiding relationships were less likely to have depressive illness following a threatening life event. Positive social support may have a direct effect on illness itself by enhancing immunological function (Thomas *et al.* 1985). Unfortunately, little is known about the effect of poor social and economic resources on older people's stress management, or the effect of dwindling social support for the very old elders who have outlived their peers. Intuitively, it seems likely that lack of these social resources limits a person's options for dealing with illness (Davies 1994). In contrast, in an earlier review of the relevant literature, Berkman (1983) cautioned that: 'there is little evidence to support the idea that the elderly are particularly fragile and vulnerable to the effects of social isolation'. However, there is some evidence from a British longitudinal study on ageing that poor economic resources, isolation, and social impoverishment carry an increased risk for physical and mental disorders in late life (Taylor 1994).

Research has suggested that an older person's social network provides an important resource for consultation about illness. This 'lay consultation' occurs both in conjunction with and independent of consultation with healthcare professionals, and appears to have an important, complementary role (Furstenberg 1985; Strain 1990). Deterioration of social resources for the older, ill person may give rise to a need for greater interaction with healthcare professionals and community-based support resources for both primary and secondary appraisal processes.

Personal perception of illness

Stress from an illness can result from various types of changes or appraisals. The illness may represent a change in circumstances, a loss, a threat, or a challenge, with each view attracting quite different responses (McCrae 1982; Folkman *et al.* 1987; Lazarus 1998). An illness may represent a major life change, perhaps moving in with others, or even institutionalization. It may signify a threat to quality of life, or a loss of independence, mobility, and sometimes life. For some, illness presents a challenge of learning to be one's own care manager and developing adaptive coping styles. Furthermore, the person's own contextual view may be quite different to the liaison clinician's view of the same stress in that person!

Whilst this contemporary view can aid in appraising the significance of an illness event, the older person also perceives the stressor from a generational or cohort view. People born in the early twentieth century differ in their world-views from those born in the post World War II period. It is useful to remember that today's older people have had lives of unprecedented rapid social and technological change that has undoubtedly shaped their world-views and how they perceive and respond to stressors (Costa *et al.* 1998). For example, the present cohort of older people were often discouraged from expressing how they felt and encouraged to adopt a stoical approach to help them cope with global adverse events. Consequently, they may respond to late-life illness in much the same way. Older people who have had particular adverse experiences such as war combat, the Holocaust, or are victims of sexual abuse may have had a lifetime of seemingly good adjustment to their traumas. Yet, with the increased vulnerability of ageing and physical illness, unresolved painful traumatic memories, suppressed for many years, may resurface (Clipp and Elder 1996).

Case study 3.1

Dr I.G. was an 80-year-old former general practitioner from a middle-class German family, with a Jewish father and Aryan mother. Her father died of a heart attack in 1940, whilst expecting to be deported to a concentration camp. As a young woman, Irena never felt safe from persecution, and most of her father's family perished in the Holocaust. She trained in medicine in Berlin in the late 1930s before her training was terminated. During the war, she was employed in the mortuary as an attendant, a job that was considered offensive and degrading but represented relative safety. After the liberation, a soldier from the occupying forces raped her, which resulted in a pregnancy. With her mother and child she became a refugee and emigrated. The small town community in her adopted country ostracized her for being a solo mother as well as an enemy alien. This discrimination diminished after she completed training in medicine and she subsequently became a very successful and respected general practitioner. Dr I.G. never spoke of her experiences with anyone, including her daughter. She was disabled by a stroke at 80 years of age that necessitated her going into a nursing home. In care, she felt imprisoned and patronized. The staff teamed her up with a German-speaking resident thinking they could converse. Dr I.G. developed a paranoid psychosis with distressing auditory hallucinations, the flavour of which pertained to her earlier adverse experiences.

Emotional and physical health status

Older people frequently present with multiple physical comorbidities. Whilst one disorder may tax an older person, several can be overwhelming (Farrell *et al*. 1995). In addition, the cumulative effect of several disease states, anatomical deformations, pain, or loss of mobility can all adversely affect mood state (Aneshensel *et al*. 1984; Arling 1987; Felton and Revenson 1987; Lindesay 1990). The cyclical relationships between physical symptoms, mood state, cognitive appraisals, and behaviours can be conceptualized within the cognitive–behavioural model of response to changes in health status (Fig. 3.1). The central role of cognitive appraisals is highlighted, as well as the interrelationships between physiological, cognitive, emotional, and behavioural functioning. More complications arise with the cognitively impaired older person who often has regressed ideas regarding illness (Reisberg *et al*. 1986), which impact on emotional and behavioural functioning, and in turn affect physical symptoms. In addition, cognitive deficits may inhibit problem-solving. These can lead to miscommunication with health professionals and caregivers. Poor health practices such as non-compliance or malnutrition may also jeopardize a person's ability to deal with problems.

Negative mood states (e.g., depression, anger, fear) complicate the appraisal of an illness by negatively influencing the person's perception of the problem itself, so that it may seem worse than the reality. The impact on cognitive processes extends to the

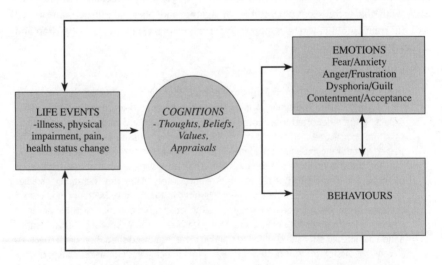

Fig. 3.1 Cognitive–behavioural model of the interaction between physical symptoms, cognitions, emotions, and behaviours.

individual's sense of personal control, motivation, and self-confidence, thus compromising the person's ability to manage the problem (Sullivan and D'Eon 1990).

Control

Illness or disease, especially when unexpected, impacts on the individual's personal sense of their ability to control what is happening to them. The 'locus of control' attribute (Rotter 1966; Wallston *et al.* 1978) identifies whether a person perceives that their personal experiences are influenced most significantly internally by themselves or by external sources, for instance healthcare professionals, deities/religious/political figures, or chance/fate/luck. Locus of control can be quite differentiated in specific areas (Schulz *et al.* 1991) such as social, economic, family, interpersonal, intellectual, or health domains. Whilst a person's innate predominate sense of control does not usually change with age, locus of control for the specific domain of health usually shows more of a trend towards external attribution with ageing than do other domains (Lachman 1991).

The significance of personal, control beliefs lies in their influence on the process of adapting to the illness and treatment. These beliefs directly influence the secondary appraisal of options for dealing with the stressor. The Amsterdam Longitudinal Aging Study found that an external locus of control is a dominant vulnerability factor for anxiety disorders in late life (Beekman *et al.* 1998), and that an internal locus of control is protective for depression in women (Van den Heuvel *et al.* 1996). A longitudinal study of changes in physical functioning for older adults found that internal health locus of control was strongly related to changes in physical functioning (Wallhagen *et al.* 1994). This relationship was present for women at all levels of baseline functioning, though only for men with low physical functioning at baseline. The authors of this study noted the limitations of locus of control as a predictor of health outcomes in older adults, based on existing evidence.

Traits, temperament, and personality

People try to make sense of what has happened to them and achieve some sense of order and continuity in their lives. Every stressful illness-event is viewed and responded to in the light of the person's subjective experience of the moment (flexible and changeable) and their accumulated experience of a lifetime (enduring and stable). This distinction has long been regarded as an important one, and is integral to a number of enduring theories of personality, coping, and psychopathology. It has been characterized in these various contexts as a distinction between appraisals and responses that are *intraindividual* versus *interindividual* (Folkman *et al.* 1986), *dispositional* versus *situational* (Schwarzer and Schwarzer 1996), and *trait* versus *state* (Johnson and Spielberger 1968).

Another way to understand the interplay between appraisals and responses that are stable but adaptive, and those that flexibly change with different circumstances is the dialectic self-concept of 'I' and 'Me'. This concept was originally proposed by the nineteenth-century American psychologist William James (1842–1910) in 1890. 'I' refers to subjective, personal, immediate, inner experience, which changes in response to immediate environmental events. 'Me' refers to the more objective accumulated experiences and characteristics that make up personal identity. These include memory, cultural characteristics, cohort experiences, previous coping, and cognitive belief schemas. A person's 'Me' identity also includes the salient social roles such as parent, worker, retiree, or even sick person. 'Me' aspects of a person are relatively consistent and stable, though they can adapt with ageing, knowledge, and experience. An illness threat to a valued 'Me' aspect will have a negative impact on a person's adjustment to the event. As evidenced by its reappearance in the twentieth century under different guises, this concept remains a useful way of understanding the stable and fluid aspects of coping and behaviour, including those of older people (Coleman 1998).

When personal beliefs, sense of control, and 'Me' aspects of personality are challenged by ageing and illness, self-value and esteem may suffer. Murrell *et al.* (1991) suggested that a strong positive sense of self is important for successful adaptation to illness, and that older people need encouraging to maintain their sense of psychological 'integrity' (Erikson 1959) in the face of physiological malfunctioning.

Stigma

If an illness makes a person different, then it is stigmatizing. For example, stroke patients appear physically different as do patients stigmatized by abnormal bodily movements, parkinsonism, or physical defects. Patients may feel humiliated by having to resort to wheelchairs or walking sticks. Sudden reliance on such aids can cause a marked loss of confidence as they indicate loss of normal adult autonomy or independence to all (Luborsky 1994).

However, many factors influence the impact of the physical stigma on the older person, including the presence of a medical diagnosis as well as the previously discussed beliefs, appraisals, and traits. Some research has suggested that an older person's self-identity is more strongly influenced by other factors when stigma is associated with a named disease and concrete physical problems (Belgrave 1990). In some cases, observable symptoms or impairments can serve to validate an illness, and thus the associated activity restrictions and need for caregiver assistance. This validation can be perceived in a positive way by some older persons, such as those with dependent personality traits and those seeking release from home, work, or family responsibilities.

The absence of a clear medical diagnosis increases the risk of negative effects from stigma, especially if medical professionals, family members, or peers view symptoms as exaggerated or unfounded. This is a common occurrence in some types of chronic pain conditions, such as myofascial pain syndromes, though it is more common in younger age groups. Another significant source for negative feelings of stigmatization is the presence of a mental health problem and involvement in psychiatric treatment.

Case study 3.2

Mr J., a 70-year-old man, was admitted following a right-sided stroke. He had a resulting speech defect, a dense hemiparesis, and he dribbled continuously. Previously, Mr J. had been a successful business man with his own major public relations company and was noted for his communications skills, ability as an entertaining raconteur, and engaging personal charisma. He had married his secretary who was 30 years his junior in his late middle age and they had a teenage daughter with whom he had a close relationship. His wife failed to hide her repugnance at his handicap and stopped visiting him. The patient felt depressed and suicidal and was also extremely humiliated at 'what he had become'.

Once an older person has appraised the illness event, their next psychological task is to manage or cope with the problems engendered by the illness.

Coping with illness

Folkman and Lazarus (1980) defined coping as:

... the variety of cognitive and behavioural efforts used by the individual to manage the specific external and internal demands that are appraised as exceeding the resources of the individual.

More simply, coping is the thoughts and actions used to restore a person's state of psychological equilibrium. It has two main functions. The first is to manage or alter the person–environment relationship that is the source of the problem, and the second is to regulate the accompanying emotional response (Folkman and Lazarus 1980; Lazarus 1980, 1998). When coping responses fail to do these two things, the person's psychological equilibrium is upset, and distress follows. This may be of such severity that it results in subnormal functioning or disability. The liaison clinician needs to assess the first parameter thoroughly and to assist the person with the second. This process is well characterized by the cognitive–behavioural model (see Fig. 3.1).

The secondary appraisal process evaluates the person's options for coping with the event (Table 3.2).

Table 3.2 Aspects of secondary appraisal and coping—COPES

Competence to perform a coping response
Outcome-expectancy of the response
Problem-focused function
Emotional-focused function
Strategies employed to deal with the stressor

Competence or self-efficacy

Self-efficacy (Bandura 1977) is the personal belief of one's competence to perform behavioural intentions or coping response. Data from the McArthur studies of successful ageing indicate that strong self-efficacy beliefs have a significant positive impact on the perception of functional disability independent of actual physical limitations (Seeman *et al*. 1999). Furthermore, strongly perceived self-efficacy seems to have an immunoenhancing effect (Wiedenfeld *et al*. 1990). Self-efficacy can suffer in an illness. Admission to hospital provides an environment that may adversely affect an older person's sense of personal control and self-efficacy (Welch and West 1995). Confidence is insufficient by itself. Older people need to believe that their actions are safe and will not compromise them. If pain or illness affects mobility and activities of daily living, the older person may prefer to accept increased dependence rather than to struggle with the difficulty of maintaining their self-reliance. Clashes may occur between patients and rehabilitation staff who believe the patient is 'not trying' hard enough at therapy, particularly physically based tasks, without staff enquiring if the patient believes the requested task is actually within their capabilities or consistent with their personal goals. Rehabilitation programmes for younger adults often emphasize personal autonomy to reduce dependency on drugs and healthcare systems, but for older people, this may be quite inappropriate. For older people, self-efficacy is often a trade-off between a need for security and preservation of personal autonomy. If the autonomous side of self-efficacy is emphasized at the expense of the security of appropriate dependency, then the result might be increased distress, more anxiety, and additional loss of confidence. Alternatively, if security is emphasized above autonomy, then the result may be premature dependency and loss of quality of life (Melding 1995).

Outcome-expectancy

Poor outcome-expectancy correlates very closely with a reduced belief in one's competency or self-efficacy (Kirsch 1985). However, outcome-expectancy is a less robust concept in coping than self-efficacy. The effectiveness of a coping strategy in someone with a chronic painful illness, appears to be determined more by that person's appraisal of their competence to perform it (self-efficacy) than by any belief in the likely success of the strategy (outcome-expectancy) (Jensen *et al*. 1992). Nevertheless, outcome-expectancy may be negatively affected by depressed mood. A depressed person may not even try to perform a coping response if they have a negative belief in their personal competence and/or the expected outcome of their coping efforts. Both self-efficacy and outcome-expectancy can improve if therapists use experiential learning, building confidence, rather than didactic teaching, handouts, or vicarious advice (Bandura 1977). If such devices are used, the messages should be clear, unambiguous, and easy to remember. Overall, people tend to do better if shown and guided through the required actions. An important caveat here is that individual circumstances and coping styles need to be assessed and considered in planning interventions, as will be discussed in the following section.

Personal control beliefs, self-efficacy, and outcome-expectancies are linked (Williams and Koocher 1998), in that an external locus or loss of personal control undermines self-efficacy and negatively affects secondary appraisal and coping. A common story in geriatric liaison is that of a previously extremely competent and capable person who 'falls apart' in the face of an illness stressor, and appears to undergo a personality change that astonishes their normal caregivers. For the first time in their lives, the person seems incapable of dealing with current problems. Typically, their life story is devoid of previous 'training' in dealing with illness and, at a time of life when their personal resources are limited, they have the 'new' experience of being personally ill. The rather disparaging term 'acopia' or 'Humpty Dumpty Syndrome' is sometimes used to describe these patients.

Case study 3.3

Miss B. had a successful career as a former principal nurse of the district general hospital and had received special community honours for her work. She was the eldest of eight children and had been brought up during the Depression on a dairy farm, with a very strong work ethic. From the age of six, she helped her mother with the younger children and assisted with milking the dairy herd. Miss B. was a keen walker and hiker, a competent musician, and, until her retirement, led a Girl Guide troop. At 75 years of age, she fractured the neck of her femur. Her rehabilitation took place in the same hospital she had administered for most of her professional life. Rehabilitation was compromised by Miss B.'s extreme distress about her impairment that led to a conviction that she was to be crippled for life. She was humiliated at being a patient and lacked confidence in her ability to deal with the physical therapy programme. The previously capable Miss B. seemed to have had a personality change and 'fallen to pieces'.

Problem- or emotion-focused coping

The aims of coping strategies are not only to solve problems, but also to modify the meanings of events for individuals and to control the accompanying stress responses. Coping efforts can focus on the problem or on the emotion that the problem engenders (Folkman and Lazarus 1980; Lazarus 1980, 1996, 1998; Folkman *et al.* 1987). Problem-focused coping efforts attempt to modify the sources of stress and direct active attention to changing health status. These efforts can be interpersonal and confrontational or intrapersonal and cognitive. Thus, problem-focused coping may be directed to the many practical problems that illnesses present for older persons, such as difficulties with normal daily activities that include dressing, transferring, and mobility, or to controlling the health problem itself. Emotion-focused coping concentrates on managing the emotional consequences of stressors such as resulting anxiety, panic, or dysphoria, without changing the realities of the situation (Folkman *et al.* 1987; Lazarus 1998).

These two functions are difficult to separate and attempts to do so may be reductionist, as many people address both problem and emotion in their coping efforts, either sequentially or simultaneously. However, either aspect may predominate in an individual's coping responses, and the differentiation can be useful in planning and implementing interventions. Some research on health-related interventions has shown that matching interventions with the individual's primary coping styles (i.e. problem- or emotion-focused) produces better symptom and psychological coping outcomes, including interventions for older persons (Martelli *et al.* 1987; Fry and Wong 1991).

Strategies for coping

Most individuals' repertoire of coping strategies is quite stable throughout their life cycle. Yet, as a person grows older, their coping repertoire becomes refined with the employment of fewer but more effective strategies (Meeks *et al.* 1989). The personal history obtained in a clinical interview will provide valuable information on an individual's previous coping responses to various life stressors.

In addition to the problem- versus emotion-focused distinction, coping strategies have been classified in other ways—such as active (or instrumental) versus passive, behavioural versus cognitive, and illness- versus wellness-focused. There is some overlap in these artificial dichotomies, and many actual coping responses seen in clinical practice are difficult to classify within these categories (DeGood 1999). Active coping strategies are more common in young people, with more passive strategies emerging as people age (Vaillant 1977; Folkman *et al.* 1987). Active strategies include problem-solving, active health behaviours (e.g. physical exercise), seeking support or social networks, information seeking, ritualizing time, and physical or mental activity for distraction or enjoyment. A recent, active, problem-focused coping phenomenon to emerge in the older generation has been their increasing use of the Internet to seek health information. There is a tendency to judge passive strategies as maladapative, though this depends greatly on the individual and the circumstance. Additionally, cognitive and behavioural strategies such as reinterpretation, mental distraction, meditation, and the use of relaxation techniques can be viewed as both passive and active. Potentially adaptive, passive strategies include acceptance, resignation, humour, and prayer.

Religious coping can span many of these categories of coping. Koenig *et al.* (1992) analysed the importance of religious belief in elderly men hospitalized with medical problems. They found that religious coping was important for 20% of subjects and that this variable was inversely related to depression scores at baseline and at 6-months' follow-up. These adaptive coping strategies do not change the nature of the problem, but they seem to reduce the emotional response. When an individual has to contend with an uncontrollable and extremely threatening stressor such as a terminal illness, or if the more active strategies have failed, then passive and more reflective styles are both effective and beneficial in controlling associated distress and depression (Folkman *et al.* 1987; Fry 1990; Kausar and Akram 1998). Indeed, under such uncontrollable adverse conditions, adaptive emotion-based coping is more beneficial than problem-focused active styles (Solomon *et al.* 1988; Collins *et al.* 1993)

Some emotion-focused, passive styles such as ignoring, escape-avoidance regression, and especially 'catastrophizing' (i.e. cognitively overestimating and compounding the significance and impact of an event or circumstance) are associated with depression, disability, prolonged illness, and poorer psychological adjustment (Brown *et al.* 1989; Keefe *et al.* 1989; Sullivan and D'Eon 1990). Catastrophizing in particular has attracted some debate in the literature, as some researchers consider this phenomenon to be an abnormal belief influencing secondary appraisal (especially self-efficacy and outcome-expectancies), rather than a coping strategy that results in poor outcome (Keefe *et al.* 1999). However, as catastrophizing does fit the Folkman and Lazarus paradigm of a coping strategy (Keefe *et al.* 1999), albeit a poor one, it is included as such in this discussion. Catastrophizing as a means of coping with a problem also correlates with strong external locus of control beliefs, particularly those invested in chance or fate (Felton and Revenson 1987; Blanchard-Fields and Irion 1988; Crisson and Keefe 1988). In addition, this style of coping is associated with a lowered sense of self-efficacy and outcome-expectancy.

Case study 3.4

Mrs R. had always been anxious throughout her life. She had married a career naval officer, and in retirement the couple lived in an immaculate house overlooking the naval dockyard. After a heavy fall, Mrs R. was admitted with a severe periosteal haematoma of her leg. She was unable to concentrate on her therapy programme and her thinking became increasingly anxious. She worried that her husband might not be able to cook his evening meal and catastrophized this into thoughts that if he lost weight he would become a vulnerable target to other women, who would want to feed him. Consequently, he might fall in love with someone else, leaving her 'in the gutter' destitute and penniless. Her husband, Captain R. a taciturn man, was unable to reassure her. Mrs R. spent most of the day in tears, her sleep deteriorated, her appetite declined, and she developed a severe mixed anxiety depression that was resistant to pharmacological treatment. The distress elicited a considerable amount of attention from her adult children.

Interventions to improve coping responses can have a substantial impact on behavioural, cognitive, emotional, and physical functioning. The cognitive–behavioural therapy (CBT) approach (see Chapter 14) is well suited for this area of intervention, as it focuses on the cognitions and behaviours that comprise the coping response. Its focus on learning, rehearsal, and the application of specific coping skills with a problem-solving approach, which tends to enhance self-efficacy, internal locus of control, and generalizability of skills. There is a large empirical literature demonstrating the effectiveness of CBT for improving coping with, and adjustment to, various acute and chronic illnesses. Other supportive, educational, analytical, and alternative interventions can also play a valuable role in enhancing the coping responses to illness (see Chapter 14).

Conclusions

Coping with illness in late life is complex, and involves a myriad of interconnecting variables that influence an older person's primary and secondary appraisal of an illness stressor and mediates the subsequent coping process. Consequently, an individual's response to an illness stressor is always unique. Coping cannot be divorced from either the emotion driving it or the person who is doing it (Lazarus 1998). The liaison clinician needs to identify whether there are any factors that might compromise coping and to identify those strengths that will assist with a good outcome. The primary variables that can compromise coping are listed in Table 3.3, the variables that can enhance coping in Table 3.4, and the Coping model is conceptualized in Fig. 3.2.

For older people, a medical disease state is only part of the story. The individual's psychological response, personal resilience, and adaptability are important elements affecting the patient's illness state. These aspects of personality are important factors in the primary and secondary appraisal of the adverse illness event, and in the individual's subsequent adaptation. Inadequate coping can lead to poorer outcomes with

Table 3.3 Variables that compromise coping with illness

Poor health status
Cognitive decline
Poor social support
The presence of depression
External locus of control (especially attributed to chance or fate)
Lowered sense of self-efficacy
Low outcome-expectancy
Predominant maladaptive, passive coping strategies—particularly catastrophizing

Table 3.4 Variables that enhance or facilitate coping with illness

Previous history of good coping skills and resiliency to stressors
Cognitive intactness
Attainment of good educational level
Good social network and resources
Internal locus of control
Religious affiliation and faith
Active or adaptive passive coping strategies
High self-efficacy
Good outcome-expectancy
Fewer complicating medical conditions
Health status not compromised by iatrogenic complications of treatment such as sedation or dehydration
Good health practices and positive compliance

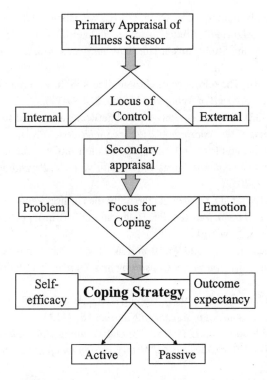

Fig. 3.2   A conceptual model of coping.

decreased functioning and the increased risk of disability. Prolonged hospitalization, reduced quality of life, and possibly premature institutionalization can unfortunately result. Understanding how older people respond, adapt, and cope and assisting them with strategies to manage their difficulties more effectively enhances the chance of a positive outcome.

References

Aneshensel, C.S., Frerichs, R.R., and Huba G.J. (1984). Depression and physical illness: a multiwave, nonrecursive causal model. *Journal of Health and Social Behaviour*, **25**, 350–71.

Arling, G. (1987). Strain, social support and distress in old age. *Journal of Gerontology*, **42**, 107–13.

Bandura, A. (1977). Towards a unified theory of behavioural change. *Psychological Review*, **84**, 191–215.

Beekman, A.T.F., Bremmer, M.A., Deeg, D.J.H., Vanbalkom, A.J.L.M., Smit, J.H., Debeurs, E., *et al.* (1998). Anxiety disorders in later life—a report from The Longitudinal Aging Study Amsterdam. *International Journal of Geriatric Psychiatry*, **13**, 717–26.

Belgrave, L. (1990). The relevance of chronic illness in the everyday lives of elderly women. *Journal of Aging and Health*, **2**, 475–500.

Berkman, L. (1983). The assessment of social networks and social support in the elderly. *Journal of the American Geriatrics Society*, **31**, 743–9.

Blanchard-Fields, F. and Irion, J. (1988). The relationship between locus of control and coping in two contexts: age as a moderator variable. *Psychology and Ageing*, **3**, 197–203.

Brim, O.G. and Ryff, C.D. (1980). On the properties of life events. In *Life-span development and behaviour* (ed. P.B Baltes and O.G Brim), pp. 33–48. Academic Press, New York.

Brown G.K., Nicassio P.M., and Wallston K.A. (1989). Pain coping strategies in rheumatoid arthritis. *Journal of Consulting and Clinical Psychology*, **5**, 652–7.

Burke, M. and Flaherty, M.J. (1993). Coping strategies and health status of elderly arthritic women. *Journal of Advanced Nursing*, **18**, 7–13.

Busse, E.W. and Maddox, G.L. (1985). *The Duke longitudinal studies of normal ageing, 1955–1980. An overview of history, design and findings*. Springer, New York.

Catell, H.R. (1988). Elderly suicide in London: an analysis of coroner's inquests. *International Journal of Geriatric Psychiatry*, **3**, 251–61.

Cavanaugh, J.C. (1998). Friendships and social networks among older people. In *Clinical geropsychology* (ed. I.H. Nordhus, G.R. VanderBos, S. Berg, and P. Fromholt), pp. 137–40. American Psychological Association, Washington DC.

Clipp, E.C. and Elder, G.H. (1996). The aging veteran of World War II. Psychiatric and life course insights. In *Aging and post traumatic stress disorder* (ed. P.E. Ruskin and J.A. Talbott), pp. 19–51. American Psychiatric Press, Washington DC.

Coleman, P.G. (1998). Identity management in late life. In *Handbook of the clinical psychology of ageing* (ed. R.T Woods), pp. 93–113. Wiley, Chichester.

Collins, D.L., Baum, A., and Singer, J.E. (1993). Coping with chronic stress at Three Mile Island: psychological and biochemical evidence. *Health Psychology*, **2**, 149–66.

Costa P.T., Yang J., and McCrae, R.R. (1998). Ageing and personality traits: generalizations and clinical implications. In *Clinical geropsychology* (ed. I.H. Nordhus, G.R. Vandenbos, S. Berg, and P. Fromholt), pp. 33–48. American Psychological Association, Washington DC.

Crisson J.E. and Keefe F.J. (1988). The relationship of locus of control to pain coping strategies and psychological distress in chronic pain patients. *Pain*, **35**, 147–54.

Davies A.D.M. (1994). Life events in the normal elderly. In *Principles and practice of geriatric psychiatry* (ed. J.R.M Copeland, M.T. Abou-Saleh, and D.G. Blazer), pp. 106–14. Wiley, Chichester.

Davies, A.D.M. (1996). Life events, health, adaptation and social support. In *Handbook of the clinical psychology of ageing* (ed. R.T. Woods), pp. 115–40. Wiley, Chichester.

DeGood, D.E. (1999). The relationship of pain coping strategies to adjustment and functioning. In *Personality characteristics of pain patients, recent advances* (ed. R.J. Gatchel and J.N. Weiberg). APA Press, Washington DC, pp. 129–164.

Eisenberg, L. (1977). Disease and illness: distinctions between professional and popular ideas of sickness. *Cultural Medical Psychiatry*, **1**, 9.

Erikson, E. (1959). 'Identity and the Life Cycle: Selected Papers'. *Psychological Issues, 1*, 1–171. International Universities Press, New York.

Farrell, M.J., Gibson, S.J., and Helme R.D. (1995). The effect of medical status on the activity level of elderly chronic pain patients. *Journal of the American Geriatrics Society*, **43**, 102–7.

Felton, B.J. and Revenson, T.A. (1987). Age differences in coping with chronic illness. *Psychology and Ageing*, **2**, 164–70.

Folkman, S. and Lazarus, R.S. (1980). An analysis of coping in a middle aged sample. *Journal of Health and Social Behaviour*, **21**, 219–39.

Folkman, S., Lazarus, R.S., Dunkel-Schetter, C., DeLongis, A., and Gruen, R. (1986). Dynamics of a stressful encounter: cognitive appraisal, coping, and encounter outcomes. *Journal of Personality and Social Psychology*, **50**, 992–1003.

Folkman, S., Lazarus, R.S., Pimley, S., and Novacek, J. (1987). Age differences in stress and coping processes. *Psychology and Ageing*, **2**, 171–84.

Fry, P.S. (1990). A factor analytic investigation of home bound elderly individual's concerns about death and dying and their coping responses. *Journal of Clinical Psychology*, **46**, 737–48.

Fry, P.S. and Wong, P.T. (1991). Pain management training in the elderly: matching interventions with subjects' coping styles. *Stress Medicine, 7*, 93–8.

Furstenberg, A.L. (1985). Older people's choices of lay consultants. *Journal of Gerontological Social Work*, **9**, 21–34.

Gurland, B.J., Wilder, D.E., and Berkman, C. (1988). Depression and disability in the elderly: reciprocal relations and changes with age. *International Journal of Geriatric Psychiatry*, **3**, 163–79.

James, W. (1890). *Principles of psychology*. Holt, New York.

Jensen, M.P., Turner, J.A., and Romano, J.M. (1992). Self-efficacy and outcome expectancies: relationship to chronic pain coping strategies and adjustment. *Pain*, **44**, 263–9.

Johnson, D.T. and Spielberger, C.D. (1968). The effects of relaxation training and the passage of time on measures of state- and trait-anxiety. *Journal of Clinical Psychology*, **24**, 20–3.

Kausar, R. and Akram, M. (1998). Cognitive appraisal and coping of patients with terminal versus nonterminal diseases. *Journal of Behavioural Sciences,* **9**, 13–28.

Keefe, F.J., Lefebvre, J.C., and Smith S.J. (1999). Catastrophizing research. Avoiding conceptual errors and maintaining a balanced perspective. *Pain Forum*, **8**, 176–80.

Keefe, F.J., Brown, G.K., Wallston, K.A., and Caldwell, D.S. (1989). Coping with rheumatoid arthritis: catastrophizing as a maladaptive strategy. *Pain*, **37**, 51–6.

Kennedy, G.J., Kelman, H.R., Thomas, C., Wisniewski, W., Metz, H., and Bijur, P.E. (1989). Hierarchy of characteristics associated with depressive symptoms in an urban elderly sample. *American Journal of Psychiatry*, **146**, 220–5.

Kirsch, L. (1985). Response expectancy as a determinant of experience and behavior. *American Psychology*, **40**, 1189–202.

Koenig, H.G., Cohen, H. J., Blazer, D.G., and Pieper, C. (1992). Religious coping among elderly, hospitalized medically ill men. *American Journal of Psychiatry*, **149**, 1693–700.

Krause, N. (1994). Stressors in salient social roles and well-being in later life. *Journal of Gerontology: Psychological Sciences*, **49**, 137–48.

Lachman, M E. (1991). Perceived control over memory ageing. *Journal of Social Issues*, **47**, 159–75.

Lang, F.R, Staudinger, U.M., and Carstensen, L.L. (1998). Perspectives on socioemotional selectivity in late life: how personality and social context do (and do not) make a difference. *Journals of Gerontology Series B-Psychological Sciences and Social Sciences*, **53B**(1), 21–30.

Lazarus, R.S. (1980). The stress and coping paradigm. In *Theoretical bases for psychopathology* (ed. C. Eisdorfer, D. Cohen, A. Kleinman, and P. Maxim.), pp. 177–214. Spectrum, New York.

Lazarus, R.S. (1996). The role of coping in the emotions and how coping changes over the life course. In *Handbook of emotion, adult development and aging* (ed. C. Malatesta-Magai and S.H. Mc Fadden.), pp. 286–306. Academic Press, New York.

Lazarus, R.S. (1998). Coping with aging: individuality as a key to understanding. In *Clinical geropsychology* (ed. I.H. Nordhus, G.R. VanderBos, S. Berg, and P. Fromholt), pp. 109–27. American Psychological Association, Washington DC.

Lindesay, J. (1990). The Guy's/Age Concern survey: physical health and psychiatric disorder in an urban elderly community. *International Journal of Geriatric Psychiatry*, **5**, 171–8.

Luborsky, M.R. (1994). The cultural adversity of physical disability: erosion of full personhood. *Journal of Ageing Studies*, **8**, 239–53.

McCrae, R.R. (1982). Age differences in the use of coping mechanisms. *Journal of Gerontology*, **4**, 454–60.

Martelli, M.F., Auerbach, S.M., Alexander, J., and Mercuri, L.G. (1987). Stress management in the health care setting: matching interventions with patient coping styles. *Journal of Consulting and Clinical Psychology*, **55**, 201–7.

Meeks, S., Carstensen, L.L., Tamsky, B.F., Wright, T.L., and Pellegrini, D. (1989). Age differences in coping: does less mean more? *International Journal of Ageing and Human Development*, **28**, 127–40.

Melding, P.S. (1995). How do older people respond to chronic pain? A review of coping with pain and illness in elders. *Pain Reviews*, **2**, 65–75.

Murphy, E. (1982). Social origins of depression in old age. *British Journal of Psychiatry*, **141**, 135–42.

Murrell, S.A., Norris F., and Hutchins, G. (1984). Distribution and desirability of life events in older adults: population and policy implications. *Journal of Community Psychology*, **12**, 301–11.

Murrell, S.A., Meeks S., and Walker, J. (1991). Protective functions of health and self esteem against depression in older adults facing illness or bereavement. *Psychology and Ageing*, **6**, 352–60.

Penninx, B.W.J.H., Vantilburg, T., Kriegsman, D.M.W., Deeg, D.J.H., Boeke, A.J.P., and Vaneijk, J.T.M. (1997). Effects of social support and personal coping resources on mortality in older age—The Longitudinal Aging Study Amsterdam. *American Journal of Epidemiology*, **146**, 510–19.

Reisberg, B., Ferris, S.H., and Franssen, E. (1986). Functional degenerative stages in dementia of the Alzheimer's type appear to reverse normal human development. In *Biological psychiatry*, Vol. 7 (ed. C. Shagass), pp. 1319–21. Elsevier Science, New York.

Roberto, K.A. (1992). Coping strategies of older women with hip fractures: resources and outcomes. *Journal of Gerontology, Psychological Sciences*, **47**, 21–6.

Rotter, J.B. (1966). Generalised expectancies for internal versus external control of reinforcement. *Psychological Monographs*, **80**, 1–28.

Schulz, R., Heckhausen, J., and Locher, J. (1991). Adult development, control and adaptive functioning. *Journal of Social Issues*, **47**, 177–96.

Schwarzer, R. and Schwarzer, C. (1996). A critical survey of coping instruments. In *Handbook of coping: theory, research, application* (ed. M. Zeidner and N.S. Endler), pp. 107–32. Wiley, New York.

Seeman, T., Unger, J.B., Mcavay, G., and de Leon, C.F.M. (1999). Self-efficacy beliefs and perceived declines in functional ability: MacArthur studies of successful aging. *Journals of Gerontology Series B—Psychological Sciences and Social Sciences*, **54**(4), 214–22.

Shock, N.W., Greulich, R.C., Andres, R., Arenberg, D., Costa, P.T., Lakatta, E.G., *et al.* (1984). *Normal human ageing: the Baltimore longitudinal study of ageing*. NIH publication 84–2450. US Government Printing Office, Washington DC.

Solomon, Z., Mikulincer, M., and Flum, H. (1988). Negative life events, coping responses and combat related psychopathology: a prospective study. *Journal of Abnormal Psychology*, **97**, 302–7.

Strain, L.A. (1990). Lay consultation among the elderly: experiences with arthritis. *Journal of Aging and Health*, **2**, 103–22.

Sullivan, M.J.L. and D'Eon, J.L. (1990). Relation between catastrophising and depression in chronic pain patients. *Journal of Abnormal Psychology*, **99**, 260–3.

Taylor, R.C. (1994). Elderly persons at risk. In *Principles and practice of geriatric psychiatry* (ed. J.R.M. Copeland, Abou- M.T Saleh, and D.G. Blazer), pp. 116–22. Wiley, New York.

Thomas, P.D, Goodwin, J.M., and Goodwin, J.W. (1985). Effect of social support and stress related changes in cholesterol, uric acid level and immune function in an elderly sample. *American Journal of Psychiatry*, **142**, 735–7.

Turner, R.J. and Noh, S. (1988). Physical disability and depression: a longitudinal analysis. *Journal of Health and Social Behaviour*, **29**, 23–37.

Vaillant, G.E. (1977). *Adaptation to life*. Little Brown, Boston.

Van den Heuvel, N., Smits, C.H.M., Deeg, D.J.H., and Beekman, A.T.F. (1996). Personality—a moderator of the relation between cognitive functioning and depression in adults aged 55–85. *Journal of Affective Disorders*, **41**, 229–40.

Wallhagen, M.I., Strawbridge, W.J., Kaplan, G.A., and Cohen, R.D. (1994). Impact of internal locus of control on health outcomes for older men and women: a longitudinal perspective. *Gerontologist*, **34**, 299–306.

Wallston, K.A., Wallston, B.S., and de Vellis, R. (1978). Development of the multidimensional health locus of control (MHLOC) scales. *Health Education Monographs*, **6**, 160–70.

Welch, D.C. and West, R.L. (1995). Self-efficacy and mastery—its application to issues of environmental control, cognition and aging. *Developmental Review*, **15**, 150–71.

Wiedenfeld, S., O'Leary, A., Bandura, A., and Brown, S. (1990). Impact of perceived self-efficacy in coping with stressors. *Journal of Personality and Social Psychology*, **59**, 1082–94.

Williams, J. and Koocher, G.P. (1998). Addressing loss of control in chronic illness: theory and practice. *Psychotherapy*, **35**, 325–35.

Wolcott, L.E. (1981). Rehabilitation and the aged. In *Topics in ageing and long term care* (ed. W. Reichel), pp. 87–110. Williams and Wilkins, Baltimore, MD.

Young, R.F. (1994). Elders, families, and illness. *Journal of Aging Studies*, **8**, 1–15.

4 A geriatrician's perspective of consultation and liaison psychiatry

Philip Wood

This chapter addresses perspectives of psychiatric consultation, primarily on geriatric wards but also medical and surgical units. In addition, the reverse role is considered, that is, the medical or surgical consultation to psychiatric wards. Issues relating to patients with medical and surgical diseases that increase the probability of psychiatric illness are also explored.

The geriatrician's approach to multiple illness in older people

For most geriatricians, it is far easier to identify the elderly patient by their ageing physiology than by their chronological age. Multiple medical disorders complicated by psychosocial issues characterize the health of hospitalized elderly people. Indeed, this complexity contributes to the concept of 'frailty'. Because multiple diseases are the rule rather than the exception, the geriatrician has had to abandon the 'unifying hypothesis' of parsimonious medicine, and instead attempt to explore the link between various diseases and their treatments. Disease processes involving multiple organs often present with a flurry of seemingly unconnected, vague yet significant signs, symptoms, or functional impairments, each of which suggests a variety of treatments. Indeed, this complex interplay makes geriatric medicine and psychiatry technicolour versions of the complementary adult disciplines. The physician and psychiatrist are continually confronted by the fascinating interaction between mind, body, and complex social issues of late life, challenging them to work together as a team to provide appropriate holistic care.

The specialty of geriatrics

Marjorie Warren (1943) is widely credited with creating the impetus for Geriatrics to emerge as a subspecialty of medicine in the UK. Her work also inspired the development of the specialty in other countries. In the 1940s the long-term care of the elderly was neglected, poor quality, and low priority. Rehabilitation was minimal, and not always well directed or led. In the United Kingdom, the nineteenth-century 'workhouses' (of Pickwickian notoriety) were reinvented as geriatric hospitals. These virtual 'geriatric warehouses' too often were the depressing last refuge of the elderly. The medical specialty of Geriatrics developed in response to these observed deficiencies in care, to provide a degree of compassion for the elderly, which at that time was lacking in the general medicine of the era.

Despite over 50 years of geriatric endeavour, sadly the situation Marjorie Warren sought to solve in the 1940s still exists in some parts of the world today. Some societies devalue old age, frailty, or those individuals who seem to be a burden on the community. In such societies, services for these people are a lower political priority, and consequently their development is lacking. As the world's population ages, the need to provide appropriate healthcare for elderly people has become increasingly important. Sick and frail elderly people have difficulty in advocating for better services on their own behalf. Consequently, the responsibility for representation and equity of healthcare for the elderly often falls on geriatric services and geriatricians.

The specialty of geriatrics has been delineated both by the types of services provided and by the characteristics of the patients treated. Evans, Hodkinson, and Mezey (1971), in a contentious paper, defined geriatrics as 'the comprehensive care of the sick over the age of 75, the service being organized by a geriatrician whose role should involve both hospital and community care'. Unfortunately, this definition has unresolved internal reference, as 'Geriatrician' is part of the interpretation! Consequently, it is necessary to define 'Geriatrician'. Traditionally, a geriatrician is a physician who looks after patients over 65 years of age, but this is a somewhat simplistic definition. Indeed, in most hospitals the majority of the 'elderly', i.e. those over the age of 65 years, are not cared for by geriatricians, but are under the care of general physicians and other specialists. How do such physicians differ from a 'geriatrician'? The prevailing view is that physicians who specialize in the care of older people consider themselves geriatricians when they have advanced training in the problems associated with late life, and have special expertise in multidisciplinary rehabilitation. Their primary focus is those elderly patients who have multiple medical problems and are frail. The foundation tenet of geriatrics is to reduce the burden of undiagnosed and untreated illness.

Referrals to geriatricians come from the total pool of elderly patients (both in- and outpatients) who fit the above criteria and whose problems match the specifications of the geriatric services. Service description and models are quite variable. Some services primarily undertake rehabilitation of the elderly; others focus on the management of multiple medical problems, be they acute or chronic. Other services focus on community care and the maintenance of long-term care institutions. Finally, some larger services take all patients over a certain age, such as 65 years, and have elements of all the above. These system differences explain the great variety of styles of 'geriatric services', geriatric 'case-mix', treatment patterns, and management outcomes.

The fundamental principles of geriatric medicine

The basic principles of geriatric medicine are:

- Sound medical practice is adhered to.
- Quality of life is valued over quantity of life.
- Good care is valued as high as cure.
- Symptomatic relief is paramount.
- Treatable conditions are identified and managed.
- The potential for rehabilitation is recognized and exploited.
- Counterproductive or futile interventions are avoided.

The geriatric multidisciplinary team

No single person is likely to be familiar with the whole range of required knowledge or skills for managing elderly patients. Geriatricians generally feel quite at ease working with other clinical professionals, such as nurses, physiotherapists, occupational therapists, speech and language therapists, or social workers. For treating most medically ill older people, the involvement of several of these disciplines will be required. Moreover, the team approach provides for a wide range of professional expertise. The geriatrician's role can be as variable as the service descriptions given above. Some services are very much 'doctor-driven', others less so. The prime responsibility of the geriatrician is medical management, maximizing the patient's medical health in order to enhance the efforts of the other team members. The medical staff may take on the role of team leader, or 'captain', much as in a sports team, with the clear recognition that the position can only expect respect and support if it is deserved, and continuously earned. Strategy, planning, and leadership are required, and an understanding and respect for each team member's part is essential. Teamwork and interpersonal skills are critical for those working in geriatric services. In many geriatric multidisciplinary teams, consensus between members, rather than command from a senior doctor, drives the team. Occasionally there are problems within a multidisciplinary team. The clinical staff is not always in agreement, interactions may be inhibited, and important impressions withheld. Open, clear communication needs active encouragement, so that the treatment goals of all members of the team are in the same direction.

'The geriatric giants'

There are four major areas of geriatric medicine which occupy a large portion of the practise of medicine in the elderly, traditionally termed the 'geriatric giants'. These include instability, incontinence, incoherence, and impairment of drug handling (especially polypharmacy). Incoherence or delirium is discussed within Chapters 9, 10, 11, 12 and 14. Postoperative delirium is discussed later in this chapter.

Instability and falls

The annual incidence of falls is approximately 30% in persons aged over 65 years, and approximately 50% in those aged over 80. The incidence is even higher in the institutionalized elderly. Falls in the elderly are common enough in the community to be mistaken for being the natural consequence of ageing. However, as most falls result from the combined effect of apparently inconsequential factors, an assessment of falls means paying close attention to the details in the patient's history. In general, the interaction of multiple causes is far more likely than a single unifying hypothesis.

Falls are caused by a complex interaction of both intrinsic and extrinsic factors. The risk increases in those with postural hypotension, sedative or multiple medication use, poor balance, abnormal gait, impairment of limb strength or range of motion, and cognitive impairment. However, about half of all falls are due to extrinsic factors such as slippery floors, loose mats, poor lighting, and so on.

One important and possibly underestimated factor associated with the increased risk of falls is the use of benzodiazepines or other psychotropic agents (Schwab et al. 2000). Numerous other factors are associated with falls, but some important ones are over 80 years of age, previous falls, restricted mobility, poor physical health and abnormal gait, cognitive impairment, and the use of restraints (Capezuti et al. 1996). Psychotropic drugs given to patients who also have one or more of these risk factors, increases the potential for falls.

Geriatricians are particularly interested in the reversible intrinsic factors, which require a thorough history, examination, and investigations to identify them (Table 4.1). While it may be tempting to attribute falls to an obvious abnormality (such as stroke), one should be prepared to keep an open mind as the potential causes of any fall can be diverse. In general, a definite loss of consciousness is not usually due to a transient ischaemic attack. A vascular event large enough to cause a fall through loss of consciousness is typically fairly substantial and does not resolve over a short period.

The 'timed up and go' test is a sensitive and specific measure for identifying community-dwelling adults who are at risk of falls (Shumway-Cook et al. 2000). In this test, those patients taking longer than 10 seconds to arise from a chair without assistance and move 3 metres demonstrate a positive test.

In some cases, one specific cause cannot be found, but it is still worth while encouraging gait, balance, and other physical exercises. A thorough review of

Table 4.1 Evaluation of the elderly person who has fallen

History	Where did the fall occur, and in what circumstances?
	Were there any associated symptoms, before, during, and after the fall?
	Did loss of continence or consciousness occur? How long did it take for the patient to recover?
	(Generally, a cardiac arrhythmia causes sudden loss of consciousness with a relatively quick recovery, whereas epilepsy can be associated with a postictal period.)
	Were there any witnesses?
	Was alcohol involved?
Physical evaluation	Observe the gait
	Search for intercurrent illness
	Check cognitive state and mood
	Timed 'up and go' test (see below for explanation)
	Nutritional status
	Drug record and medications (include non-prescription, previously prescribed, or acquired from other patients)
	Cardiac parameters:
	Pulse rate and volume
	BP and postural drop
	Aortic stenosis, heart failure, carotid bruits
	Neurological:
	Focal neurological abnormalities such as hemiparesis and peripheral neuropathy
	Parkinson's disease and parkinsonian symptoms.
	Cervical spondylosis and basilovertebral insufficiency
	Vestibular disease
	Hearing
	Vision, acuity, peripheral fields/inattention
	Musculoskeletal:
	Weakness in the legs
	Arthritic hips and knees
	Examination of feet and footwear
Laboratory and other investigations	Urea and electrolytes (look for low sodium levels, abnormalities in potassium), glucose (?dehydration/hypoglycaemia)
	Liver function tests (check for elevated γGT)
	FBC (anaemia)
	ECG (arrhythmia, prolongation of PR interval, abnormal QRS complex, ischaemic changes)
	Carotid sensitivity (generally reserved for specialist indication)

γGT, gamma glutaryl transferase; FBC, full blood count; ECG, electrocardiogram.

medication and alcohol use should be undertaken, and it may be worthwhile considering treatment of any nutritional deficiencies with vitamin D and multi-nutrient supplements. Occasionally, the provision of mobility-assistant devices such as a walking stick or frame may be necessary following the appropriate assessment by a competent physiotherapist. Sometimes patients may need advice on footwear and orthotic devices. Whenever possible the safety of the home should be reviewed by an occupational therapist so that obstacles can be removed, uneven and slippery surfaces corrected, heating ensured, lighting optimized, and handrails provided. Falls can have serious medical consequences for older people, as illustrated by the following case study.

Case study 4.1

Mrs K., a 78-year-old woman, lived alone in her own home and managed well until she fell and fractured the left neck of her femur. She developed an acute confusional state that left her mildly dehydrated. She was admitted to an orthopaedic ward that managed her confusion with a mixture of benzodiazepines and psychotropic drugs. Surgery was delayed for 3 days because of her confusion. The medical staff also noted the possibility of a perioperative myocardial infarction, with mild left ventricular failure. At 5 days post-surgery she was able to weight-bear and was transferred to a geriatric assessment and rehabilitation unit. She had incipient pressure areas on her sacrum and her heels. The geriatricians re-established contact with the psychogeriatric liaison team. They assessed the patient as having an acute delirium. The geriatrician and psychiatrist managed her together. Her fluid balance, diuretic use, and other medications were adjusted. The psychotropic medications were slowly withdrawn and the patient carefully remobilized. The psychiatrist established contact with the family and the neighbours, who reported a history suggestive of premorbid, mild cognitive impairment.

Comment   This elderly lady's case demonstrates the ease at which a delirium can develop in the perioperative state because of a variety of factors. There may be a primary or a secondary myocardial event, dehydration, electrolyte imbalance, or oversedation with painkillers or psychotropic drugs. Whatever the aetiology, the patient's condition can rapidly become unstable, both psychologically and medically. Such patients may not get the necessary attention on an acute surgical ward. The background history of her cognitive state may be pivotal in the ongoing expectations for the extent and rate of her improvement. The liaison between the psychiatrist and geriatrician helps to focus on areas of medical and nursing management.

Urinary incontinence

Urinary incontinence is not the inevitable consequence of ageing, or even dementia, despite being present in about one-third of those in acute-care settings, and half of those in long-term care institutions (Johnson and Busby-Whitehead 1997). Continence is a complex function, depending on mobility, cognition, motivation, manual dexterity, and muscular control of the lower urinary tract. While there may well be significant age-associated changes in the urinary tract, more important is that a loss of continence in an elderly person may well be due to factors outside the urinary tract, and therefore be amenable to medical intervention. Geriatricians disentangle these contributions, and alleviate those that are amenable to treatment. One of the most effective times to intervene in loss of continence is when it first

Table 4.2 Causes of transient incontinence

Constipation	May cause both urinary and faecal incontinence
Obstruction	More common in males e.g. prostatic hypertrophy, although uterine prolapse and cystocoele can also impact on continence
Nocturia	Excessive urinary output at night, such as from the effects of caffeine, alcohol, glucose or due to shift of postural oedema
Tablets	A very long list that includes, diuretics, anticholinergics, antipsychotics, antidepressants, sedatives/hypnotics, narcotics, alpha-blockers and alpha-agonists, calcium antagonists, and alcohol
Infection	A common cause of a change in continence. Note that asymptomatic infection does not necessarily cause incontinence, even though it is quite common
Neuro-psychiatric	Stroke, epilepsy and encephalopathy
Electrolyte and metabolic disturbances	Fluid and electrolyte disturbances, low serum sodium, hypoglycaemia, and the hyperosmolar effect of hypergylcaemia can cause confusion with loss of continence
Environment	Disorientation and misinterpretation of surroundings, poor mobility and need to access a distant toilet can lead to loss of continence
Confusion	Confusion from a variety of causes but especially in delirium can cause a loss of continence. Confusional states superimposed on dementia can cause incontinence, which should resolve if the cause of the confusion is correctable
Endocrine	Atophic urethritis/vaginitis characterised by vaginal wall smoothing, friability, telangectasia, petechiae or erosions. May respond if treated with estrogens (contraindicated by breast or uterine cancers).

starts. This is to avoid the 'transient' causes becoming persistent. The causes of transient urinary incontinence are listed in Table 4.2.

Of the persistent causes of urine incontinence, most lie within the urinary tract itself. These relate to the over- or underactivity of the detrusor muscle, stress incontinence, and urethral obstruction. As the full exploration of this topic is beyond this text, the reader is referred to excellent review articles on this subject (Resnick 1995).

Those involved in the care of the elderly can initiate an incontinence evaluation, before expert advice is sought (Table 4.3). Whilst medical causes predominate in

Table 4.3 Evaluation of the incontinent elderly patient

History	• Pattern
	    • Diurnal, nocturnal or in relationship to medications etc.
	• Type of incontinence
	    • Urge, stress, overflow, reflex, or mixed
	• Frequency, severity, and duration of urination
	• Any associated symptoms e.g. small leaks, incomplete voiding, dysuria, haematuria, or pain
	• Functional limitations such as mobility, manual dexterity, cognitive function, motivation
	• Alteration in bowel/sexual function
	• Medications, especially those listed as contributing to transient causes of incontinence (see Table 4.2) and also over the counter medications that could cause a continence problem
	• Other disease states such as diabetes, cancer, acute illness, neurological conditions, arthritis, previous radiotherapy etc.

Physical examination	• Physical conditions
	    • postural hypotension,
	    • oedema,
	    • heart failure
	• Stress incontinence. (Test when bladder is full).
	• Direct examination of voiding with particular emphasis on force and continuity of stream or any strain
	• Palpation of bladder for post void volume
	• Pelvic examination
	    • atrophy,
	    • urethritis,
	    • pelvic musculature,
	    • prolapse,
	    • sensation
	• Rectal examination
	    • sphincter tone and reflexes,
	    • prostate
	    • faecal impaction
	• Neurological examination
	    • sensatioin
	    • evidence of 'saddle' anaesthesia
	    • evidence of stroke
	    • mental status
	    • cognitive status
	    • affect
	    • mobility

Laboratory investigations	Routine • Voiding record (continence chart) • Urinalysis and culture • Metabolic screen (U&Es, Calcium, glucose) • Urine cytology Specialised investigations when indicated • Renal ultrasound in those males with larger residual volumes (reflux nephropathy) • Uroflowmetry if overflow obstruction suspected • Urodynamic evaluation when empiric therapy is either considered potentially dangerous, has previously failed, or surgery is contemplated • Cystoscopy

Based on Resnick, N.M. and Yalla, S.V. (1985). Management of urinary incontinence in the elderly. *New England Journal of Medicine*, **313**, 800–5.

some individuals, some situations may represent 'inappropriate urination' rather than urinary incontinence. For example, does the patient urinate in the bedroom rather than the toilet (a representation of confusion and disorientation), or does the patient have an urge incontinence? The only way to disentangle this is by obtaining a detailed history, assembling the facts, and evaluating the probabilities.

The most important part of the evaluation is the history and the voiding record. Whenever possible, staff should be encouraged to detail the frequency, location, volume, and factors associated with episodes of both continence and incontinence. For example, if a patient seems to maintain continence in their own familiar environment with the toilet being 30 or so metres away, yet becomes incontinent in the ward when the toilet is only 15 metres away, this could represent geographical disorientation. Medication records are practically important, especially those for new prescription medications, or even non-prescription agents such as cold remedies. For example, the anticholinergic effects of phenothiazines may cause urinary retention in susceptible individuals. Analgesics such as codeine may cause constipation and new episodes of both faecal and/or urinary incontinence.

A thorough physical examination should place emphasis on heart conditions (increased urinary excretion at night), bladder volume, pelvic and rectal examination, and a general neurological examination including perineal reflexes and sensation. The most important laboratory investigation includes screening for infection. More sophisticated renal and pelvic ultrasound may be necessary. Urodynamics are often reserved for those patients in whom the diagnosis remains in doubt or where the risk of empirical therapy exceeds the benefit.

Treatment strategies will need to be tailored to the individual. For the person with depression and urge incontinence, a tricyclic antidepressant might be a good choice. However, such a prescription would be unwise if the patient has urinary retention, and a serotonin reuptake inhibitor is a better choice. The combined smooth muscle relaxant and anticholinergic agents, such as oxybutynin, causes increased confusion in some susceptible individuals. Urinary infection requires appropriate antibacterial treatment. Behavioural reasons for inappropriate urination can be targeted with behavioural strategies.

Faecal incontinence

Despite this being a common reason for requesting placement in a nursing home, faecal incontinence is often treatable and continence recoverable. A history of laxatives use or abuse is often very helpful. Passive faecal incontinence or soiling is usually associated with dysfunction of the anal sphincter or with impacted stool in the rectum. Faecal urgency and incontinence occurs in patients with an irritable bowel, or diarrhoea from other causes. A rectal examination will reveal evidence of haemorrhoids, prolapse, or fissures, as well as providing important information on anal tone, sensation, reflexes, consistency of stool, and the presence of palpable masses. Generalized tenderness may well be associated with colitis. In some cases, more sophisticated investigations including colonoscopy, imaging, and physiological testing may be necessary, but these should be reserved for specialist interpretation.

In the majority, by simple attention to faecal consistency, regular toileting, and, occasionally, stimulation of defecation with suppositories will be all that is needed to improve faecal continence. The reader is directed to more detailed reviews, such as that by Kamm (1998), for further information.

Polypharmacy

Polypharmacy, or multiple drug use, is common in older people. The main risk of polypharmacy is adverse drug reactions (ADRs). There are a number of reasons for these. First, there is a higher incidence of coexistent illnesses, and the elderly see the doctor more often. Second, the elderly have had a longer period of exposure to a wide variety of treatments, and accumulate long lists of medications. Third, altered pharmacokinetics and pharmacodynamics increase the possibility of side-effects. Finally, the risk of drug-associated toxic delirium steadily increases with age.

The majority of ADRs are often predictable as they are usually dose-dependent and reverse with drug withdrawal or dose reduction. There remain a smaller percentage of ADRs that are bizarre, unexpected, and possibly immunologically mediated.

Increasing age is associated with an increasing risk of ADRs, but the most important factor is the number of medications. A good rule of thumb is that for less than 5 drugs the risk is approximately 5%; between 5 and 10 drugs, 10%; between 11 and 15 drugs, 25%; and more than 16, 50% of patients will suffer an ADR (May *et al.* 1977).

There are a number of approaches to this complex subject. A few simple principles are worth highlighting that may reduce the attendant risks of polypharmacy:

1. An accurate diagnosis is essential to guide specific and tailored therapy. One mistake is to treat the side-effects of one drug with another. It is important to ask which drugs can be stopped? Are there good indications to continue the drugs?

2. Clearly define the risk–benefit ratio with any new drug. Is the expected endpoint worth achieving when the risks are taken into account?

3. Clarify the expected outcomes from the use of the drug. If after a reasonable period the expected outcome is not achieved, re-evaluate and if necessary stop the drug.

4. Communicate the potential side-effects and appropriate responses if they should occur to the patient. For example, postural hypotension following the initiation of an antidepressant may be expected. The patient should be instructed to take adequate fluids, and get up slowly and carefully. Similar information should be shared with the carer.

5. Simplify drug regimens whenever possible.

6. Arrange close follow-up.

7. Record the reasons for the use of the specific drug, and when changes to dose occur.

8. Monitor drug levels, this can help reduce ADRs.

9. Pay attention to poor compliance caused by dose administration containers, blister packing, etc.

10. Encourage patients to bring all medications to the clinic, and if visiting the patient at home, ask to review all medications.

Medical illness associated with psychiatric complications in the elderly

The spectrum of medical diseases is different from that seen in younger patients. Many diseases gain their full momentum in late life. The old aphorism that 'it is more likely that the patient has a common condition with an uncommon presentation, rather than a common presentation of a rare condition' remains axiomatic.

Ischaemic heart disease

The most common cause of death in the elderly (National Center for Health Statistics 1993) is ischaemic heart disease, which accounts for 38.6% of all deaths. The presentation of cardiovascular disease may not be as obvious as in younger people. In some, the 'presentation' is completely silent. Several issues influence the presentation. First, if other age-related changes or disease such as osteoarthritis limit the patient's mobility, they cannot walk far or fast enough to exceed the myocardial oxygen demands. Thus, warning symptoms of exertional angina are restricted or absent. As a result, myocardial events may be unexpected and occur when illness or delirium stresses the patient. Second, the characteristic expression of the disease may be different. Dyspnoea may be the major complaint rather than classical angina. The 'silent' myocardial infarction is really a misnomer as careful history taking will often reveal symptoms, albeit non-classical ones, at the time of the likely event. Third, symptoms may reflect more than one cause, e.g. orthopnoea or exertional dyspnoea may be a reflection of poor left ventricular compliance as well as angina or congestive heart failure.

Psychiatric syndromes following myocardial infarction include a characteristic depression. The stated prevalence ranges between 20 and 50%, with males who have coexistent medical conditions being most at risk (Schleifer et al. 1989; Ahto et al. 1997). There is substantial clinical evidence that depression after an acute coronary event and mortality are strongly related. Fortunately, outpatient cardiac rehabilitation can decrease the prevalence and severity of depression (Milani and Lavie 1998). Platelet viscosity may represent a link between these events, as this increases in depression and reduces with serotonin-reuptake inhibitor (SSRI) medications (Nair et al. 1999).

Stroke

Stroke is a common condition, with cerebrovascular disease accounting for 8.1% of deaths in those aged 65 or over (National Center for Health Statistics 1993). The prevalence of non-fatal stroke is even higher. There is an array of neuropsychiatric syndromes following cerebrovascular accidents, and the interested reader can find a good account of these in Bogousslavsky *et al.* (1995).

In medical terminology, 'stroke' is a heterogeneous category of illness that describes brain injury, usually sudden, caused by vascular disease. A transient ischaemic attack (TIA) is merely a very small stroke; defined as a vascular event that resolves within 24 hours. There is nothing peculiar to a TIA, as compared with stroke, in terms of risk factors or prognosis. It is prudent to explore with the patient, and often the relatives, what they understand by the terms 'stroke' or 'TIA'. Some patients and relatives have very limited insight into potential consequences, or have unrealistic expectations following profound strokes. Some patients misinterpret the significance of their illness because of neuropathological reasons. Depending on the area of the brain affected by the vascular insult, poor insight, lack of attention, indifference, and denial may complicate rehabilitation. Similarly, frontal lobe involvement may mean emotionalism, odd speech, and semantic or expressive language problems (Starkstein and Robinson 1997).

Visuospatial disorders can complicate both left and right parietal lobe strokes, although those associated with left hemisphere disorders tend to be more florid and long-lasting. There may be visuospatial neglect manifested by:

- reading difficulties (books and clocks);
- writing on one side of the page, or writing drifting off away from the affected side;
- 'losing' objects that are on the affected side but not appreciated;
- getting lost, because of a failure to recognize the need to take a turn towards the affected side;
- failing to shave or dress the affected side;
- accidents caused by bumping into or knocking off objects on the affected side.

The prevalence of poststroke neuropsychiatric syndromes (Table 4.4)

The most common poststroke psychiatric syndrome is a mood disorder, the prevalence being between 10 and 40% (Eastwood *et al.* 1989). A broad spectrum of problems may be manifest. Some workers describe an association between the left hemisphere stroke and major depressive syndrome (House 1987), but, in general, such an association is weak. Patients often have a degree of cognitive impairment. Poststroke depression may overlap with an adjustment disorder, with depressed mood brought on by the unexpected stress of the cerebral event, and it may be difficult to distinguish one from another. In other patients, there is apathy, social

Table 4.4 Neuropathological correlates of neuropsychiatric syndromes

Neuropsychiatric syndrome	Neuropathological correlates	Prevalence (Per cent) following stroke
Major Depression Disorder	L) Dorsolateral frontal cortex and basal ganglia; enlarged ventricles	10
General Anxiety Disorder		
with depression	L) Frontal cortex	20
without depression	R) Parietal cortex	7
Mania	R) Hemisphere, or bilateral orbitomedial frontal cortex, basotemporal, basal ganglia, and thalamus	rare
Psychosis	R) Parietal-temporal-occipital junction	rare
Neuropsychiatric symptoms		
Apathy		
with depression	L) Dorso-lateral frontal cortex and basal ganglia	11
without depression	Posterior internal capsule	11
Anosognosia	R) Hemisphere and enlarged ventricles; frontal lobe dysfunction	24–43
Catastrophic reaction	Anterior cortical lesion	19
Emotional lability	Bilateral injury	20

withdrawal, and pathological emotional indifference associated with denial. This is often termed anosognosia, the term coined by Babinski. Anosognosia is not related to the presence of sensory deficits (Starkstein and Robinson 1992) and does not preclude the clinical expression of depression. In general, the location of the stroke does not assist in delineating depressive syndromes, although a consensus is developing that the closer the stroke's proximity to the frontal pole, the more severe is the depression.

Patients may present with emotionalism or emotional lability following stroke and consequently are thought to be depressed. Furthermore, patients show their emotions (often tearful, more rarely laughter) much more easily than previously. As emotional lability is often distressing to both the patient and carers, the symptom needs to be explored. Is the emotionalism in proportion to the patient's mood state? Patients will often state that they are less able to control the expression of their emotions, but, in reality, they are coping better than is outwardly evident. In such instances, support and encouragement may well be the only input needed.

Mania following stroke is fortunately extremely rare. More common are the overly enthusiastic patients, who feel they should be doing more for themselves. Such patients are often lacking in insight or understanding into the nature of their condition, or have overoptimistic ideas concerning their rehabilitative progress. They are at risk because they attempt activities before they have the physical capabilities to do so. Such patients need firm but consistent advice regarding the strategy and long-term goals for safe and secure movement. Focusing the patient's energy into appropriate activities such as personal exercises, and providing extra short sessions of rehabilitation therapy will often be all that is necessary to keep such patients satisfied.

A stroke in the frontal lobe often results in major changes in critical elements of the person's personality. There may be apathy, inability to appreciate others' feelings, loss of emotional expression, failure to recognize friends or family, minimization or denial of deficits, loss of musical appreciation, disinhibition, or sarcasm. Carers and relatives may well need repeated explanations of the nature of the disorder to help them come to terms with these distressing changes.

In some individuals, their response to stroke can only be understood in the light of their personal circumstances. For example, the stronger partner in a relationship may suddenly become dependent, or a patient who has a conflict-laden partnership faces dependence upon a perceived aggressor. Such 'no win' situations need to be accepted and worked through with the rehabilitation team.

Carcinoma

The liaison psychiatrist needs to be aware of the direct and indirect effects of a neoplastic disorder on mental health. Even the most common carcinomas, such as those of the breast, prostate, bowel, and lung, present with a bewildering variety of strange symptoms in late life.

Effects of local neoplasia

The direct effects of primary or secondary tumours may present with focal neurological signs, or raised intracranial pressure. However, whenever sufficient doubt exists as to the possibility of a tumour explaining the patient's current situation, prudence would dictate that a computed tomography (CT) or magnetic resonance imaging (MRI) scan be obtained to substantiate that possibility. There are numerous syndromes associated with variously placed intracranial tumours. For more detail, the reader is referred to *Brain and Bannister's clinical neurology* (Bannister 1992). However, a few highlights warrant brief mention. The classical presentation of a frontal lobe tumour is a change in mental status and personality, occurring in 90% of patients, with frank dementia in 70%. Focal neurological signs may be absent (Cummings and Benson 1992). About 50% of patients with frontal lobe tumours develop seizures, usually of the focal motor (Jacksonian) type. Changes in personality with psychosis, anxiety, or even hallucinations (auditory, simple olfactory, or gustatory) occur in patients with temporal lobe tumours, sometimes with bizarre partial complex seizures and other psychomotor disturbances. Parietal lobe tumours may produce somato-sensory disturbances and a non-dominant or neglect syndrome, sometimes with minimal signs of weakness. Occipital lobe tumours will often produce contra-lateral, homonymous visual-field deficits, or simple visual seizures and poorly formed visual hallucinations. Tumours in the boundary of the temporal and occipital lobe may produce difficulties with the identification of objects, faces, or environments. Deep midline tumours may rarely cause bizarre 'psychiatric' phenomena, including rage attacks, memory loss, confusion, emotional lability, personality changes, and depression.

Treatment effects

The treatments of neoplasia also have neuropsychiatric effects. Local surgery, anaesthetics, chemotherapy, and radiotherapy all have significant effects on neuro-endocrine, metabolic, and physiological systems. Radiation and chemotherapy may cause leucoencephalopathy, with delayed demyelination of the central nervous system, which can occur between 3 months and 5 years post-therapy. Symptoms include memory impairment, cognitive decline, tremor, gait disturbance, ataxia, and long track signs. Methotrexate is the most common agent causing delayed demyeli-nation, although other agents have also been associated with the condition. The combination of radiotherapy and chemotherapy is particularly potent (Johnson *et al.* 1985).

Remote effects of neoplasia

The remote effects of carcinomas may present well before the primary source is localized. Autoimmune mechanisms or circulating polypeptide fragments are the probable cause of the 'paraneoplastic' syndrome (Dalmau *et al.* 1999). The commonest form of cancer associated with the syndrome is the small-cell carcinoma of the lung, although tumours of the breasts, ovary, prostate, kidney, and multiple myeloma may also be responsible for the syndrome. Abnormalities may occur from the cerebral cortex to the peripheral nerves. The central nervous system problems include encephalitis with perivascular lymphocytic infiltration, microglial pro-liferation, astrocytosis, and patchy loss of nerve cells. The syndrome is characterized by memory disturbance with cognitive decline, depression, anxiety, personality change, hallucinations, and fluctuating alertness, which may add up to a rapidly progressive dementia. Magnetic resonance imaging demonstrates increased signals on the T_2-weighted images in the frontal and temporal lobe. Cerebrospinal fluid assay shows elevated protein, increased IgG, and mild lymphocytic pleocytosis. Postmortem, anti-Hu antibodies are found in the nuclei of neurons (Posner 1992).

Vasculitides

Temporal arteritis is a systemic vasculitis seen predominantly in the elderly population. Women are affected twice as often as men. Symptoms of pain and proximal muscle stiffness overlap with those of polymyalgia rheumatica, a condition that coexists in 50% of patients with temporal arteritis. Headache, depression, dementia, and stroke syndromes are far less common, but they may lead to the involvement of psychiatric services. Treatment with steroids is often required in high doses, and this may be associated with steroid-induced psychosis.

Systemic lupus erythematosis affects multiple organ systems and produces neuro-psychiatric phenomenon in 40–75% of cases. Occasionally these are the first symptoms of the illness. Over 60% of patients develop memory and cognitive deficits, with impaired attention being very common. The disorder may present like a 'chronic delirium', but also have features of psychosis or anxiety, depression and hypomania. Neurological problems including seizures, strokes, and supranuclear palsies are also frequent (Moore 1997). Treatments include steroids, non-steroidal anti-inflammatory drugs, and immunosuppressive agents, all of which can produce psychiatric symptoms (Kovacs *et al.* 1993).

Another, albeit relatively uncommon, collagen vascular disease is Behçet's syndrome. It can be associated with a dementia syndrome and associated emotional disturbances do occur. Features are similar to the demyelinating disorders and vasculitides.

Surgical conditions and procedures associated with psychiatric complications

There are many surgical conditions associated with an increased frequency of psychiatric manifestations. The most common is delirium, which occurs in the immediate postoperative period or associated with an acute illness. In general, the risk of suffering a delirium rises if there is a pre-existing reduction in cognitive performance (Gustafson *et al.* 1988).

Anaesthesia and postoperative confusion

Modern anaesthesia is safe and effective. However, postoperative confusion develops in about 8–10% of cases, according to some studies (Tsutsui *et al.* 1996). Most deliria develop within the first 2 days postoperatively. The effects of the primary condition requiring surgery, pain, and analgesics add up to a potent cocktail that results in delirium in susceptible people. In a recent study of postoperative patients, Lynch *et al.* (1998) controlled for known preoperative risk factors; for example, age, alcohol abuse, cognitive function, physical function, serum chemistries, and type of surgery. They found that higher pain scores at rest were associated with an increased risk of delirium over the first three postoperative days (adjusted risk ratio 1.20, $p = 0.04$). Neither pain on movement nor maximal pain experienced was associated with delirium. The method of postoperative analgesia, types of opioid or cumulative dose were not associated with an increased risk of delirium. In contrast, effective control of postoperative pain reduced the incidence of postoperative delirium.

The elderly are particularly prone to the effects of hypoxia and hypotension. Even though blood pressure and oxygen saturation are commonly monitored during surgery, postoperatively these may fall precipitously, particularly if the patient is dehydrated or in pain. In a prospective study, major surgery was associated with both severe constant and episodic hypoxaemia on the second postoperative night. The patients had decreased mental function on the third day but not on the seventh day after operation, indicating that there was a degree of recovery. In patients undergoing major surgery, a significant relationship between the postoperative mental test score and oxygen saturation was found. However, there was no relationship between mental function and other perioperative variables (age, premedication dose, duration of operation, and opioid dose) (Rosenberg and Kehlet 1993).

Cardiac bypass

Cardiac bypass for the correction of valvular and ischaemic heart disease is increasingly undertaken on elderly patients. Unfortunately, there is an increased prevalence of neurological and psychological illness in the immediate postoperative period. Despite a number of prospective trials, debate on the extent of any long-term risk remains unresolved, but appears low. In one prospective controlled trial, 47 non-surgical control subjects were compared with 65 elderly cardiac bypass and 25 cardiopulmonary bypass subjects. The surgical patients showed some generalized impairment of neuropsychological abilities following surgery. At follow-up testing, there was no evidence of residual impairment among most surgically treated patients. In contrast, some showed greater improvement compared to initial test scores than did control subjects. However, the performance of 10 surgical patients (11%) declined for half of the neuropsychological variables between preoperative and follow-up testing. The neurobehavioural outcome was unrelated to the type of operation (coronary bypass versus intracardiac), or to factors connected with the cardiopulmonary bypass procedure (duration, aortic occlusion time, hypotension, arterial carbon dioxide tension, minimum haematocrit value, minimum temperature). The only predictor of negative outcome was advanced age. The authors conclude that although neurobehavioural impairment is common during hospitalization after cardiac operations, the prognosis for eventual full recovery is favourable, but less so among the oldest elderly (Townes *et al.* 1989).

A strong clinical perception is that those patients with deteriorating cognitive performance before surgery may be at increased risk for further decline. Often, elderly patients present with a history of sudden decline in cognition postoperatively. Perhaps the patient's covert cognitive impairment was unmasked by the operation, or attention was drawn to the deficit, which otherwise would have gone unnoticed.

The pathological mechanisms causing such damage are debatable, but may be due to microemboli, altered pH, changes in cerebral blood flow autoregulation, or dislodgement of atheroma from the ascending aorta. Precariously balanced boarder-zone areas of perfusion in the brain may also be susceptible (Murkin 1999).

Transcranial Doppler and retinal fluorescein angiography have provided further evidence of the presence of microemboli during cardiac surgical manipulations (Murkin 1999), and the frequency and severity of central nervous system complications in elderly patients undergoing cardiopulmonary bypass (CPB) may be greater than previously thought. Whilst the majority of CPB patients do not experience perioperative stroke, a high incidence of subtler central nervous system dysfunction may persist for up to 1 year after surgery.

Urological procedures

Postoperative confusion after urological procedures such as transurethral resection of the prostate (TURP) is common. A transient deterioration in the Mini Mental State Examination (MMSE) score occurs 2 hours after TURP in two-thirds of the patients. Fluid absorption is the factor most strongly associated with the change in MMSE status during TURP, while the preoperative health status and the choice of anaesthesia (general or spinal) have no influence (Nilsson and Hahn 1994). Associated with the fluid absorption is a lowering of the serum sodium level and, in susceptible individuals, pulmonary congestion.

Hip surgery

Postoperative delirium occurs in 30–50% of patients with hip fracture (Berggren *et al.* 1987; Furstenbug and Mezey 1987). Electrolyte disorders and hypotension account for the majority of such cases (Millar 1981). These contribute to a high mortality. A recent Scandinavian study instituted an intensive intervention programme to increase functional outcome. This co-operative venture between geriatricians and orthopaedic surgeons consisted of staff education, individual care plans, improvements in the ward environment, active nutrition, improved continuity of care, and the prevention and treatment of complications. Results showed a reduced incidence of delirium as well as other postoperative complications. A greater proportion of the subjects regained independent walking ability and could return to their previous living conditions on discharge (Lundstroem *et al.* 1999).

The vast majority of people progress through rehabilitation with relative ease. Those referred on to specialized rehabilitation services, such as geriatrics, are usually patients with multiple medical problems, those having difficulties in gaining maximal capacity, or those with complications. Some patients may have psychiatric difficulties pre-dating their operation, and may need the advice of psychiatrists for this alone. Some patients have excessive difficulties with rehabilitation. A traumatic fracture of any bone can lead to significant pain and associated functional decline. This may be quite catastrophic for some patients or severely disruptive to their normal functioning. Losses of independence, status, and control may need a listening ear, support, and validation as adjustment to such events is akin to grief.

Cataract surgery

Cataract surgery is extremely effective, and enjoys a 95% success rate in most series (Powe *et al.* 1994). However, the neuropsychiatric sequelae are less well studied. The patient may have experienced mild confusion before surgery, to which sensory impairment from cataracts may have contributed. Studies have shown that, in many elderly, there are significant impairments on the first postoperative day, predominantly in memory but also in other cognitive tests. A short period of 'black patch' delirium is much more common in elderly people (Chaudhury *et al.* 1992). These problems generally resolve within 3 days (Burrows *et al.* 1985) and are unlikely to predispose to cognitive deterioration in the year postsurgery. A high depression score before surgery is a significant predictor of postoperative depression following cataract surgery (Billig *et al.* 1996).

Sleep disturbance

Sleep disorders appear to be consistently associated with increasing age. The prevalence is high in the community, at approximately 16% for males and 31% for females over the age of 50. It is even higher in the inpatient setting. The common misconception is that sleep requirements decrease with age, but many elderly people feel unable to achieve the quality and quantity of sleep required for optimal functioning.

Whilst many sleep disorders occur in aged patients, the predominant ones are due to:

1. *Primary medical conditions*:
   - orthopnoea, associated with respiratory or cardiac conditions;
   - pain.

2. *Treatment of underlying medical problems*:
   - stimulating drugs such as decongestants, beta agonists, and theophyllines.
   - levodopa and other dopaminergic agents can cause nightmares.
   - mis-timing of diuretic intake can cause nocturia with sleep disturbance.

3. *Daytime sleepiness and disruption of sleep pattern*:
   - overtreatment with sedatives, prolonged action of hypnotics, or accumulation of long-acting benzodiazepine medications.

4. *Alcohol overuse*

5. *Sleep-related movement disorders*:
   - periodic movements are stereotyped twitching movements of the legs during sleep, occurring every 20–40 seconds and lasting from 4 or 5 minutes to 4 hours at a time. The movements disrupt sleep maintenance. They occur in approximately 12% of insomniacs, although a similar figure of prevalence exists in the normal population (Miles and Dement 1980).
   - sleep myoclonus—a disorder that increases with age.
   - restless leg syndrome, which patients describe as a deep discomfort within the lower legs alleviated only by frequently moving them. This can be so disruptive that they are unable to sit for long periods to watch television, or relax for any extended period. The irresistible urge to move the legs is difficult for the patient to explain, and neurological abnormalities are absent. Treatments are often short-lived in terms of efficacy, although levodopa, benzodiazepines, and clonazepam have all been partially effective.

6. *Narcolepsy and sleep apnoea*:
   - this is also associated with sleep myoclonus. The disorder sometimes responds to benzodiazepines, and any improvement in sleep is due to the increase in arousal threshold.

7. *Dementia*:
   - 'sundowning' syndrome. This involves nocturnal delirium-hallucinations, delusions, bizarre ideation, disorientation, and often confused wandering just before or even at the time of sleep. Treatment (McGaffigan and Bliwise 1997) is difficult, as hypnotic medications have minimal effect and may make the problem worse. Trials of sedative antipsychotics, chlormethiazole, hydoxyzine, or other atypical sedatives have variable effects. Good nursing strategies, which encourage daytime activity, orientation to time, and allow some activities to occur in bright daylight, have a reputation of being effective.
   - sleep–wake reversal in advanced dementia.

8. *Delirium*

9. *Psychiatric disorders*:
   - depression
   - mania
   - anxiety disorders
   - psychosis.

10. *Noise*

Why refer to liaison psychiatry?

Psychological and psychosocial factors affect many aspects of disease presentation, but their magnitude and impact are often difficult to establish. Most physicians and surgeons lack the time or skill to disentangle the impact of the patient's personality or psychosocial factors on pathology. The psychiatrists intuitive capacities, along with specialist training and new perspectives brought to bear on the patient's presentation are valuable. Sometimes, the physician or surgeon merely requires confirmation that they have correctly observed a condition, otherwise considered to be within the domain of the psychiatrist, and that their management is accepted practice. On other occasions, the physician or surgeon will wish to ensure that psychosocial issues have not been overlooked.

What information does a geriatrician want from liaison psychiatry?

The reason for referral and the type of advice needed should be clearly stated. The psychiatrist's responsibility in this matter is to try to adhere to the questions asked; or should this prove impossible, clarify what is thought to be the question and then attempt to answer it. Case discussions with the attending team are useful.

Primarily, the geriatrician wants to understand the diagnosis within the patient's context, and have some guidance on management, prognosis, and follow-up of the psychiatric disorder. Geriatricians appreciate advice on treatments, such as cognitive or behavioural therapy that require specialist skills. Most referrers want to know how to relate to abnormal and bizarre behaviours and to understand what these behaviours represent.

Second, geriatricians may be discharging patients back to the care of community carers or teams, where the patient will require the support of community mental health services in addition to geriatric care. These situations create uncertainty, and liaison requires careful planning. A whole series of questions may arise, such as: 'How do we contact the carer or psychiatric team?' 'Who can authorize such a service?' 'How often does the community mental health team call?' 'Who would normally get the feedback from such a service, especially if things were to go wrong?' 'Will there be a double-up of visitors in the community, increasing the risk of breakdown in the line of communication and responsibility?' Reinstitution of previous support networks after a long admission can be fraught with hazards.

Third, geriatricians are concerned about patients who have known psychiatric conditions. The patient's symptoms or treatment may be unfamiliar, and the attending staff wishes to be reassured that the patient's condition will not deteriorate by their interventions. Potential interactions with or peculiar adverse events of medications such as antipsychotic agents, especially the newer drugs, are also of concern. Furthermore, the attending staff may worry that their discharge plans or placement options may destabilize the patient's psychiatric state and cause more problems. This is especially true for those elderly people returning to their own home, where there is a worry that loneliness and isolation may increase the risk of depression, or even suicide. Sometimes the social support networks are sufficient for the physical needs, but inadequate for the psychological health of the person. Such issues are often beyond the average geriatric medical services.

Finally, geriatricians may request advice or expert assessment of questions relating to competency, testamentary capacity, application to the courts for guardianship and other medicolegal areas. These issues are time-consuming and often complex and are dealt with in Chapters 5, 15, and 16.

Why do delays sometimes occur before referring patients to psychiatry services?

Perceived delays in referrals are an irritating factor for liaison services. Appreciation of the perspective of the referrer may help understanding of this problem:

1. *Acute medical and surgical issues demand a higher priority*:
   - psychiatric conditions may not be at the forefront of the attending team's list of differential diagnoses.

2. *Underestimation of the impact of psychiatric problems*:
   - the attending team hopes the problems will resolve within the time course of the illness. In many cases, this is indeed the case and no further intervention is needed.

3. *Evolution of psychiatric issues during the medical admission*:
   - some psychiatric issues tend to evolve during the course of an admission and the pace of development outstrips the ability of the attending team's ability to cope. This is especially true when discharge plans are disrupted, or expected improvement does not eventuate. The psychiatrist can be involved in the disease cycle later than is optimal, and ongoing treatment is delayed. The patient suffers unnecessarily, and the psychiatrist is in the difficult position of having to advise a delay in discharge while the psychiatric condition is assessed and stabilized. This may lead to tension between the various team members and increases the pressure to transfer the patient from one team to another.

4. *Involvement of multiple medical teams or delays in referral to geriatrics from another team*:

  • the psychiatry referral may have been made soon after the transfer to another team, but this still occurs relatively late in the total patient episode.

5. *Shortage of psychiatrists of old age*:

  • expected delays in psychiatric assessment and the prospect of a prolongation of inpatient care may influence the attending team's willingness to refer.

6. *Funding constraints*:

  • in some parts of the world, there may be financial considerations and lack of funding for psychiatric consultation, or ongoing follow-up. A worldwide shortage of qualified psychiatrists may preclude many elderly people from gaining appropriate assessment and care of complicating psychiatric problems.

7. *Patient factors*:

  • the elderly often view consultation with a psychiatrist with great suspicion, because psychiatric illness has been stigmatized. Patients may fear a referral to a psychiatrist as meaning that someone 'thinks I am crazy', causing them to worry about possible incarceration in a mental institution. Referrers are often aware of the patient's anxiety and may be unduly influenced by their reluctance, thus delaying an appropriate referral.

8. *Pure bad management!*:

  • no one is perfect, and delays in referrals result from inexperience, pressure of work, and lapses of memory.

What are the expectations of the geriatrician?

In the author's opinion, consultation is an exchange of views to help reach a decision. There is a tendency for consultations to be a solitary experience, with messages, often cryptic and indecipherable, left in the notes. In preference, consultation with a member of the referring team to discuss the issues is advisable. A brief letter in the notes is useful. The best consultations are a mixture of both personal contact and succinct notes, with any new and relevant points raised—for instance, an overlooked historical detail, or signs or symptoms that have been uncovered.

In wards where there are numerous cross-referrals, case conferences are useful for full discussion. The presence of a psychiatrist in these case reviews can be invaluable, although for many services the logistics of this approach are difficult to establish.

Case study 4.2

Mr P., a 66-year-old 'graduate' schizophrenic had lived in a residential home for 30 or more years. He had received no formal input from psychiatrists for some years. For 10 years before his admission, he had an increasingly severe tardive dyskinesia. In the year before admission, he suddenly lost 43 kg in weight. Mr P was admitted to a geriatric ward for assessment and treatment and was seen by a geriatric liaison psychiatrist. The psychiatrist was already aware of this patient's physical condition but was concerned with his overall psychiatric disorder. The geriatrician and psychiatrist agreed to 'share the care' of this patient from the first day of the patient episode, and both saw the patient on ward rounds together.

Comment   In such cases, it may be very difficult to conclude in which domain, psychiatric or medical, the final diagnosis belongs. Obviously, the prime need is to investigate for medical causes of the weight loss. Multiple investigations may be required. A severe tardive dyskinesia may be the sole cause of his weight loss, due to the difficulties with swallowing, and a change in medication may be all that is required. Accordingly, close supervision by a psychiatrist may be prudent. Changing or altering his psychiatric medication may destabilize the psychiatric problem, or the physical condition itself may alter the pharmacokinetics of the psychotropic medication and cause toxicity or serious side-effects. Joint care can minimize such difficulties.

Geriatric liaison to psychiatric wards

The psychiatrist consulting to the geriatric ward often finds rich psychiatric phenomena; the geriatrician who consults to the geriatric psychiatry inpatient ward finds an area just as rich in interesting and varied medicine.

An ideal arrangement is one of reciprocity, in that a geriatrician consults to a psychiatry inpatient unit. The full range of medical conditions is often seen, and approximately one-third of the inpatients could have problems warranting review by a physician. In the first instance, the general geriatrician is often the best person to initially review the patient, deal with the immediate matters, and then call in other specialists as required. Due to the frequency of medical problems where an opinion may be required, a semiformal 'ward round' may be the best way to cope with the load, rather than an *ad hoc* approach. Ideally, the same team or consultant, to avoid mixed advice and to reduce confusion as to who is responsible, should deal with any urgent medical problems arising between ward rounds. No formal research has been reported on such an arrangement, but it is likely that much of the benefits are the result of the various interests of the participants, as well as the model of care.

Table 4.5 shows 135 successive consultations to an old age psychiatry inpatient unit by the author. Approximately 10% of patients referred had medical pathology in more than one organ system.

Eventually patients are discharged and long-term care issues become prominent. Sharing the care of some long-term patients in joint appointments at a combined clinic has some merit, and decreases the need for the patient to have to travel or be accompanied by a carer. It also encourages the joint decision-making process, exchange of important details, and decreases the possibility of contradictory advice and medications.

Table 4.5 Geriatric liaison to an old age psychiatry ward. Breakdown of referrals by organ system

Organ system	Cases (%)
Cardiac	18.5
Respiratory	10.4
Drug	5.2
Electrolyte	9.6
Urological	11.8
Neurological	14.8
Skin	5.2
Bone	4.4
General	3.7
Gastrointestinal	11.8
Opthalmological	1.5
Haematology	3

Special areas of co-operation between geriatrics and psychiatry

There are several special areas where teamwork between geriatricians and psychiatrists can enhance aspects of the care of older people. Pain clinics (Helme *et al.* 1989) and memory clinics (Fraser 1992) are good examples of how the multi-disciplinary approach is very effective. In addition, multidisciplinary perspectives enhance the teaching of students of all disciplines.

The older person's pain clinic

Many diseases associated with late life are painful. Yet, few geriatric pain clinics have been described (Helme *et al.* 1989, 1997), and are probably in short supply (Harkins and Price 1992). As access to adult pain clinics is often limited for elderly people, specialized geriatric pain clinics would seem to be sorely needed (Harkins *et al.* 1995). The multidisciplinary perspective can be useful for dealing with postoperative acute pain in frail older people, cancer pain in terminal illness, chronic musculo-skeletal pain, and abnormal pain behaviours. The multidimensional model of pain is composed of sensory–physiological–emotional–behavioural elements and holistic management requires geriatric, psychiatric, physical therapy, and psychological expertise. The treatment principles of adult pain clinics—such as education, adequate pharmacotherapy, physical therapy, cognitive strategies, coping behaviours, and psychological therapies—are just as applicable to older age groups (Helme *et al.* 1997). Development of specialized pain clinics to deal with the high morbidity of painful disease in late life would seem an important area for shared interest.

Memory clinics

In the last 15 years, there has been a proliferation of memory clinics throughout the world. Early examples exist in both the USA and UK. Memory clinics represent a good example of co-operation between medical, neurological, psychiatric, and other services (Wright and Lindesay 1995).

The pattern of memory clinics falls into two major groups. The first is service-based, the clinic comprising psychiatrists and a neurologist or geriatrician with support from neuropsychology and other specialties. The second is a more research-based system, with a similar complement of highly specialized staff but with a greater focus on research. There are mixes of both types. In both styles of clinics, the emphasis is on high-quality diagnosis and the initiation of appropriate management. Some have strong links into the community, through field workers, community nurses, and social workers, and have a focus on patient and carer education (Monitz-Cook et al. 1998).

Patient progress through memory clinics falls into two major styles. The first is a vertical model system by which the patient sees all members of the team, possibly in a series of scheduled outpatient reviews. The second is a more 'horizontal' model. Each team member assesses an individual patient and internally refers, if necessary, to other disciplines. The benefit of the former model is that a detailed profile of the person in all domains is recorded, but at a high labour-intensive and time cost. Most clinics follow proscribed approaches to patient interview and examination with standardized tools used for neuropsychometric testing. In some services, a routine set of investigations, including CT head scan or MRI, are performed irrespective of indication, in others, the indication for any individual investigation has to be fulfilled before proceeding (Barry and Moskowitz 1988; Wright and Lindesay 1995).

As with all geriatric services, co-operation and communication between team members is essential. Transfer of information to community-based field workers may be an essential component of such clinics. This may be achieved through combined multidisciplinary meetings with each patient discussed, or, less commonly, through reports from the contributing team members. The combined insight of the clinic team guides the choice of appropriate services available for patient care.

So why do memory clinics exist?:

1. Most have a standardized approach to detailed assessment, with good capacity for clinical audit.

2. They can provide a sophisticated 'one stop shop' for patient assessment, treatment, and clinical advice.

3. They provide a focus for a relatively neglected area of medicine.

4. They facilitate research and training opportunities.

5. Memory clinics provide a stimulating intellectual environment for each of the contributing team members.

Teaching and training students

Students often best appreciate the concepts and mechanisms of the multidisciplinary team approach experientially. Systems rarely stand still and the team concept is as much dependent on personalities and team interactions as on procedures. Learning by 'immersion' is often the best way for students to gain experience. In many services, students integrate into the team. The student can readily see the integration of care, and the links, means, and pitfalls of communication. Students have a subtle impact on the services, as the necessity to teach encourages staff to think more about what they do, why they do what they do, and how they do it. Teaching also encourages learning, and learning encourages research. By these means, the overall quality of service shifts in a positive direction.

Summary

Medical services for older people are often a rich source of referrals to liaison psychiatric teams. In many service settings, this has led to both formal and informal arrangements between disciplines. Such an arrangement provides a clear example where good co-operation between services makes for a satisfying work environment as well as high-quality care. Much of this work is challenging due to the considerable range of influences on the patient's welfare. It is therefore necessary that those working in the field have a well-rounded understanding of the medical, psychiatric, social, and spiritual influences on the health of the patient. Fortunately, most geriatricians as well as psychiatrists are used to a team approach, and are open to interdisciplinary co-operation to improve the management of their elderly patients.

References

Ahto, M., Isoaho, R., Puolijoki, H., Laippala, P., Romo, M., and Kivela, S.L. (1997). Coronary heart disease and depression in the elderly—a population-based study. *Family Practice*, **14**, 436–45.

Bannister, R. (1992). *Brain and Bannister's clinical neurology*. Oxford University Press, Oxford.

Barry, P.P. and Moskowitz, M.A. (1988). The diagnosis of reversible dementia in the elderly—a critical review. *Archives of Internal Medicine*, **148**, 1914–18.

Berggren, D., Gustafson, Y., Eriksson, B., Bucht, G., Hansson, L.I., Reiz, S., *et al.* (1987). Post operative confusion after anaesthesia in elderly patients with femoral neck fractures. *Anesthesia and Analgesia*, **66**, 497–504.

Billig, N., Stockton, P., and Cohen-Mansfield, J. (1996). Cognitive and affective changes after cataract surgery in an elderly population. *American Journal of Geriatric Psychiatry*, **4**, 29–38.

Bogousslavsky, J., Caplan, L., and Barnett, H. (ed.) (1995). *Stroke syndromes*. Cambridge University Press, Cambridge.

Burrows, J., Briggs, R.S., and Elkington, A.R. (1985). Cataract extraction and confusion in elderly patients. *Journal of Clinical and Experimental Gerontology*, **7**, 51–70.

Capezuti, E., Evans, L., Strumpf, N., and Maislin, G. (1996). Physical restraint use and falls and nursing home residents. *Journal of the American Geriatrics Society*, **44**, 627–33.

Chaudhury, S., Mahar, R.S., and Augustine, M. (1992). Black-patch delirium: a two year prospective study. *Indian Journal of Behaviour*, **16**, 5–14.

Cummings, J.L. and Benson, D.F. (1992). *Dementia: a clinical approach* (2nd edn). Butterworth, Stoneham, MA.

Dalmau, J., Gultekin, H.S., and Posner, J.B. (1999). Paraneoplastic neurologic syndromes: pathogenesis and physiopathology. *Brain Pathology*, **9**, 275–84.

Eastwood, M.R., Rifat, S.L., Nobbs, H., and Ruderman, J. (1989). Mood disorder following cerebrovascular accident. *British Journal of Psychiatry*, **154**, 195–200.

Evans, G.J., Hodkinson, H.M., and Mezey, A.G. (1971). The elderly sick—who looks after them? *Lancet*, **1**, 260–2.

Fraser, M. (1992). Memory clinics and memory training. In *Recent advances in psychogeriatrics* (ed. T. Arie), pp. 105–15. Churchill Livingston, Edinburgh.

Furstenbug, L. and Mezey, M.D. (1987). Mental impairment of elderly hospitalised hip fracture patients. *Comprehensive Gerontology*, **1**, 80–5.

Gustafson, Y., Berggren, D., Braennstroem, B., and Bucht, G. (1988). Acute confusional states in elderly patients treated for femoral neck fracture. *Journal of the American Geriatrics Society*, **36**, 525–30.

Harkins, S.W. and Price, D.D. (1992). Assessment of pain in the elderly. In *Handbook of pain assessment* (ed. R. Melzack and D. Turk), pp. 315–31. Guilford, New York.

Harkins, S.W., Lagula, B.T., Price, D.D., and Small, R.E. (1995). Geriatric pain. In *Chronic pain in old age: an integrated biopsychosocial perspective* (ed. R. Roy), pp. 127–63. University of Toronto Press, Toronto.

Helme, R.D., Katz, B., Neufeld, M., Lachal, S., Herber, T., and Corran, T.M. (1989). The establishment of a geriatric pain clinic: a preliminary report of the first 100 patients. *Australian Journal on Ageing*, **8**, 27–30.

Helme, R.D., Bradbeer, M., Katz, B., and Gibson, S.J. (1997). Management of chronic non-malignant pain in the elderly. Experience in an outpatient setting. *In Handbook of pain and aging* (ed. D.I. Mostovsky and J. Lomranz), pp. 241–66. Plenum, New York.

House A. (1987). Depression after stroke. *British Medical Journal Clinical Research*, **294**(6564), 76–8.

Johnson, B.E., Becker, B., Goff, W.B. II, Petronas, N., Krehbiel, M.A., Makuch, R.W., McKenna, G., Glatstein, E., and Ihde, D.C. (1985). Neurologic, neuropsychological and computed cranial tomography scan abnormalities in 2- to 10-year survivors of small-cell lung cancer. *Journal of Clinical Oncology*, **3**, 1659–67.

Johnson, T.M. and Busby-Whitehead, J. (1997). Diagnostic assessment of geriatric urinary incontinence. *American Journal of Medical Science*, **314**, 250–6.

Kamm, M.A. (1998). Faecal incontinence. *British Medical Journal*, **316**, 528–32.

Kovacs, J.A., Urowitz, M.B., and Gladman, D.D. (1993). Dilemmas in neuropsychiatric lupus. *Rheumatic Diseases Clinics of North America*, **19**, 795–814.

Lundstroem, M., Edlund, A., Lundstroem, G., and Gustafson, Y. (1999). Reorganization of nursing and medical care to reduce the incidence of postoperative delirium and improve rehabilitation outcome in elderly patients treated for femoral neck fractures. *Scandinavian Journal of Caring Sciences*, **13**, 193–200.

Lynch, E.P., Lazor, M.A., Gellis, J.E., Orav, J., Goldman, L., and Marcantonio, E.R. (1998). The impact of postoperative pain on the development of postoperative delirium. *Anesthesia and Analgesia*, **86**, 781–5.

McGaffigan, S. and Bliwise, D.L. (1997). The treatment of sundowning. *Drugs and Aging*, **10**, 10–17.

May, F.E., Stewart, R.B., and Clough, L.E. (1977). Drug interactions and multiple drug administration. *Clinical Pharmacology and Therapeutics*, **22**, 322.

Milani, R.V. and Lavie. C.J. (1998). Prevalence and effects of cardiac rehabilitation on depression in the elderly with coronary heart disease. *American Journal of Cardiology*, **81**, 1233–6.

Miles, L.E. and Dement, W.C. (1980). Sleep and ageing. *Sleep*, **3**, 1–220.

Millar, H.R. (1981). Psychiatric morbidity in elderly surgical patients. *British Journal of Psychiatry*, **138**, 17–20.

Monitz-Cook, E., Agar, S., Gibson, G., Win, T., and Wang, M. (1998). A preliminary study of the effects of early intervention with people with dementia and their families in a memory clinic. *Aging and Mental Health*, **2**, 199–211.

Moore, P.M. (1997). Neuropsychiatric systemic lupus erythematosus. Stress, stroke, and seizures. *Annals of the New York Academy of Sciences*, **823**, 1–17.

Murkin, J.M. (1999). Etiology and incidence of brain dysfunction after cardiac surgery. *Journal of Cardiothoracic and Vascular Anesthesia*, **13**(Suppl. 1), 12–17.

Nair, G.V., Gurbel, P.A., O'Connor, C.M., Gattis, W.A., Murugesan, S.R., and Serebruany, V.L. (1999). Depression, coronary events, platelet inhibition, and serotonin reuptake inhibitors. *American Journal of Cardiology*, **84**, 321–3.

National Center for Health Statistics (1993). *Advanced report of final mortality statistics 1990. Monthly Vital Statistics Report.* **41**, No. 7. Public Health Service, Hyattsville, MD.

Nilsson, A. and Hahn, R.G. (1994). Mental status after transurethral resection of the prostate. *European Urology*, **26**, 1–5.

Posner, J.B. (1992). Pathogenesis of central nervous system paraneoplastic syndromes. *Revues in Neurology*, **148**, 502–12.

Powe, N.R., Tielsch, J.M., Schein, O.D., Luthra, R., and Steinberg, E.P. (1994). Rigor of research methods in studies of the effectiveness and safety of cataract extraction with intraocular lens implantation. Cataract Patient Outcome Research Team. *Archives of Ophthalmology*, **112**, 228–38.

Resnick, N.M. (1995). Urinary incontinence. *Lancet*, **346**, 94–9.

Rosenberg, J. and Kehlet, H. (1993). Postoperative mental confusion—association with postoperative hypoxemia. *Surgery*, **114**, 76–81.

Schleifer, S.J., Macari-Hinson, M.M., Coyle, D.A., Slater, W.R., Kahn, M., Gorlin, R., *et al.* (1989). The nature and course of depression following myocardial infarction. *Archives of Internal Medicine*, **149**, 1785–9.

Schwab, M., Roder, F., Aleker, T., Ammon, S., Thon, K.P., Eichelbaum, M., *et al.* (2000). Psychotropic drug use, falls and hip fracture in the elderly. *Aging (Milano)*, **12**, 234–9.

Shumway-Cook, A., Brauer, S., and Woollacott, M. (2000). Predicting the probability for falls in community-dwelling older adults using the Timed Up & Go Test. *Physical Therapy*, **80**, 896–903.

Slater and Good (1991).

Starkstein, S.E. and Robinson, R.G. (1992). Neuropsychiatric aspects of cerebral vascular disorders. In *The American Psychiatric Press textbook of neuropsychiatry* (2nd edn) (ed., S.C. Yudofsky and R.E. Hales), pp. 449–72. American Psychiatric Press, Washington DC.

Starkstein, S.E. and Robinson, R.G. (1997). Neuropsychiatric aspects of stroke. In *Textbook of geriatric neuropsychiatry* (ed. S.E. Coffey and J.L. Cummings), pp. 458–75. American Psychiatric Press, Washington DC.

Townes, B.D., Bashein, G., Hornbein, T.F., Coppel, D.B., Goldstein, D.E., Davis, K.B., *et al.* (1989). Neurobehavioral outcomes in cardiac operations. A prospective controlled study. *Journal of Thoracic and Cardiovascular Surgery*, **98**, 774–82.

Tsutsui, S., Kitamura, M., Higashi, H., Matsuura, H., and Hirashima, S. (1996). Development of postoperative delirium in relation to a room change in the general surgical unit. *Surgery Today*, **26**, 292–4.

Warren, M.W. (1943). A case for treating the chronic sick in blocks in a general hospital. *Lancet*, **i**, 822–3.

Wright, N. and Lindesay, J.E.B. (1995). A survey of memory clinics in the British Isles. *International Journal of Geriatric Psychiatry*, **10**, 379–85.

Section 2:
Assessment

5 The assessment

Brian Draper and Pamela Melding

Summary

Assessment is the linchpin of quality service delivery in geriatric liaison psychiatry. Assessment commences at the time of referral when urgency is established through a triage process. The reasons for referral, which may be overt and covert, should be established. The medical record should be read before the patient interview to obtain a more detailed understanding of the issues. While it is critical that collateral information be obtained from family, caregivers, and nursing staff, circumstances may determine whether this occurs before, during, or after the patient interview. The geriatric liaison psychiatrist must be aware of potential barriers to communication with the older patient, including whether she/he has been informed of the referral, whether there are sensory impairments, poor language skills, performance anxiety, and transference/counter-transference issues. Interviewing techniques need to be adapted to older people. In the liaison setting, rapport may be established by initially focusing on the medical problem that led to hospitalization. A standard approach to psychiatric interview should then be followed with a format that may include symptom checklists. Mental status examination should invariably include a detailed cognitive assessment, suicide risk, and, where indicated, competency. Standardized cognitive, depression, delirium, and behavioural screening instruments may be useful. The assessment should culminate in a written report detailing the conclusions drawn from the consultation process, with a focus on the facilitation of good patient outcomes.

Psychiatric assessment of older people—the principles

Assessment in geriatric psychiatry includes the gathering of information about a patient that enables identification of psychiatric symptoms, description of behaviour, identification of psychosocial problems, measurement of functional capacity, and determination of relevant medical conditions. The liaison psychiatrist combines these to construct a prioritized problem list, formulate a psychiatric diagnosis, and to devise a management strategy.

The referral process

Triage

A major priority is to establish the urgency of the case by conducting a risk-assessment screen at the time of referral. Although a formal written referral letter should be expected in all cases, in urgent cases the risk assessment will often be conducted over the phone or in face-to-face discussion. The assessment should include the domains of harm risk to the patient or to others, risk within the medical context, and potential harms within the ward environment, to allow an appropriate triage of the case (Table 5.1).

Table 5.1 Risk assessment screen

A. Harm assessment	
The levels of risk of harm to self or others are:	
Low	No thoughts/actions of harm towards self and/or others.
Mild	Occasional thoughts of harm towards self and/or others; occasional, apparently unintentional dangerous behaviours, e.g. wandering, rummaging, uncooperative with care.
Moderate	Current thoughts of harm towards self and/or others with no, or only vague, plans; or frequent, apparently unintentional, dangerous behaviours. No history of impulsive harm.
Severe	Well-formed plans of harm towards self and/or others; or vague plans with a history of impulsive harm; or current life-threatening behaviours, e.g. refusal to eat, persistently refusing treatment.
Extreme	Actual harm towards self and/or others has occurred recently.
B. Medical context assessment	
The nature of the patient's medical and psychiatric condition will also have an impact upon the urgency of the assessment. The following levels of severity can be identified:	
Low	Chronic, stable medical and psychiatric conditions, e.g. request for opinion regarding diagnosis or management.
Medium	Stable medical condition complicated by an acute, distressing psychiatric disorder, e.g. poststroke major depression.
High	Unstable medical condition complicated by an acute or chronic psychiatric disorder, e.g. delirium.

Table 5.1 Risk assessment screen (cont.)

C. Ward environment assessment

The capacity of a ward to manage behaviours often depends on the suitability of its design and the purpose of the ward. The following levels can be identified:

Good	Ward has design features that allows safe wandering, staff is experienced in the management of the elderly, has a low utilization of monitoring/intravenous devices, e.g. geriatric rehabilitation, special-care nursing homes.
Fair	Ward may not be secure in design; or staff may not be as experienced in the care of the elderly; or frequent utilization of monitoring/intravenous devices, e.g. acute medical wards, orthopaedics ward, standard nursing home.
Poor	Ward may have little security; or staff inexperienced in the management of the elderly; or high utilization of monitoring/intravenous devices, e.g. postoperative surgery.
Very Poor	Ward is mainly devoted to intensive resuscitation and maintenance of critically ill patients, e.g. intensive care units, general emergency rooms.

This risk assessment allows for a more accurate triage of referrals.

Three categories of referral can be identified:

Emergency	Requires an immediate response as there is high risk due to a combination of the patient's risk of harm, the ward environment, and the medical context. Examples include threats of self-harm or violence; aggressive patient in emergency room.
Urgent	Requires a same-day response as the combination of the patient's risk of harm, the ward environment, and the medical context indicates a moderate risk, e.g. refusal to eat on medical ward; depressed patient in intensive care.
Non-urgent	The assessment should be undertaken as soon as practicable, usually within 72 hours of referral. Examples include assessment of financial competency on geriatric rehabilitation ward, opinion on diagnosis of medically stable patient in orthopaedics ward.

In situations where there is a multidisciplinary service, the triage process will also assist in deciding which team member is most suited to undertake the initial assessment. For example, a nurse may be the best person to undertake referrals where the main issue is nursing management of a behavioural problem in a medical ward, particularly if the problem had been identified by a nurse who is a member of the referring team. The majority of referrals, however, will require a psychiatric opinion, although a supervised trainee may undertake the initial assessment.

Establishing the reason for referral

Generally, a referral letter will mention a problem and pose questions to be answered by the liaison team. Psychiatric phenomena arise in a context of pathophysiological change, that interacts with the person's idiosyncratic psychological functioning and the environmental response. Miscommunication between referring team members, lack of understanding of psychiatry, or the dynamics of systems and personal assumptions can confuse the real issues so that these are sometimes not identified in the initial referral letter. A successful liaison consultation is highly dependent on the clinician's skill in identifying the actual reasons for the referral and addressing the real issues in the management plan.

In this respect, the first question to ask is who is the initiator of the referral? Team members vary in their focus and, generally, doctors are more concerned with diagnosis or treatment, the occupational therapist with aspects of rehabilitation, social workers with family issues and placement, and nursing staff with behaviour problems. It is useful to clarify the expectations of the referring team. Does the referrer want the geriatric liaison psychiatry team to give advice, treat a psychiatric problem simultaneously with medical treatment, take over management, sanction discharge, or do a competency assessment?

The next question is what is the cited problem? The referral letter may identify a problem as a diagnostic issue, an interpersonal relationship problem, or a placement issue. Is this the correct problem, or is the cited problem camouflaging much deeper covert issues? Such a referral often requires more time to be dedicated for the assessment so that covert and overt problems can be explored.

An important question to answer is who is the focus of the referral? Most referrals identify an index patient as the focus. During the assessment process, it may become clear that the true focus is a family member, a staff system, or even the referrer. Patient behaviour may test the personal skills or resources of staff for a variety of reasons. Challenging incidents involving patients with delirium or dementia may expose ward-staff systems problems, while staff may find some patients offensive because of their previous behaviour or history, for example a medically ill paedophile. A patient problem may lead to staff disagreements or poor team functioning as in the following case study.

Case study 5.1

Mr V. was a 65-year-old heavy smoking, highly intelligent, single man who had run a successful music school for many years, until he was hospitalized because of a leg ulcer and peripheral vascular disease. Whilst in hospital he developed gangrene of the toes. Within a month, he had both legs amputated. Mr V.'s rehabilitation was extremely stormy. Attempts to transfer or discharge him were met with complaints to hospital authorities and intense anger at staff. He insisted that he could not maintain his music school and that the hospital had to look after him for the rest of his life. Several months of impasse resulted before the referral to geriatric liaison psychiatry, which requested assessment for possible depression. He refused to see the geriatric liaison psychiatrist who, realizing there were some strong opinions surrounding the patient, held a case conference with the entire ward staff. This discussion indicated no objective evidence of depression, but revealed some split attitudes of the staff towards the patient. There were those who felt intensely sorry for him, those who were frightened of him, and those that were very angry at his intransigence. After a full discussion of all the issues, together they formulated a discharge plan that gave him opportunities to ventilate his grief and anger over his disability. The discharge date was set for 2 weeks later when a backup support system was in place. The patient was furious when told of his intended discharge, but once he realized this was non-negotiable, he returned home. Within a week he had his car modified, started driving again, and had reopened his music school.

Use of interpreters

The triage should also establish whether there is a need for an interpreter. In countries that have a high immigrant population, many older migrants are non-English speaking. Some have joined their children, who migrated earlier, on family reunion schemes. Often in these circumstances there have been mounting health problems or recent bereavements that have precipitated the migration. Concern of the children for their elderly parents' welfare is often the reason for the migration, rather than the desire of the parent. Other patients are refugees from one of the many world conflicts. Adjustment to a new culture and language, loss of social network, in addition to pre-existing problems or traumas makes for a complex mix of issues.

Such an assessment requires the use of a professional interpreter, preferably with mental health training, who can assist the consultant with an understanding of both language and culture (Shah 1997). A pre-interview meeting with the interpreter is required to establish rapport and identify the focus of the interview. Sometimes, the interpreter has been involved earlier in the medical admission and has already established a relationship with the patient. If this has happened, it is important to ensure that the patient agrees with the choice of the same interpreter.

Family members should only act as interpreters in emergencies. The patient may not want to give full information in front of a family member. In addition, family members lacking experience in health interpretation may give inaccurate or personally biased interpretations of sensitive material. Some family members find the reluctance of the clinician to use them as translators upsetting, but a careful explanation of the reasons usually resolves the situation.

Case study 5.2

Mrs T., an 87-year-old, non-English speaking, Russian widow, was admitted to the geriatrics ward due to a progressive decline in self-care, lethargy, and weight loss. She was referred for psychiatric opinion for assessment of depression. Since admission, she refused food and was very withdrawn. An assessment with a Russian interpreter was arranged in combination with a family interview. Mrs T. refused to talk when interviewed with the interpreter alone. When the family were called in she became more at ease, though she still spoke monosyllabically and avoided eye contact. The interview established features of depression, along with her evident trust and rapport with her family. The spoken English of some family members was limited and the interpreter was invaluable in obtaining important historical information. Mrs T. had migrated from Russia 9 months earlier at the behest of her children, due to their concerns that she had become depressed following the death of her sister in Russia. Mrs T. had never entirely settled in to her new country and missed her friends in Russia.

Examining the medical record

Before interviewing the patient, it is best to read the medical record to understand the sequence of events leading up to the referral. Some clinicians prefer to do this after the interview, but this may lead to a failure to focus on the main issues and to check specific incidents noted in the file. Integrated, single-record files, to which all multi-disciplinary staff contributes, assist in this process. Often the nursing, social work, and other paramedical reports are of great value, particularly in the description of nocturnal behaviours, social circumstances, and the findings of recent physical examinations. Frequently, the picture painted by a range of health professionals over days to weeks is quite different to that described by the referral letter.

The patient may previously have been seen by psychiatry, old age psychiatry, community aged care, or welfare services. Information gleaned from these sources may save considerable time in the interview. For example, if the referral relates to the diagnosis of dementia or delirium then knowledge of a previous assessment may be critical. If the patient came to hospital by ambulance, the ambulance officer's report may provide additional insights into the home situation. The medical record can provide information on the patient's hospital presentation, physical health, and functional capacity. Review of all investigations is mandatory, for both results and any possibly overlooked important investigations, for example lithium levels or computed tomography (CT) scan reports.

The interview setting

Where the clinician sees the patient may determine the quantity and quality of information collected. It is best to conduct the interview in a quiet private office. In liaison psychiatry, however, often the only possibility is the bedside due to the patient's medical condition, lack of alternative quiet rooms, or reluctance of the patient to co-operate. In these circumstances, quieten the room by turning down the volume on radios and televisions. Obtain privacy in a shared room by the use of curtains or, if possible, asking the other patients to move. Attempt to minimize interruptions by informing ward staff that an interview is in place and by use of a 'do not disturb' sign.

Despite all best efforts, the bedside interview setting is far from ideal, particularly from the privacy perspective, and this may inhibit the patient on critical issues such as suicidal ideation. It may be one of the reasons the expression of suicidal thoughts diminishes so rapidly in hospital after a suicide attempt (Nowers 1993).

Family and caregiver participation

It is a basic tenet in geriatric psychiatry to interview family, informal caregivers, and other informants in order to obtain collateral information. This is of critical importance when the patient is cognitively impaired. In the cognitively intact patient, information about the patient's previous coping styles and reactions to physical illness is often invaluable.

Whether the informant interview occurs before or after the patient interview varies according to the situation and the personal choice of the consultant. Family interviews prior to the patient interview may provide important insights about the patient. However, there are ethical objections to this approach unless the patient is clearly too confused to give competent consent to a request for an interview with family members. Furthermore, it may inadvertently bias the clinician in the patient interview, particularly if there have been any family conflicts. Conducting the patient interview first avoids these pitfalls but the interviewer may miss some important issues.

Some clinicians attempt to have the family available in the hospital at the time of the patient interview to facilitate integration of the family interview into the assessment. Occasionally, the patient may specifically request an interview with a family member present. In general, it is preferable to interview the patient alone as the presence of family or friends can be distracting to both the patient and interviewer.

It is crucial to assess the level of caregiver stress present in the family. Many geriatric admissions to medical wards are for social reasons—the ubiquitous 'acopia'—when caregivers are unable to continue to provide care due to stress. A major question to determine is the extent to which family members agree about the main care issues. An interview with the family and the patient together can help to ascertain family functioning and pinpoint potential problems. The usefulness of this approach depends on time constraints and the capacity of the family to tolerate it. If caregiver stress is a significant issue, it is wise to involve the ward social worker so that extra community services, respite care, future caregiver support, and placement options can be considered.

Consultation with the nursing and clinical staff

It is also a good idea to discuss the patient with nursing staff before the interview to get their current concerns and whether there have been any recent changes. In many cases, nursing observations of mood and neurovegetative symptoms clarify depressive illness or identify specific signs and symptoms for ongoing scrutiny. Close observation of patient behaviours or responses to unfamiliar environments may be invaluable in assessing cognitive impairments. Tactful exploration of staff–patient interactions may highlight systems or interpersonal issues.

Ward nursing staff may also request to be present at the interview. Providing that there do not appear to be any issues regarding patient–staff conflict and the patient agrees to their presence, this may be beneficial for the nursing staff's understanding of the patient's problems. If the clinician suspects that there is conflict between patient and staff, the initial interview should be with the patient alone to lessen any inhibition when discussing sensitive issues.

The patient interview

Barriers to communication with older people

Several factors may adversely influence the effectiveness of communication with older patients. In a hospital setting, an initial barrier is whether the patient has been informed of the intended consultation. Older patients are less likely to be informed than younger patients are about psychiatric referral (Pérez *et al.* 1985). The liaison service should insist that all referred patients be informed of the intended consultation. Some patients may be very indignant if not informed, others may be very embarrassed, some will simply forget. Usually the experienced clinician is sufficiently able to calm and reassure the patient about the purpose of the referral to allow the interview to occur. Occasionally the patient is so enraged that the interview needs to be rescheduled until the referring consultant has spoken with the patient.

Many older patients have sensory deficits that facilitate misperceptions. These deficits may be enhanced in bedside interviews and require compensation. For hearing-impaired patients, it seems almost universal that if the patient has a hearing aid, it is either not in use, not available, or there is a flat battery! A hearing wand is an invaluable and inexpensive aid for the clinician in these circumstances. Visual impairments are less problematic in the interview, but certainly require recognition and acknowledgement.

For many older patients the hospital experience itself may be very anxiety-provoking, though they may not openly mention it. The insensitive use of routine cognitive screens on older patients in a general hospital by medical and nursing staff may accentuate anxiety and cause resentment. A common complaint by patients is that, 'the doctor kept asking me to remember 'apple', 'table', and 'penny' as if I were stupid'. Some errors made in these cognitive screens are due to unrecognized performance anxiety. Mild cognitive impairments may be purely anxiety-related and in such patients, it may be best to defer a diagnosis of a possible early dementia until more information is available.

It is important to be aware that the patient may be unable to communicate clearly due to their anxiety. They may worry about being incorrect and withhold important information. Much reassurance is required to overcome this. Older people take longer to respond to questions and the interviewer should resist the temptation to pressure the patient into answering before they are ready.

Transference and counter-transference issues may contribute to communication barriers (Blazer 1989, p. 280). The older patient may perceive the clinician unrealistically, e.g. may view the clinician as the idealized child who can provide care to the impaired parent. If this occurs, there are dangers of splitting between the clinician and the patient's family. This may manifest itself in resentment from the offspring and a sense of competition. Similarly, the clinician can perceive the older patient incorrectly because of their own preconceived fears of ageing and death or previous negative experiences with their parents.

Interviewing techniques with older people

There is no standard interview for older people and it is essential to be flexible. Development of rapport is a priority to facilitate free exchange of information in a trusting atmosphere. The length and depth of the interview will depend on the patient's capacity to tolerate it, and the clinical circumstances. Sometimes, two or three short interviews may be necessary if the patient fatigues. Patients with severe cognitive impairment and behavioural disturbance are particularly prone to tire easily, thus limiting an interview in scope. However, even short interviews allow sufficient observation to start behavioural monitoring.

Information to be elicited

Presenting complaint

There are often multiple perspectives about what constitutes the 'presenting complaint' in liaison psychiatry. For example, the patient is usually concerned with their physical health, the staff with the patient's behaviour or response to treatment. However, the initial focus should be the patient's understanding of the reason they are in hospital. Discussion of the medical aspects of the admission is often less threatening and enables the patient to develop some trust in the interviewer, before proceeding to more personal topics. An informal manner and interest in the patient's viewpoint helps to develop rapport. Usually the patient will describe the medical problems that led to admission with varying degrees of accuracy depending on their cognitive status. This also allows the consultant to determine the patient's orientation at the same time without appearing to be conducting a test.

The next stage is to address the issues that resulted in the psychiatric referral. If the problem relates specifically to a psychological disturbance, e.g. depression, delusions, anxiety, etc., the standard approach to the psychiatric interview is recommended. In essence, the presenting symptoms are clarified in the patient's own words to determine the nature, onset, duration, change over time, diurnal variation, and the precipitating and relieving factors. Older people are prone to seek somatic explanations for their symptoms and this is particularly the case in general hospital settings. Thus, psycho-logical symptoms may be attributed to a physical illness that may mislead the clinician if accepted without question (Knauper and Wittchen 1994). Blazer (1989, p. 265)

Table 5.2 Interviewing older people

Approach the older patient with respect; call them 'Mr', 'Mrs', or 'Miss' unless the patient invites you to do otherwise.
Identify yourself and say why you are seeing the patient.
Establish whether there are any sensory deficits that require compensation, e.g. use a hearing wand or 'reverse stethoscope'.
Where possible, attempt to conduct the interview with the patient comfortably seated in a quiet room.
Be 'low key', friendly, and conversational to reduce anxiety and improve rapport. Use touch appropriately to reassure the patient.
Pace the interview so that patient has sufficient time to give answers.
Speak clearly and slowly.
Use short questions, avoid questions that include more than two alternatives for the patient to remember.
Use clarifying questions: – directive questions, e.g. 'How long have you felt depressed?' 'How old are you?'
Establish precise areas of deficits in cognitively impaired patients, and in other patients where specific information is needed.
Ask for descriptions in the 'patient's own words': – non-directive questions, e.g. 'How do you feel?' and this is important for those patients suffering from functional disorders to allow for a better understanding of their experiences. Also useful in cognitively impaired patients to aid rapport, as well as validating their own experiences.
Acknowledge the patient's perception of the problem. It may differ considerably from that provided by observers and may seem improbable. Often patients are acutely aware that others do not believe them and they require some level of reassurance.

recommended that a relatively structured format be used to check common symptoms such as depressed mood, loneliness, helplessness, hopelessness, guilt, worthlessness, anxiety and phobias, diurnal variation, obsessions, anorexia, sleep problems, lethargy, weakness, anhedonia, poor concentration and memory, thoughts of death and suicide, suspiciousness, hallucinations, and delusions. Suicide attempts, compulsive behaviours, and social withdrawal require specific enquiries.

In many cases, the patient has been symptomatic before admission. It is important to establish the treatment history of the current episode, including response and adverse effects to treatments. Most patients will grant permission to approach their treating physician in the community for such information.

If the presenting problem relates to the patient's behaviour, disclosure of staff concerns to the patient depends on the type of behaviour involved. For example, if the behaviour is 'food refusal', then a reasonably direct explanation is appropriate. A circumspect approach is more appropriate for aggressive behaviour to allow the clinician to assess the level of dangerousness present. Even when the patient is insightless about their behaviour, it is important to allow the patient to give their version of events. Often this provides the clinician with an opportunity to test the patient's awareness and judgement. In the psychotic patient, such inquiry will often reveal misperceptions, hallucinations, and delusions.

Case study 5.3

Mrs W-G. was admitted to an old age psychiatry ward following a stroke suffered soon after the death of her husband. The stroke left her unable to speak. The patient had no children or close relatives but several friends from her local church who were most concerned to hear from the ward staff that Mrs W-G was refusing to eat, behaviour they thought 'out of character'. The patient was referred to a speech therapist who was able to ascertain from the patient that she had been unable to swallow any solid food, even a biscuit, for many years and that all her food had to be pureed. Although she had visited her GP on numerous occasions to seek help for the problem, no cause was ever found, and the patient learned to 'live with it'. She told the therapist that she was very self-conscious of this and wouldn't eat in front of anyone apart from her late husband. Consequently, no one else in her family or social network knew about the problem. Fortunately, with this information the problem was immediately dealt with and she made a good recovery. Sometimes food refusal is just the inability to eat the food as presented.

Sometimes, it becomes clear that the staff or other patients have provoked the behaviour. Information gleaned from the patient should be checked with the staff, in part to inform them of the patient's concerns as well as to assist in developing a management plan. If there are serious concerns about staff behaviour, this necessitates diplomatic exploration of the problems with senior ward management.

Past psychiatric history

It is important to establish details of previous episodes and their response to treatment. This should include similarities with the current episode, frequency of occurrence, precipitants, adverse effects of treatment. and degree of recovery. Exploration of the patient's attitudes towards their condition and treatment not only assesses abnormal belief systems but highlights potential problems with compliance.

Family history

This should particularly focus on parents, siblings, and offspring to ascertain any genetic risk factors. A history of dementia, 'senility', 'hardening of the arteries', psychiatric hospitalization or treatment, and depression should be covered.

Medical history, medication, and alcohol/substance use

Most of the relevant medical history should be available in the medical file. Some commonly overlooked issues in the medical history include head injuries and the use of over-the-counter drugs. Details of alcohol and substance use are often missing or inaccurate, and review of the quantity, frequency, and duration of use is essential in all patients. A history of medical, psychiatric, or social problems resulting from alcohol overuse should induce the liaison psychiatrist to explore further.

Case study 5.4

Mrs M. had a 30-year history of bipolar affective disorder in remission, but her admission to a geriatric rehabilitation ward followed surgery for a fractured neck of the femur. She initially made a good recovery after surgery, but after a few days on the rehabilitation ward she presented with symptoms of a possible delirium with some hypomanic features. The usual screening tests did not find a cause. Her husband told the consultant that she had caught a cold in the orthopaedic ward and been left with an irritating cough. Mrs M. had asked him to bring in several bottles of her favourite cough mixture and the nurses had allowed her free access to this proprietary medication. The consultant asked the pharmacy to check the contents, the analysis showed that it not only contained codeine but also considerable alcohol. The staff was further shocked to learn that, despite being an inpatient, Mrs M. had a blood alcohol well above that legal for driving!

Personal history and premorbid personality

This should be considered in terms of life stages (i.e. childhood, adolescence, young adult, middle age, old age) and issues (i.e. losses, illnesses, traumas, relationships, education, work, retirement, achievements, ambitions, regrets). The detail required depends upon the patient. Knowledge of how the patient has habitually coped in stressful circumstances across the life cycle assists in understanding the current problem in context. Mistrust or suspiciousness of hospital staff might result from a history of abuse, child or family violence, neglect, maltreatment, or severe trauma. Some older people have lived through extraordinary circumstances that affected their development, such as the Holocaust, earthquakes, or various world conflicts.

Issues relevant to old age to be pursued include perceptions of health; adjustment to spousal or peer deaths and retirement; fears of nursing home placement, dependency, or death; and relationships with spouse, children, and grandchildren. A key issue to elicit is who supports the person and is interested in their welfare. This person may or may not be the primary caregiver. Particular attention to the quality of the relationship with this primary caregiver is important, as this will affect management plans. Many patients are concerned they are a burden on their families. Even patients with significant cognitive impairment may be sensitive to the family dynamics and can give insights about whether their spouse or child is feeling stress. Of course, the depressed patient may exaggerate the burden.

An examination of personal history also contributes to the assessment of the patient's personality and intelligence, particularly when combined with information from other sources.

Social history

This should include occupation, activities, hobbies, and interests as well as informal and formal social networks. Isolation is of particular importance. The nature of the patient's living arrangements, whether the patient lives alone or with family, on the ground floor or up many flights of stairs are important items to consider. Older people have a tendency to both overstate and understate their circumstances so collateral information is imperative. A general idea of the patient's financial situation is needed to assist in discharge planning, especially if residential care is an option.

Functional capacity

Referrals from geriatric medical services will invariably have adequate functional assessments from the ward occupational therapist (OT), who often complete a Barthel Index (Mahoney and Barthel 1965) or similar functional assessment routinely. Unfortunately, other referring consultants in medical or surgical wards do not focus on this critical aspect of assessment of the elderly to the same extent. Where such information is missing, the consultant should check a few activities of daily living (ADL) with the patient or nursing staff. These activities can include toileting, bathing, feeding, transferring, walking, and instrumental activities of daily living (IADL), e.g. housework, telephone, cooking, shopping, finances, laundry. If ADL functioning is suspect, an OT assessment is helpful.

The mental status examination

The mental status examination commences at the first contact with the patient and continues throughout the interview and sometimes beyond it. The examination should encompass all the observed behaviours of the patient and all the interactions with the examiner. Even before the interview takes place, the clinician may observe an agitated patient pacing the corridors of the ward, and the patient's response to the clinician's initial contact provides further information. Most of the examination occurs through the history taking and the clinician should use appropriate moments in the interview to ascertain the presence or absence of mental phenomena.

Appearance and behaviour

Simple observation of older patients in a hospital setting reveals considerable data. For example, the use of bed rails, restraints, and ill-fitting hospital gowns invariably announces a patient with cognitive impairment and associated behavioural disturbance. Food-stained pyjamas may indicate difficulties with self-care. The clinician should note the patient's physical status. Is the patient dehydrated? Do they appear in any pain or discomfort? Does the patient appear alert and aware of their surroundings? Does the patient require intravenous therapy?

Other features to note include level of activity, e.g. psychomotor retardation, and involuntary movements, e.g. tremors. Non-verbal communications—gestures, posture, and facial expression—may give clues to issues unspoken. The patient's attitude to the interview, the interviewer, and their hospital admission may give clues to the diagnosis, e.g. a psychiatric interview often irritates the somatically focused patient. Often, to the chagrin of the nursing staff, sporadic behaviours are not always observable during the examination but the clinician should note any actually observed.

Mood and affect

The entire interview is an opportunity to assess mood and affect. Affect is the feeling tone that accompanies the patient's verbal and non-verbal expression, and this may vary during interview. Features of affect to note include type(s), range, appropriateness, and control. For example, emotional lability is common post-stroke; constricted, flattened affect may be associated with Parkinson's disease.

Mood is a more sustained state that underlies the affect throughout the course of the interview. Probes include, 'How do you feel inside?' 'Do you feel sad now?' 'How are your spirits?'

The patient may volunteer depressive symptoms or need encouragement to discuss any present. Patients with debilitating medical illnesses can have sleep, appetite, energy, and motivational disturbances without being clinically depressed. In such patients, the cognitive triad of Aaron Beck (1976) is a useful, quick screen— how does the person feel about themselves, their current environment, and their future (Blackburn and Davidson 1995, p.23). Negative answers to these questions should prompt further exploration for negative cognition such as hopelessness, guilt, nihilism, etc. Denial of subjective affective disturbance may be misleading, particularly as 'non-dysphoric' depression is common in old age (Gallo et al. 1997). Such patients may complain of lack of enjoyment or pleasure in their life but attribute this to their physical condition. Contrary to popular opinion, older people do not pay chronic symptoms, aches, and pains excessive attention as they get older but tend to minimize them as 'ageing'. When they do, somatic concerns often mask underlying depression (Lipowski 1990).

Thought process

Thought process abnormalities include disturbances in thought-stream, for example: flight of ideas in manic disorders; retardation in melancholic depression. Formal thought disorder might be less common in the elderly (Blazer 1989, p. 272). Examples include the rambling, incoherent speech associated with delirium and poverty-of-thought content in dementia.

Content of thought

In older people, poverty of thought content may be confused with poverty of speech. Poverty of thought content occurs when there are adequate words but limited ideas. In contrast, poverty of speech occurs when very few words convey adequate ideas. Poverty of speech may be a cultural characteristic or due to a stoical or taciturn personality, and as such is a normal phenomenon in the absence of other symptoms of mental illness. Pathological poverty of both speech and content of thought can occur in dementia and depression in older people.

Disturbances of thought content may range in severity from preoccupations to delusions. Older people may become preoccupied with certain themes, e.g. the state of their health, and conversation will seem to invariably return to the same issues without prompting from the interviewer. In a depressed patient, such ruminations indicate areas of concern that the management plan should address.

Obsessions are recurrent ideas or images that cannot be voluntarily dispelled. They are often associated with a subjective feeling of compulsion together with a desire to resist and a sense of distress. The development of new obsessions in old age may occur in several contexts, e.g. in association with major depression or an early dementia. It is important to differentiate perseveration of themes due to cognitive impairment, from depressive ruminations and obsessional preoccupations

Misinterpretations are common in the hospitalized elderly. The hospital environment is full of features likely to increase their occurrence. For hearing and visually impaired older people who may also be confused, the murmur of corridor conversations and electronic noises from pagers and hospital equipment provide fertile material for ideas of reference and persecution. This may be accentuated by the unfamiliar surroundings at night, regular nursing observations, medical procedures, poor lighting, or the need to share a room with strangers.

Delusions are false unshakeable beliefs that are out of keeping with the patient's culture or education. They occur in approximately 30% of patients with dementia at any given time, with delusions of theft and suspicion being most frequently reported (Allen and Burns 1995). For an older person with early dementia, a false belief of theft when they mislay something may be less psychologically threatening than a correct perception that their memory and intellect are failing.

Misidentification syndromes are also common in dementia, and failure to recognize close relatives or the assertion of being acquainted with strangers should alert to this possibility. In the hospital setting, suspicions about the motives of staff form the basis of many delusions in patients with dementia, particularly when there is comorbid delirium.

Cognitively intact patients are prone to having more systematized delusions that might incorporate persecutory themes of being monitored by the hospital staff, technical equipment, or involve accusations of medical negligence. Psychotic depression occurs frequently in the elderly (Brodaty et al. 1997), with mood-congruent delusions of guilt, poverty, sin, nihilism, and hypochondriasis prominent.

Hypochondriacal delusions, often relating to bowel complaints, may result in multiple medical investigations before the medical team seeks a psychiatric opinion.

Perceptions

Hallucinations (false sensory perceptions without external stimuli) and illusions (actual sensory perceptions of external stimuli misinterpreted or distorted by the patient) are common in hospitalized older patients, for reasons similar to those previously described for the occurrence of delusions. Visual hallucinations and illusions are particularly common in delirious and dementing patients, often accompanied by fear and suspiciousness. Common examples include the illusion that cracks in the ceiling are spiders, or that water is running down walls. Patients may have hallucinations of small people or 'gypsies' camping in the room. It is often not entirely clear whether these are hallucinations or illusions. If a patient cannot give sufficient detail, the examiner may be unable to determine adequately whether or not there was a real stimulus. Patients can be convinced of the reality of the 'intruders', but then describe them as wearing 'clothing similar to the wallpaper to fool me'.

Auditory hallucinations are more characteristically encountered in patients with schizophrenia and may involve comments attributed to the hospital paging system, radios, or intercoms. Another common symptom, frequently described as a hallucination, is 'machinery noise', which is usually accompanied by the secondary delusion that someone (usually their neighbour) is using 'the machine' to spy on them. As many patients with late-onset schizophrenia are also hearing-impaired, it is more likely that the machinery noise is tinnitus, misinterpreted by the patient. Severely depressed patients may experience command hallucinations that encourage self-harm. Olfactory and tactile hallucinations may also occur.

It is also salutary to note that sometimes the alleged misperceptions of cognitively impaired patients are real.

Case study 5.5

An 85-year-old woman with mild dementia described in detail the cockroaches that were crawling over her bed, through her food, and up the wall. An intern presumed she was hallucinating and asked for a psychiatry consultation. As the psychiatrist introduced himself, he noted the cockroaches crawling over the bed...!

Insight and judgement

Information obtained from the examination and collateral sources enables the liaison psychiatrist to assess the patient's insight and judgement. Insight refers to the degree of awareness and understanding the patient has about their mental disorder and the need for treatment. Judgement refers to the patient's decision-making capacity, which is based on their understanding and appreciation of the consequences of their choices (Molloy *et al.* 1999, p. 4). Often judgement is only subtly affected in older patients and can only be properly assessed with access to a broad range of information. Appraisals of insight and judgement are crucial elements in competency assessments, which will be discussed in more detail later in the chapter.

Cognitive assessment

Cognition is passively observed throughout the interview. The primary concern is the level of consciousness, as impairment confounds assessment of all other domains of cognitive function. How attentive is the patient? Do they lose track of your questions? Is the patient easily distracted? How aware is the patient of their immediate environment?

As the patient gives their history, language skills should be assessed, in particular word-finding difficulties and paraphasic errors are recorded. Significant problems with aphasia will confound the rest of the assessment. The personal history also allows for passive assessment of remote memory, e.g. when providing personal history the examiner should attempt to get precise dates of anniversaries, ages of children, days in hospital, etc. without expressing any concern when details are obviously lacking or inaccurate (Silver and Herrman 1996, p. 237).

Many clinicians are hesitant about conducting structured cognitive examinations due to fear of insulting or irritating the patient. Most patients are very co-operative if properly informed of the purpose of the interview. One approach is to tell the patient, 'I would like to check your memory and concentration. We ask everyone the same questions. Some of the questions will be easy and others will be harder. I would like you to answer all the questions no matter how easy or hard they are.'

Whether or not the examiner chooses to use a standardized cognitive screening test is a personal choice. Whatever approach is used, the precise responses of the patient should be recorded. The following areas of cognition should be assessed:

Attention and concentration

If, during the passive examination, the patient has been noted to be inattentive, intellectually impaired, or poorly educated, the initial approach should be to use a relatively easy task. Immediate recall of three simple words (that can be later used to check short-term memory recall) is a test of attention. Forward and reverse digits are more complicated tests. Simple tests of concentration include counting backward from 20 and reciting the months of the year backward from December. More complex tasks include counting backward from 100 by 3 (serial 3s) and then serial 7s. These tasks are tests of more than concentration as they also involve calculating skills. Patients who make errors on serial 7s but do not demonstrate any other signs of poor concentration, should be given further calculating tasks to clarify. In all these tests, any perseveration of responses should be noted.

Orientation

The beginning of the interview is an opportune time to check orientation by asking name, age, and date of birth. Orientation to time and place is checked hierarchically from information that is general to specific. The usual hierarchy for place is state/province, city, suburb, hospital, ward/floor, while for time it is year, season, month, date, day, and time of day.

Memory

There are many dimensions of memory function including immediate recall, recent or short-term memory, remote or long-term memory, semantic memory, visual memory, and verbal memory. At the bedside, memory testing should be simple, but sufficient to establish any need for more extensive testing in a more suitable setting. The three words used to test attention also serve as a test of immediate memory. The number of trials required to learn the words should be recorded. Providing that the patient has been able to learn the words, short-term recall can be checked 3 minutes later. Alternatively, the patient can be asked to remember a name and address, with short-term recall again being checked 3 minutes later. Both spontaneous and cued recall should be recorded. Cued recall may be semantic (e.g. a type of fruit), or phonetic (e.g. t. . .t. . .). Asking general knowledge questions, appropriate to the person's education and culture, can check remote memory. Common examples include asking the name of the prime minister/president, the previous prime minister/president, or details of important world events of the last 50 years.

When the patient has severe hearing impairments, visual memory tests can be substituted by showing the patient three simple objects (e.g. book, comb, and wallet) and obtaining immediate and short-term recall after hiding them. Any errors in identifying the objects may suggest a peripheral visual impairment, nominal aphasia, or visual agnosia.

Throughout memory testing, the examiner should note any confabulation, as evidenced by the presentation of bizarre or incorrect information to general questioning. Its presence suggests a frontal disorder occurring in conjunction with disturbances of learning new material (Cummings and Benson 1992, p. 33).

Speech and language

Speech is the mechanical art of expression and should be assessed in terms of rate, quantity, and quality. Mood disorders in particular may affect speech patterns, with depressed patients having flat, monotonous speech and manic patients having rapid, pressurized speech. Spontaneous speech should be monitored throughout the interview, particularly when asked to read a simple sentence. The patient should be asked to say three syllables, 'puh', 'tuh', and 'kuh' separately and then to put them together as a single word 'puhtuhkuh'. This allows the examiner to assess the quality of respiration, phonation, resonance, and articulation (Cummings and Benson 1992, p. 25). The presence of dysarthria usually suggests a subcortical dysfunction.

Language is symbolic communication. A total of six language functions can be checked: spontaneous verbal output, comprehension, repetition, naming, reading, and writing (Cummings and Benson 1992, p. 25). The fluency of spontaneous verbal output should be monitored, particularly the melody (prosody). Paraphasic errors include the substitution of incorrect words or syllables. Asking the patient to follow a series of commands can check comprehension (and short-term memory). For example, 'Take the piece of paper in your left hand, fold it in half, and put it on the table', or to point to various objects in the room in a hierarchy of difficulty. These tests of comprehension may be difficult to interpret if the patient is apraxic or aphasic. Repetition of spoken language is initially tested when the patient is asked to immediately repeat three words earlier in the cognitive assessment. A more complex task is to repeat 'no ifs, ands, or buts'.

Asking the patient to identify various categories of objects in the room (confrontational naming) should test naming. The production of names can be checked with semantic and phonetic word-generation tasks that are timed over a minute. A cognitively intact older person should be able to generate 11 words in one minute. The interviewer should ask the patient to read a sentence out loud and then to follow the instruction contained in the sentence, e.g. 'Touch your knee with your elbow'. This tests reading ability and comprehension. Getting the patient to write a spontaneous sentence of their choice assesses writing and comprehension. The sentence should contain a noun and a verb and make sense, but spelling errors should be ignored. Knowledge of the patient's premorbid literacy is important.

Visuospatial function

Asking the patient to copy and draw assesses constructional ability. The copying of two- and three-dimensional diagrams such as circles and cubes should be followed by the more difficult task of clock drawing. With the clock drawing test, some examiners prefer to give the patient a clock outline and then get the patient to place the numbers and set the time (usually 10 minutes past 11 o'clock). Others prefer the patient to initially attempt the outline and to only assist if the patient is incapable. Clock drawing is a very useful and simple test that not only tests visuospatial construction, but also visual memory, planning ability, and comprehension. In addition, clock drawing detects evidence of unilateral neglect, perseveration, and executive dysfunction (Fig. 5.1). The drawing may be scored in various ways (Brodaty and Moore 1997).

Praxis

Ideomotor apraxia is the inability to carry out purposeful movements on command and usually indicates dominant, parietal lobe dysfunction. Tests include buccal–lingual commands (e.g. puffing out cheeks), limb commands (e.g. combing hair,

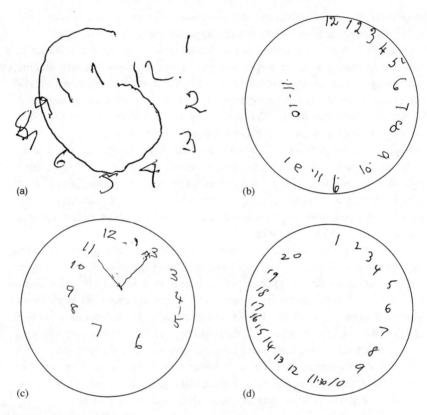

Fig. 5.1 Examples of clock drawing. A, Severe visuospatial disorganization. B, Neglect; time written, no hands. C, Mild visuospatial disorganization. D, Perseveration.

lighting a match), and whole-body activities (e.g. standing, walking to the door and back again). Dressing apraxia is an important variant and can be tested by getting the patient to put on/take off various pieces of clothing.

Gnosis

Asking the patient to name each of the fingers checks for finger agnosia. If the patient fails this test, they are asked to show the finger named by the examiner and then asked to indicate and name other body parts. Anosognosia is present when the patient neglects or ignores parts of the body, or even denies ownership of the part.

Executive function

Executive function involves the frontal lobes and their interconnections with cortical and subcortical structures. Some aspects of frontal lobe function are assessed by the

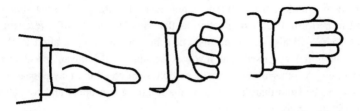

Fig. 5.2   Examples of Luria test—palm, fist, side.

previously mentioned tests of attention, concentration, verbal fluency, visuospatial function, insight, and judgement. Perseveration is often apparent during the interview. Tests of motor sequencing may also elicit perseveration, e.g. go/no-go testing where the patient is asked to tap once when the examiner taps twice and to tap once when the examiner taps twice, or the Luria hand side–fist–palm test (Fig. 5.2). A quick indication of ability to sort and change response 'set' can be achieved by asking the patient to sort coins in several different ways, for example in value, colour, or size.

Abstract thinking can be difficult to assess due to educational and cultural factors that impact upon performance. For this reason, proverb interpretation has limited utility. Comparisons and differences between simple objects such as lemon and apple, or child and dwarf, may detect concrete thinking, but again interpretation is difficult in patients from diverse backgrounds. Another technique involves showing the person a simple action drawing of a girl, a cat, and a bird, then asking the patient to tell the interviewer a story about what is happening in the picture (Royall *et al.* 1993).

Neuropsychological assessment

The liaison psychiatrist's main task is to delineate any problems in cognitive functioning that need to be addressed in the management plan. Detailed neuropsychological testing is indicated where there are subtle deficits to be quantified, and to more accurately describe the pattern of deficits to assist in diagnosis and management. However, the tests are complex, may take several hours to complete, and are outside the province of brief assessment within the clinical liaison context. When required, it may be more appropriate to arrange testing after discharge.

Physical examination

Although it may seem strange to include this in the psychiatric assessment of a patient in a medical setting, there will be occasions when it is important for the psychiatrist to check for physical, particularly neurological, signs. For example, if the psychiatrist suspects dementia with Lewy bodies, an examination for signs of parkinsonism should ensue. This does not mean that the psychiatrist should feel obliged to perform a full examination as that should be left to the referring consultant. There will also be occasions when the patient's co-operation is obtained through an initial approach that involves examining the pulse, blood pressure, abdomen, etc. At other times, the patient's physical condition may appear to be at serious variance from that described by the referring consultant and so a check of relevant features may be appropriate.

Special assessments

Assessment of suicide risk

Older people have a high rate of successful suicide, particularly men. Suicidal ideation has been reported in 13% of the hospitalized elderly and needs exploration in all patients (Shah *et al.* 1998). A graduated approach should commence with queries about 'whether life is worth living', thoughts of death and euthanasia. Sensitively presented questions to determine if there is any passive and active suicidal ideation follow, together with an exploration of any potential plans or active intentions. Patients assessed because they have made a suicide attempt need special attention. Attempts vary in dangerousness, but the person's perception of the risk is of prime importance. Did the person believe that five diazepam tablets or cutting a wrist would cause death? Was the method used researched for lethality or was it impulsive? Had the person made their plan well in advance and waited for the right opportunity to implement it? Did family or friends interrupt them in their attempt? If so, was this interruption a relief or an annoyance? The interviewer should assess if the person made provision for the (postsuicide) future, such as drawing up wills, leaving notes, or funeral instructions. Is the person prepared to try again or have they changed their mind? Are there significant cognitions of hopelessness, worthlessness, or pessimism about the future? It is also useful to gauge if there are religious, cultural, or personal prohibitions to suicide that may restrain a further attempt. Specific suicide risk factors should always be checked out. These include male gender, single status, depression, past suicide attempts, sleep disturbance, chronic pain, and social isolation (Draper 1995). The suicidal older patient is further discussed in Chapter 11.

Competency assessment

The ethical issues surrounding assessment of competency are discussed in detail in Chapter 15. Assessment of competency is a special area of expertise for the geriatric liaison psychiatrist. A patient's competency may be in question for a variety of reasons. In the medical setting, refusal to accept treatment or treatment recommendations, requests to discharge against medical advice, or dysfunctional behaviour may hasten referral for assessment of competency. A common reason for such a request occurs when the patient opposes placement into supervised residential or sheltered care, or desires to go home to a risky situation.

Lack of competency to make decisions affecting a person's own property, self-care, or welfare may be global and total, but is much more likely to be situation-sensitive or task-specific (Ryan 1996). A person may be competent to make a will but not to drive a car, or vice versa. Tests of competency need to be more stringent as the complexity of the specific task in question increases.

The specific areas that need to be assessed in determining a person's competency (Appelbaum and Grisso 1988; Ryan 1996) are as follows:

1. Does the person know what specifically has to be decided? If about treatment, do they know exactly to what they are consenting or not consenting. For appointment of a power of attorney, do they understand the powers of the attorney, what assets or properties are to be managed, and what rights they have or not have if they wish to rescind the decision.

2. Has the patient a disorder of cognition, mood, perception, or thought that influences the person's decision-making capacity for the task or tasks in question. Are there delusions or depressive cognitions biasing decision-making? Has the person hallucinatory voices giving contrary advice?

3. Is the process of decision-making based on a sound starting premise and is the reasoning process internally consistent? The interviewer needs to explore these aspects very carefully with open-ended directive questioning, and may have to explore backwards from the final point until the starting premise is reached. 'So, what made you decide that?' or 'How did you come to that conclusion?' If the starting premise is erroneous, then does the decision change if this is corrected or does the patient refuse to accept an alternative scenario?

4. Could there be any undue influence being brought to bear on the patient's decision-making, from a relative, caregiver, or other person? This issue needs tactful exploration, starting from, 'Has anyone been giving you advice on this?' or 'Have you discussed this (decision) with anyone?'

5. The interviewer needs to assess if the proposed decision is in keeping with the person's previous long-term goals and values (dispositional autonomy). Whilst dispositional autonomy always needs to be taken into account, it should also be noted that people are allowed to change their minds (Ryan 1996).

6. Can the person clearly communicate their wishes? If unable to speak, can the patient communicate their decisions clearly in writing or using picture cue cards.

7. Can the person assess the benefits and risks of each option open to them and foresee consequences of the final decision for themselves and others if they are affected by it. This tests a person's executive function and is a crucial part of the competency assessment. Probes such as, 'So if this (decision or consequence) happens, how do you think this would affect you?'

Table 5.4 Checklist for competency assessments

Decision to be made
- Comprehension of decision
- Understanding of rights
- Perception of risks and benefits of options
- Logical starting premise
- Internally consistent reasoning process
- Able to foresee consequences of decision
- Undue influence or coercion
- Insight and judgement
- Dispositional autonomy and previous decision making trends

Communication
Able to clearly communicate wishes either verbally or by using aids

Mental disorder
- History and premorbid functioning
- Depression
- Mania
- Hallucinations
- Delusions
- Other mental disorder

Cognitive Disorder
- Memory and new learning ability
- Orientation
- Attention and concentration
- Other cognitive deficits
- MMSE or other structured test
- Executive functioning

The patient may arrive at a decision that may be contrary to one the interviewer might make under the same circumstances, for example to refuse treatment or leave hospital. That standard should not be the arbiter of the patient's competency. People can and do make silly decisions and, indeed, many that do are otherwise technically competent people. Most clinicians can even recognize examples of such people in their own social or professional sphere! The important standard is whether the decision is understandable, rational, and logical according to the person's previous and current functioning. Ryan (1996) suggests that a person is fully competent if they meet minimal standards of understanding required to make an autonomous decision. The person is partially competent if the patient fails to meet the standard of logical deliberation but makes choices consistent with long-term values and principles. Patients are fully incompetent if unable to make decisions with either concept of autonomy.

Table 5.4 provides a schema for competency assessments. Legal aspects of competency are covered in more detail in Chapter 16.

Case study 5.6

Mrs A. was an 85-year-old widow from a residential care home admitted with a sudden deterioration in her mental state and confused behaviour at night. Until 2 years previously she had been fit enough to take a daily swim in the sea. Over the last year, she had become increasingly immobile, and her friends noticed some decline in her memory and functioning. The geriatric team made a diagnosis of delirium and early cognitive impairment. The cause of the delirium was a strangulated hernia. Mrs. A. declined surgical treatment. A competency assessment was sought as the condition was life-threatening but reversible.

The interview took place when she was quite lucid, with her family present. Mrs A. was quite aware of the decision required, what the likelihood of non-treatment would be, and the deleterious effect for her and her family. She had no depressive or psychotic symptoms and although she had some cognitive deficits, these were not impinging on the task in hand. Her family was clear that her decision was 'just like her' and consistent with her previous behaviour. She was deemed competent to make this autonomous decision, and she died a few days later in the hospice with her family present.

Standardized screening instruments in liaison psychiatry

Some interviewers like to use standardized screening instruments. These have several advantages. Providing interviewers are properly trained in their use, they can be replicable, comparable, and useful to monitor change and may aid research. There are currently dozens of instruments available to measure many aspects of geriatric psychiatry practice. However, in the liaison setting, the brief bedside instruments are the more practicable to assist with diagnosis, assess severity, or monitor change. For a full discussion of the range of measurement scales currently used in geriatric psychiatry, the reader is referred to Burns *et al.* (1999).

Several brief instruments are useful for the liaison psychiatrist to have in their repertoire.

Cognitive scales

The Mini-Mental State Examination (MMSE) (Folstein *et al.* 1975) is probably the most widely used bedside cognitive instrument used in geriatric populations. It consists of 12 items in six domains of cognition that include orientation, registration, attention and concentration, recall, language, and praxis. The scale is scored out of 30 and takes 5–10 minutes to complete. The standardized Mini-Mental State Examination (sMMSE) has more explicit instructions on how to administer each item in order to improve interrater reliability and objectivity (Molloy *et al.* 1991). However, neither version of the MMSE examines executive functioning, and additional tests, such as clock drawing or trail making, should be used to investigate these aspects.

The 10-item Abbreviated Mental Test Scale (AMTS), with scores of seven and under indicating the presence of significant cognitive impairment, is a simple and useful scale for cognitive screening (Hodkinson 1972).

The Executive Interview (EXIT) (Royall *et al.* 1993) is a brief bedside instrument that examines executive functions in some detail. A score of 10 or more indicates a frontal lobe dysfunction. It takes a trained interviewer about 15 minutes to administer. The scale covers memory, abstract thinking, word fluency, echolalia, echopraxis, frontal lobe release signs, and pattern recognition.

Depression scales

The Geriatric Depression Scale (GDS) is a self-rated scale that is available in 15- and 30-item versions (Yesavage *et al*. 1983). It is easy to follow and takes about 5–10 minutes to complete. While the GDS may be useful to detect depression in a cognitively intact healthy population, it is less reliable in the cognitively impaired (Burke *et al*. 1989) or in the physically ill (Rodin and Voshart 1986).

Objective scales may be more useful in monitoring treatment response. The Hamilton Depression Rating Scale (HDRS) is based on an objective semi-structured interview and takes about 20 minutes to complete (Hamilton 1960). The HDRS comes in 17- and 21-item versions, with the 17-item version being the most widely used. The HDRS focuses on affective and somatic symptoms of depression, and thus may be more applicable to patients who do not have confounding medical illness. Alternatively, the Montgomery Åsberg Depression Rating Scale is a 10-item instrument that has more emphasis on affective and cognitive symptoms of depression and may be more applicable to a medically ill population (Montgomery and Åsberg 1979).

In dementing individuals, the Cornell Scale for Depression in Dementia is useful (Alexopoulos *et al*. 1988). The Cornell scale is interviewer-rated and combines observed and subjective information on mood-related signs, behavioural disturbance, physical signs (appetite and energy), cyclic functions (diurnal variations, sleep pattern), and ideational disturbance.

Behaviour scales

Many scales measure behaviour in dementia. The most widely used is the BEHAVE-AD (Reisberg *et al*. 1987), a 25-item scale that covers delusions, hallucinations, paranoid behaviours, activity disturbances, aggressiveness, agitation, and affective and diurnal rhythm disturbances. However, in a liaison setting, the Disruptive Behavior Rating Scale (DBRS), a 21-item scale that includes physical and verbal aggression, screaming, agitation, wandering, and distress, may be more appropriate (Mungas *et al*. 1989). This scale takes a caregiver nurse only 10 minutes to complete and is not reliant on family or other informants.

Delirium scales

The Confusion Assessment Method (CAM) (Inouye *et al*. 1990) was designed to enable a non-psychiatrist clinician, given a little training, to detect delirium in medical populations. Consequently, it is very useful in the liaison context. The CAM consists of the nine operational criteria of DSM-IV, including the cardinal features of fluctuation, attention span, disorganized thinking, and level of consciousness. The Delirium Index (DI) (McCusker *et al*. 1998) is a variant of the CAM. This instrument is a 7-item, 3-point severity rating scale based on direct observation of the patient. It is designed for use with the MMSE.

Other scales

Other brief scales that might be useful in a liaison context include the Abnormal Illness Questionnaire (Pilowsky 1978) for patients with somatization disorders or chronic pain complaints. If caregiver stress is suspected, the General Health Questionnaire (Goldberg and Williams 1988) is a useful screen for significant depression, anxiety, or psychological distress. In addition, the Ways of Coping Questionnaire (Vitaliano et al. 1985) might also be useful for identifying coping problems in patients or caregivers.

The consultant's report

The written psychiatric record is the official permanent record of conclusions drawn from the consultation process (Garrick and Stotland 1982). This report, to the referring consultant, should address the specific questions posed by the referral.

How extensive should the report be? Many other health professionals involved in the case may read the report, so confidentiality of delicate information is essential. The components of the report include an identifying statement, succinct history, examination, problem list, formulation, and recommendations.

The identifying statement is a summary of the patient's condition in the context of the request for referral. For example, a 76-year-old man who is referred for assessment of 'aggression towards nurses', is found by the psychiatrist to have moderately severe Alzheimer's disease complicated by persecutory delusions of harm from the nursing staff. He irritably resists their attempts to assist him during personal care by pushing them away, but does not strike them. The identifying statement might read, 'This patient with a moderately severe dementia of Alzheimer type, is uncooperative and resistive during personal care due to his delusional beliefs that the nurses are trying to harm him'.

Only relevant aspects of the history and mental status examination need be reported. This will vary from case to case, but should include the main clinical features, past psychiatric history, and relevant personal history in summary form. Relevant negative data should be cited.

The diagnostic formulation should be geared to the case. It does not necessarily need to be tied to a specific diagnosis or differential diagnosis. Diagnoses are usually based on a diagnostic system, either DSM-IV or ICD-10. The liaison psychiatrist may need to keep in mind that referring consultants often have only a limited understanding of psychiatric diagnostic systems.

Some referrals are about difficult situations and here the diagnosis is less relevant. The problem-oriented approach allows the consultant to outline the relevant issues from the assessment that may require attention. A prioritized problem list constructed from a biopsychosocial perspective provides a summary of concerns. These are often best linked with management recommendations, e.g. a patient whose symptoms of fatigue and anorexia are not adequately explained by depression may have further medical review recommended.

Outcomes of assessment

The assessment process can generate many outcomes. Sometimes the referral letter explicitly requests that the liaison psychiatrist take responsibility for initiating management. More frequently, the extent to which the liaison psychiatrist is expected to institute management is unclear and may require direct contact with the referring consultant if there are urgent problems that need addressing. Other outcomes might be to advise on or institute psychopharmacotherapy. Some patients will require psychotherapy. A ward may need guidance to set up a behavioural management programme. The liaison psychiatrist may need to be involved in discharge planning or assisting with appropriate placement. Some patients may require not only transfer to a psychiatric unit but also legal restraint or committal proceedings. In addition, the liaison psychiatrist may have to take an advocacy role for the patient by recognizing and dealing constructively with ageist attitudes accentuated by the patient's mental disorder.

Although, a very time-consuming pursuit, a good geriatric psychiatry liaison assessment can have great benefits for everyone in the system. The patient and their families have the chance to tell their story in detail, to feel heard, and to have their problem treated. The ward or caregiving staff have their issues shared, and the consultant and referring consultant have the opportunity to work together co-operatively and hopefully facilitate mutual respect and understanding between two different systems.

References

Alexopoulos, G.S., Abrams, R.C., Young, R.C., and Shamoian, C.A. (1988). Cornell Scale for depression in dementia. *Biological Psychiatry*, **23**, 271–84.

Allen, N.H.P., Burns, A. (1995). The noncognitive features of dementia. *Reviews in Clinical Gerontology*, **5**, 57–75.

Appelbaum, P.S. and Grisso T. (1988). Assessing patient's capacities to consent to treatment. *New England Journal of Medicine*, **318**, 1635–8.

Beck, A. (1976). *Cognitive therapy and the emotional disorders*. International Universities Press, New York.

Blackburn, I-M. and Davidson, K. (1995). *Cognitive Therapy for Depression and Anxiety. A Practitioner's Guide*. Blackwell Science, Oxford.

Blazer, D.G. (1989). The psychiatric interview of the geriatric patient. In *Geriatric psychiatry* (ed. E.W. Busse and D.G. Blazer), pp. 263–84. American Psychiatric Press, Washington DC.

Brodaty, H. and Moore, C.M. (1997). The clock drawing test for dementia of the Alzheimer's type: a comparison of three scoring methods in a memory disorders clinic. *International Journal of Geriatric Psychiatry*, **12**, 619–27.

Brodaty, H., Luscombe, G., Parker, G., Wilhelm., K., Hickie, I., Austin, M-P., *et al.* (1997). Increased rate of psychosis and psychomotor change in depression with age. *Psychological Medicine*, **27**, 1205–13.

Burke, W.J., Houston, M.J., and Boust, S.J. (1989). Use of the Geriatric Depression Scale in dementia of the Alzheimer's type. *Journal of the American Geriatrics Society*, **37**, 856–60.

Burns, A., Lawlor, B., and Craig, S. (1999). *Assessment scales in old age psychiatry*. Martin Dunitz, London.

Cummings, J.L. and Benson, D.F. (1992). *Dementia: a clinical approach* (2nd edn). Butterworth-Heinemann, Boston.

Draper, B. (1995). Prevention of suicide in old age. *Medical Journal of Australia*, **162**, 533–4.

Folkman and Lazarus (1980).

Folstein, M.F., Folstein, S.E., and McHugh, P.R. (1975). 'Mini Mental State': a practical method for grading the cognitive state of patients for the clinician. *Journal of Psychiatric Research*, **12**, 189–98.

Gallo, J.J., Rabins, P.V., Lyketsos, C.G., Tien, A.Y., and Anthony, J.C. (1997). Depression without sadness: functional outcomes of non-dysphoric depression in later life. *Journal of the American Geriatrics Society*, **45**(5), 570–8.

Garrick, T.R. and Stotland, N.L. (1982). How to write a psychiatric consultation. *American Journal of Psychiatry*, **139**, 849–55.

Goldberg, D.P., and Williams, P. (1988). *A user's guide to the General Health Questionnaire*. Windsor: NFER-Nelson.

Hamilton, M. (1960). A rating scale for depression. *Journal of Neurology, Neurosurgery and Psychiatry*, **23**, 56–62.

Hodkinson, H.M. (1972). Evaluation of a mental test score for assessment of mental impairment in the elderly. *Age and Ageing*, **1**, 233–8.

Inouye, S.K., van Dyck, C.H., Alessi, C.A., Balkin, S., Siegal, A.P., and Horwitz, R.I. (1990). Clarifying confusion: the Confusion Assessment Method. *Annals of Internal Medicine*, **113**, 941–948.

Knauper, B. and Wittchen, H.U. (1994). Diagnosing major depression in the elderly: evidence for response bias in standardized diagnostic reviews? *Journal of Psychiatric Research*, **28**, 147–64.

Lipowski, Z.J. (1990). Somatization and depression. *Psychosomatics*, **31**, 13–21.

McCusker, J., Cole, M., Bellavance, F., and Primeau, F. (1998). Reliability and validity of a new measure of severity of delirium. *International Psychogeriatrics*, **10**, 421–33.

Mahoney, F.I. and Barthel D.W. (1965). Functional evaluation: the BARTHEL index. *Maryland State Medical Journal*, **14**, 61–5.

Molloy, D.W., Alemayehu, E., and Roberts, R. (1991). Reliability of a standardized Mini-Mental State Examination compared with the traditional Mini-Mental State Examination. *American Journal of Psychiatry*, **148**, 102–5.

Molloy, D.W, Darzins, P., and Strang, D. (1999). *Capacity to decide*. Newgrange Press, Troy, Ontario.

Montgomery, S.A. and Åsberg, M. (1979). A new depression scale designed to be sensitive to change. *British Journal of Psychiatry*, **134**, 382–9.

Mungas, D., Weller, P., Franzi, C., and Henry, R. (1989). Assessment of disruptive behaviour associated with dementia: the Disruptive Behaviour Rating Scales. *Journal of Geriatric Psychiatry and Neurology*, **2**, 196–202.

Nowers, M. (1993). Deliberate self-harm in the elderly: a survey of one London borough. *International Journal of Geriatric Psychiatry*, **8**, 609–14.

Pérez, E.L., Silverman, M., and Blouin, J. (1985). Psychiatric consultation to elderly medical and surgical inpatients in a general hospital. *Psychiatric Quarterly*, **57**, 18–22.

Pilowsky, I. (1978). A general classification of abnormal illness behaviours. *British Journal of Medical Psychology*. **51(2)**, 131–137.

Reisberg, B., Borenstein, J., Franssen, E., Salob, S.P., Steinberg, G., Chulman, E., *et al.* (1987). BEHAVE-AD: a clinical rating scale for the assessment of pharmacologically remediable behavioural symptomatology in Alzheimer's disease. In *Alzheimer's disease: problems, prospects and perspectives* (ed. H.J. Altman), pp. 1–16. Plenum Press, New York.

Rodin, G. and Voshart, K. (1986). Depression in the medically ill: an overview. *American Journal of Psychiatry*, **143**, 696–705.

Royall, D.R., Mahurin, R.K., and Gray, K.F. (1993). Bedside assessment of executive cognitive impairment: the executive interview. *Journal of the American Geriatrics Society,* **40**(12), 1221–6.

Ryan, S.P. (1996). Competence and the elderly patient with cognitive impairments. *Australian and New Zealand Journal of Psychiatry*, **30**, 768–73.

Shah, A.K. (1997). Interviewing mentally ill ethnic elders with interpreters. *Australian Journal on Aging*, **16**, 220–1.

Shah, A.K., Dighe-Deo, D., and Chapman, C. (1998). Suicidal ideation among acutely medically ill elderly inpatients. *Ageing and Mental Health*, **2**, 300–5.

Silver, I.L. and Herrmann, N. (1996). Comprehensive psychiatric evaluation. In *Comprehensive review of geriatric psychiatry—II* (2nd edn), (ed. J. Sadavoy, L.W. Lazarus, L.F. Jarvik, and G.T. Grossberg), pp. 223–50. American Psychiatric Press, Washington DC.

Vitaliano, P.P., Russo, J., Carr, J.E., Maiuro, R.D., Becker, J. (1985). The ways of coping checklist: revision and psychometric properties. *Multivariate Behavioural Research*, **20**, 3–26.

Yesavage, J.A., Brink, T.L., Rose, T.L., Lum, O., Huang, V., Adey, M., *et al.* (1983). Development and validity of a geriatric depression screening scale: a preliminary report. *Journal of Psychiatric Research*, **17**, 37–49.

6   Affective disorders

Mavis Evans and Patricia Mottram

Summary

This chapter provides an overview of affective disorders in a general hospital setting. Pertinent diagnostic issues are covered with particular reference to common depressive signs and symptoms. Diagnostic pitfalls are considered, such as the effects of culture, comorbid depression and dementia, depressive pseudodementia, and somatization. The role of depression screening instruments is reviewed. Important management issues are reviewed in the context of the prognosis of depressive disorders. Guidelines for management are provided. The diagnosis and differential diagnosis of manic disorders is examined. Management issues are considered.

Introduction

Depression can adversely affect an older person's subjective rating of their health, which may lead to the increased presentation of somatic complaints at primary-care or emergency medical facilities. Missing a diagnosis of depression may result in unnecessary investigations, increased likelihood of hospital admissions, or even admission to residential care (Evans 1995).

Depression causes increased morbidity and mortality, and may increase the length of hospital stay (Verbosky *et al.* 1993). Psychiatric intervention increases the recovery rate, reduces the duration of stay, and lessens the need for residential care after discharge, thus reducing the overall cost to society (Strain *et al.* 1991). Depression usually responds well to treatment, so improving the quality of life and possibly reducing the mortality rate. Antidepressant treatment is effective, safe even with comorbid physical disease, and cost-effective when compared with the costs of untreated disease (Bruce 1997; Badger 1998). Continuing follow-up to identify and treat any relapses will further improve the prognosis of late-life depression (Baldwin and Jolley 1986; Burvill *et al.* 1991).

Diagnostic issues

While major depression, as defined by DSM-IV or ICD-10, is obviously important to diagnose, psychiatrists in clinical practice tend to recognize a continuum of the severity of symptoms. In the elderly, particularly those with concurrent physical problems, the full criteria for major depression are often not reached. Despite this, psychiatrists will often initiate treatment for elderly patients with significant depression that does not fulfil the strict diagnostic criteria because of the significant morbidity and loss of quality of life caused by the symptoms.

Depressed mood can be secondary to serious physical illness. Furthermore, the biological features of depression may be difficult to distinguish from those of a physical illness or somatization of the depressed mood. A reactive depression or adjustment disorder with depressed mood (DSM-IV) may develop due to the admission itself, in response to a diagnosis such as malignancy, following a disabling stroke, or in fearful anticipation of future residential placement. These situations require appropriate supportive treatment rather than psychotropic medication. Secondary depression occurring in response to an illness or its consequences must be distinguished from a primary depressive illness, sustained over time, which developed before the admission or illness. This latter condition requires the same treatment as that prescribed for the clinically depressed elderly person without physical illness. Therefore, it is important to seek collateral information about the severity of the patient's mood-state before admission.

Problems of adjustment are particularly salient in the management of older people with chronic illness who have slight chance of recovery. However, such an adjustment disorder can progress into a depressive illness that, if diagnosed, will respond to appropriate treatment with improvement in the quality of life for the patient and their carers. Consequently, important aims for clinicians treating elderly people are to minimize disability and pain, slow progression of disease, and enable psychosocial support for the person. It is important to be wary of concepts such as: 'of course they're depressed, they're old and ill'. Patients with secondary adjustment-type depression tend to have less suicidal thoughts but have more feelings of helplessness, pessimism, and anxiety (Lloyd 1985). Features of anxiety can contribute to diagnostic difficulty.

Before making a diagnosis of depressive illness (Table 6.1):

1. Ensure the common physical causes of depressive symptoms have been excluded or optimally treated, for example anaemia, thyroid dysfunction or other endocrine disorders, organ failures, malignancies, neurological disorders, and chronic pain from any cause.

2. Check the medication. The elderly are likely to be on multiple medications. Some, for example beta-blockers, digoxin, or major tranquillizers, are central nervous system depressants. Drug interactions may also cause problems. Discussion with a pharmacist is always valuable.

3. Do not forget that alcohol is also a depressant, and unless specifically questioned many elderly patients will not consider their regular 'nightcap' worthy of mention. Alcohol abuse or dependence is not uncommon in the elderly population.

Signs and symptoms of depression

Depression and dysphoria

Depressed mood or sadness are not always easily identified. Some patients deny such feelings when questioned, whereas complaints of not coping, anxiety, or irritability are more frequent (Shulman 1989). Such patients may complain of the biological features of depression, e.g. sleep, appetite disturbances, or loss of energy. However, they will usually acknowledge a loss of interest or pleasure in their daily activities if questioned. Examples of such questions are: ' Is there anything you enjoy?' and 'Is there anything you look forward to?' Depressed mood is not an absolute requirement for the diagnosis of depressive illness in either DSM-IV or ICD-10 so additional criteria are required. It cannot be emphasized too often that elderly patients can be severely depressed in the absence of overt depressed mood.

Crying

This is rare, particularly in men, in the current cohort of elderly people who have been brought up not to show their feelings. Crying may therefore point to a deep depression where the patient no longer cares how others perceive them. However, crying may also point to associated lability of mood resulting from cerebral ischaemia and be a false symptom of depression.

Anxiety/agitation

Some degree of associated anxiety or irritability occurs in the majority of depressed elderly patients, often associated with low self-esteem and decreased ability to cope.

Sleep disturbance and diurnal variation

Early morning wakening is often present in the depressed elderly patient but may be rationalized into, 'I don't need as much sleep as I used to'. Patients may attribute sleep disturbance to problems in reinitiating sleep after going to the toilet, or being woken by ward activities or other patients whilst in hospital. Patients who sleep during the day may only require a short sleep at night. A full sleep history should identify these problems. There is no required amount of sleep for elderly people, some genuinely do seem to cope well with 4–5 hours per day, whilst others, particu-

Table 6.1 Links between depression and physical illness

1. Physical illness causing depression
- Direct cause, e.g. malignancies, especially head of pancreas and oat-cell carcinoma of the lung
- Effect of pain or disability, initially starting as adjustment disorder
- Loss of health, independence, ultimately life itself. Can be hypothesized as a bereavement reaction
- Fear of loss of independence or dignity; of becoming a 'burden' on loved ones, financial or otherwise; of the mode of dying
- The sick role as a means of coping with life stress, often a lifelong mechanism

2. Depression causing physical illness
- Poor nutrition or reduced mobility leading to poor physical health
- Delayed recovery may result in longer hospital admissions and transfer to residential care
- Medication non-compliance or non-attendance for outpatient clinics or investigations, causing worsening of the physical problem
- Depression increases mortality of the associated physical disease[a]

3. Effect of somatic medication on mood
- Drugs that depress mood, e.g. β-blockers, digoxin, major tranquillizers, cimetidine, chemotherapy, etc.
- Mood altering, e.g. steroids
- Sedating, e.g. antihistamines, antiemetics, analgesics, causing difficulty in coping with ADLs, increasing stress, and precipitating depressed mood
- Unpleasant side-effects, e.g. chemotherapy producing persistent nausea and anergia, can lead to secondary depression

4. Effect of psychotropic medication on physical state
- Falls due to postural hypotension and dystonias
- Dry mouth leading to soreness under dentures, difficulty eating a balanced diet
- Blurred vision causing problems with reading instructions on prescriptions or for food preparation, etc.
- Sedation causing difficulty in coping with everyday living
- Nausea and other gastrointestinal upset leading to poor diet
- Acute confusional states can be precipitated, especially with TCAs in those with existing cognitive problems
- Risk of drug interactions, e.g. fluoxetine and diuretics causing hyponatraemia

5. Common aetiological factor
- Bereavement
- Medication, for example steroids can cause depression and increased risk of GI bleeds

6. Coincidental
- Depression is common—over 10% prevalence among those over 65 years living in the community; physical illness is found in up to 40%, minor problems (e.g. non-symptomatic arthritis) are virtually pervasive

7. Acute severe illness causing resolution of depression
- Acute severe physical illnesses may lead to resolution of depression[b]

[a]Evans *et al.* 1999; [b]Deahl 1990.
ADL, activities of daily living; GI, gastrointestinal.

larly if physically ill, may sleep during both the day and night. It is useful to enquire if the patient feels mentally refreshed on waking at whatever time in the mornings. Do they waken ready to face the day, enjoying a time of quiet before others also wake, or is this a lonely unpleasant time, full of fears of the future and desire to return to the oblivion of sleep? The initial insomnia or restlessness of associated anxiety may cause fatigue and further difficulties in coping with activities of daily living.

Appetite changes

A change in appetite and weight is a cardinal symptom of depression (Spitzer *et al.* 1978), and is also symptomatic of many physical diseases. If a physical cause that could explain the anorexia, such as malignant disease or organ failures, is not *easily* detected, depression should be considered in the differential diagnosis. Recognition and successful treatment of a masked depression may avoid the use of invasive investigations such as gastroscopy or barium studies (Evans 1995). Increased appetite and weight gain occasionally occur in physically ill elderly people. Some patients indulge in 'comfort eating' in response to feeling depressed, with its importance as a symptom of mood disorder being unrecognized by the patient or physician.

Low energy

Complaints of tiredness are common. These complaints may be due to physical disease or to sleep disturbance rather than depression. Alternatively, symptoms wrongly identified as depressive may mask underlying physical problems. Correct attribution of fatigue to a physical rather than a psychiatric cause requires a value judgement by the clinician as to how much fatigue could be associated with any physical problem. The concept of 'enough energy to do what you want to do' implies acceptance of physical problems and associated limitation of activity. In contrast, the elderly person who fails to come to terms with the limitations of their physical illness will often complain of low energy. This association is possibly a reason for the correlation of low energy with depression in the physically ill elderly (Evans 1996).

Social isolation

An elderly depressed person may be unwelcoming or irritable to visitors. They may refuse to join in social conversations on the ward, stay by their bed rather than go into the day room, or turn their back on social contact, often physically as well as metaphorically. Although the social isolation may be 'self-inflicted', the elderly depressed patient will view it subjectively as further 'proof' of being unwanted or a burden on others, thus perpetuating depressive ideation. This social isolation is not that of a housebound patient, who may still receive visitors or make telephone calls.

Nor is it the same as the isolation due to sensory difficulties, especially poor hearing or other causes such as culturally appropriate behaviour or language problems. The self-imposed isolation of depression is different to these socioenvironmental circumstances. Irritability may disrupt or strain relationships so that necessary help is withdrawn. Importuning behaviour can estrange relatives and neighbours who withdraw all assistance when they feel the demands are becoming too heavy. Conversely, a sense of worthlessness or feelings of 'being a nuisance' or 'a burden to others' may lead to a failure to request help, and the need denied by the patient or unrecognized by carers (Evans and Mottram 2000).

Physical retardation

Thyroid function tests must be investigated to eliminate a physical cause of retardation before making a diagnosis of depression. In people with severe retarded depression, slowing of movements and thoughts can lead to increased difficulty coping with the activities of daily living, poor or no diet, and ultimately cessation of eating and drinking. Reduced mobility can progress to no movement at all, leading to the development of pressure sores. The condition when severe is life-threatening. Clinicians may prescribe ECT (electroconvulsive therapy) in this situation, as speed of response is essential when retardation is severe.

Cognitive deficits

Depression in older people can cause cognitive deficits. Deficits in language and memory processing are relatively common, but are often not explainable just by retardation or lack of motivation; moreover, they are not always fully reversible with treatment (Katona 1994). Poor concentration and attention associated with depression can lead to faulty registration of memory or difficulty in recall. A depressed patient with memory problems will often improve with cues, as the memory problem is one of accessing rather than loss of information (Kindermann and Brown 1997). Treatment with tricyclic antidepressants (TCAs) can make memory deficits worse and even precipitate acute confusion due to the centrally acting, anticholinergic side-effects of this class of drug (Moscowitz and Burns 1986). Sometimes, the cognitive deficits in the depressed older person are severe enough to be pseudodementia (see below).

Whether depression is a prodromal feature of dementia, an aetiological factor causing cognitive impairment (perhaps through raised cortisol levels), or if the dementing process is causing depression, the clinician should be aware of the close links between these conditions in the elderly (Roose and Devanand 1999).

Suicidal ideas

Feelings of life not being worth living and wishing to die can sometimes occur in the absence of depressed mood (Jorm *et al.* 1995). They should always be taken seriously. In the study, by Jorm *et al.* (1995) other factors linked with the wish to die included not being married, poor subjective health, disability, pain, sensory impairment, and living in a nursing home or hostel. These factors are also common in the development of depressive illness. Fleeting suicidal thoughts, or the wish not to waken from sleep, are common in the elderly, especially those who are physically ill or disabled. Completed suicide is not rare—age and physical disease are risk factors. Recorded suicides are probably an underestimate. Not all suicidal activity in the elderly is obvious, for example non-compliance with medication such as digoxin or steroids, necessary for treatment of their physical conditions, can lead to death from 'natural causes'.

Behavioural disturbances

Many forms of behavioural disturbance are seen—from irritability and even aggression towards relatives and carers, histrionic importuning or screaming, to staged falls that appear to be a plea for attention. Low self-esteem, energy, and motivation can lead to poor personal hygiene, and the development of urinary and faecal incontinence.

Diagnostic pitfalls

Cultural context

When the patient is from a different ethnic group than the clinicians, signs and symptoms must be seen in the context of that person's cultural context. Different cultures, religions, and social groupings can have unique ways of expressing distress. Relatives and carers are the best source of information about the patient's social norms. Ignoring sociocultural differences, such as the social isolation from strangers of a devout Moslem woman, or the belief in witchcraft in someone of African origins, can lead to a mis- or missed diagnosis.

Depression and dementia

Community studies show that depression is much more common than dementia (more than 10% over 65 years of age compared with 5% over 65 years, respectively) (Copeland *et al.* 1987), but both are common conditions and so may occur in the same patient coincidentally.

Depression may be the presenting feature of a dementia, particularly Alzheimer's disease, occurring as much as 2 years before diagnosis (Jost and Grossberg 1996). Such depression is often resistant to treatment and a cognitive deficit is usually present, although initially mild. In a community study of depression with cognitive impairment, patients had nearly a threefold increased risk of developing dementia, mostly Alzheimer's disease (Devanand *et al.* 1996). A similar follow-up of inpatients with severe depression, comparing those with and without cognitive impairment, showed a fivefold increased risk of dementia during a 3-year follow-up, regardless of the amount of initial improvement in cognition with treatment of the depression (Alexopoulos *et al.* 1993).

Low mood is also common in the early stages of any dementia where there is some preserved insight, and has established links with cerebrovascular disease (Starkstein and Robinson 1989). Wragg and Jeste's (1989) review of the literature reported that depressed mood was present in 40% of patients with Alzheimer's disease, with 20% of patients meeting the criteria for a diagnosis of depressive illness.

Depressive pseudodementia

The condition of pseudodementia is a severe, melancholic, depressive illness that presents with impaired concentration, poor memory, retardation, and decreased function in activities of daily living. Missing the diagnosis of pseudodementia leads to increased morbidity, mortality, and possibly necessitates residential placement with permanent loss of a person's previous home and independence. In contrast, recovery of normal function can result from effective treatment.

An important factor in differentiating pseudodementia from dementia is that the severity of cognitive impairment tends to fluctuate in depressed patients, remaining constant or worsening in the evenings in demented patients. Memory loss in the depressed patient is pervasive, recent and remote events are forgotten, and there is marked variation of performance on tasks of similar difficulty. The patient often gives up with 'I don't know' or 'I can't' responses. Demented patients will try, using memory prompts such as lists and calendars, but they can become very distressed by failure. Biological symptoms of appetite and weight loss, diurnal variation, sleep disturbance, and headache are more typical of depression rather than dementia. The patient with pseudodementia often has a previous history of depression. A stressful life event, such as bereavement, onset of a new physical problem, moving to a smaller house or into care, is often the precipitant (Baldwin 1999).

With recognition and treatment of the depression, the cognitive deficit is at least partially reversible. However, an 8-year follow-up (Kral and Emery 1989) of 44 patients with pseudodementia found that 39 of them had developed Alzheimer's disease during the study period. This study indicates that the long-term prognosis for a patient with depressive pseudodementia is poor and that there seems to be an increased risk of eventually developing irreversible dementia.

Somatization

Somatization as a concept is becoming increasingly recognized. Lipowski (1988) defined somatization as: 'The tendency to experience and communicate somatic distress and somatic symptoms unaccounted for by relevant pathological findings, to attribute them to physical illness, and to seek medical help for them'. Unnecessary investigations and unwanted treatment side-effects can lead to iatrogenic disease. In addition, the underlying and undiagnosed depressive illness may become chronic (Unutzer *et al.* 1997).

There is an unfortunate tendency among some health professionals to attribute 'difficult to diagnose' symptoms, or physical symptoms in those patients known to have a psychiatric diagnosis, to somatization (see Chapter 8). Yet, routine screening of psychiatric referrals may find severe anaemia, thyroid disorders, and malignancies. In a series of 100 depressed elderly people, 46% had a comorbid physical diagnosis (Sweer *et al.* 1988).

Hypochondriasis

Hypochondriasis is commonly associated with both depression and anxiety disorders in the elderly population. It differs from somatization in the active seeking of medical investigations and reassurance for normal bodily sensations. It may be part of a lifelong maladaptive behaviour. However, in the elderly, genuine physical problems must be excluded before diagnosing hypochondriasis or somatization. Unfortunately, such investigations can confirm the hypochondriacal fears of the patient. That such patients are depressed is inferred from their good response to standard treatments for depression (Jacoby 1981).

Stigma of diagnosis

Elderly patients may actively deny depressed mood due to perceived stigma ('I've nothing to worry about', 'There's nothing to upset me') both of the depression itself and of the need for help with psychiatric problems ('I'm not mental'). The patient perceives the biological features such as poor appetite or disturbed sleep as acceptable reasons to request help. The elderly are more likely to seek help from physicians rather than from services and professionals with explicit mental health labels (Bruce 1997). This highlights the need for primary-care and general hospital physicians to be familiar with the spectrum of depressive symptoms.

Is there a place for screening scales in the assessment of depression?

Screening scales are of most use when there is a risk of missing a disorder. It is cost-effective to use scales if the condition is:

◆ relatively rare but has serious consequences if missed;

◆ common but has an appreciable degree of morbidity.

Screening scales are more useful if a treatment is available, as there is little point encouraging staff to identify a condition if there is no treatment. Effective treatment and an improvement in the patients identified by such instruments gives positive feedback to staff that encourages further use of case-finding scales. In medical wards, as staff are usually unfamiliar with psychiatric symptoms, may not know how to weight particular symptoms, or they may have difficulty eliciting sensitive information such as suicidal thoughts or plans, they may finding case-finding scales especially useful.

Both the 15-item Geriatric Depression Scale (GDS) (Sheik and Yesavage 1986) and the 15-item Evans Liverpool Depression Rating Scale (ELDRS) (Evans 1993*a*) have been validated in the physically ill and frail elderly. The GDS may be difficult to use in the hospital setting. Questions such as, 'Do you think it is wonderful to be alive right now?' can be inappropriate to ask someone after, for example, a disabling stroke. The ELDRS was initially developed for use on geriatric medical wards. contains five items designed to identify associated features such as isolation, sleep disturbance, and irritability, thus aiding diagnosis in patients who are consciously or subconsciously denying problems. The carer or primary nurse answers these questions.

If the general hospital staff is to undertake a screening programme, support for identified patients and the staff involved must be easily obtainable. Scales, whilst helpful, are only part of the liaison process. Training in treatment strategies must occur first.

Prognosis and treatment of depression in elderly, medically ill patients

Depressed older patients use more hospital inpatient and outpatient services and have greater medical costs, but do not receive more mental health services (Koenig *et al.* 1989; Koenig and Kuchibhatla 1998; Druss *et al.* 1999). Many older people with depression do not need to be treated by a psychiatrist; indeed a 20–30% prevalence of depression on medical wards would overwhelm the majority of services. In theory, a physician could treat many patients with depression quite appropriately. However, a substantial number of depressed patients are undiagnosed, misdiagnosed, or untreated (Koenig *et al.* 1992, 1997*a*; Jackson and Baldwin 1993; Crawford *et al.* 1998).

Failure to treat depression is not entirely the fault of the physician. Patients who believe that their depressive symptoms are secondary to their physical condition may refuse treatment, and are more likely to 'give up' and request euthanasia (Koenig and Breitner 1990; Knauper and Wittchen 1994; Hooper *et al.* 1996). This may contribute to 'do not resuscitate' orders being given, sometimes at the request of families (Wasserman 1989; Philpott 1990). The assessment of depression as a normal psychological reaction to the illness does not mean that treatment is unnecessary. Yet, the evidence suggests that often this is the result. Even when treatment is provided, sub-therapeutic doses of the less appropriate antidepressant agents, such as tertiary amine tricyclic antidepressants (TCAs), are common (Koenig *et al*. 1997*a*).

All the above reasons contribute to the poor prognosis for depression in elderly medical inpatients. A retrospective audit of the outcome of antidepressant therapy in medical wards found a response rate of around 40% (Popkin *et al*. 1985). Cole and Bellavance (1997) performed a meta-analysis of the naturalistic outcomes of depression in eight studies of elderly medical inpatients. At 3 months or less, 18% of patients were well, 43% were depressed, 22% were 'other' diagnoses (e.g. dementia) and 22% were dead. At 12 months or more 19% were well, 29% were depressed, and 53% were dead. Patients with poorer outcomes had deeper depression, physical illness that was more serious, and pre-admission symptoms of depression. In contrast, the study that reported the best outcomes was one in which all depressed patients were treated and followed up by the investigator (Evans 1993*b*).

Guidelines for the management of depression

The optimal management of depression includes strategies to improve case identification, diagnostic accuracy, and the use of appropriate treatments (Table 6.2). Details of the use of antidepressant drugs, ECT, and non-pharmacological strategies are covered in Chapters 12, 13, and 14.

As the average length of stay in medical wards is less than 2 weeks, most depressed patients are likely to be discharged before they respond to treatment. Therapy needs to continue for at least 8–12 weeks before reviewing efficacy, as a response in elderly people can be slow (Georgotas and McCue 1989). Thus, it is imperative that appropriate follow-up is arranged. For some this will necessitate transfer to a geriatric psychiatry ward, particularly for those with severe depression. For patients well enough for discharge, follow-up could be through a specialist ambulatory clinic, community geriatric psychiatry service, or primary care, although the latter may be best reserved for those patients who have already achieved a good response. The extent to which the poor prognosis of depressed, physically ill, hospitalized patients may relate to inadequate follow-up is unknown. An assertive approach to community follow-up is worthwhile, with appointments arranged by the geriatric liaison service and review mechanisms in place to limit the possibility of missed appointments. Patients need monitoring for at least 6 months following remission, and maintenance antidepressants to be continued in high enough doses to prevent relapse.

Case study 6.1

Mrs J., an 83-year old widow with a history of severe osteoarthritis and congestive cardiac failure, collapsed at home and was admitted to hospital. She had a urinary tract infection (UTI) but, despite responding to antibiotic treatment, she remained listless, withdrawn, and unmotivated. Depression precipitated by the UTI was suspected and she was referred to the liaison psychiatrist. This assessment revealed that Mrs J. had experienced symptoms of major depression with prominent self-neglect, anorexia, weight loss, and social withdrawal over the previous 3 months. She had worried excessively about her ability to live independently with the worsening of her arthritis, and this appeared to have precipitated the depression. A combination of antidepressant therapy, supportive psycho-therapy, rehabilitation, and the arrangement of appropriate community services allowed Mrs J. to successfully return home.

Many of these patients have a poor prognosis for their physical conditions, and significant fluctuations in health status may adversely affect their mood state (Geerlings *et al.* 2000). So, irrespective of the intensity of follow-up, incomplete remissions and relapses are likely to occur, sometimes in association with readmission to medical wards.

Bipolar affective disorder and mania

The features of mania in the elderly are the same as those seen in younger patients, such as irritable mood or euphoria, rapid and voluble speech. Flight of ideas and pressure of speech also occur occasionally. Disturbed behaviour occurs with over-spending, social and sexual disinhibition, hyperactivity, and belligerence towards family and/or others. Persecutory ideas, delusions and grandiosity, or religiosity are characteristic. Unpredictable changes in appetite and libido are common, as is the reduced sleep with activity rather than the lying awake found in depression.

Diagnosis is not difficult, but mania can be mistaken on hospital wards for delirium. In a study by Broadhead and Jacoby (1990) 35 young (under 40 years of age) and 35 old (more than 60 years) patients were assessed using the Modified Mania Rating Scale (Blackburn *et al.* 1977), no major differences were found between the presentation of the two groups. The incidence of depressive symptoms was no higher in the older group, but they were more likely to develop a depressive illness after recovery from the manic episode.

Late-onset bipolar illness is associated with a lower rate of familial illness than the early-onset form and greater medical and neurological comorbidity (Young 1997). An association of mania and physical illness in old age has been repeatedly described in the literature (Shulman and Post 1980; Robinson *et al.* 1988; Chawla and Lindesay 1993; Young 1997; Cassidy *et al.* 1999). Medical treatments have also been associated with manic episodes—hormone replacement therapy (Young *et al.* 1997), following surgery using lidocaine (lignocaine) (Clark and Clunie 1996), anti-depressant medication or its withdrawal (Boerlin *et al.* 1998). Other drugs cited include steroids, painkillers, and antibiotics.

Management of manic episodes

Acute management of manic elderly patients often requires admission to hospital unless strong family support is available. Neuroleptics, lithium, carbamazepine, or

6.2(a) Management strategies for late-life depression—identification

Strategy	Rationale	Caveats
Encourage the routine use of depression screening instruments (e.g. Geriatric Depression Scale-15, Evans Liverpool Depression Rating Scale) in geriatric medical wards	Evidence of increased recognition, treatment, and appropriate referral of depressed elderly patients when used[a]	False-negatives may occur when patients are uncooperative, somatasize, or are very withdrawn[b]
Provide education about depression in the elderly to all health professionals on medical wards, e.g. in liaison ward rounds	Better knowledge of depression may increase recognition, treatment, and appropriate referral of depressed elderly patients[c]	Educational sessions need to be repeated regularly due to staff turnover and decay of learnt information

[a]Shah and De 1998; [b]Rodin and Voshart 1986; [c]Anderson and Philpott 1991

Table 6.2(b) Management strategies for late-life depression—diagnosis

Strategy	Rationale	Caveats
Ensure the common physical causes of depressive symptoms have been excluded or optimally treated	Depressive symptoms secondary to general medical conditions often spontaneously resolve when the illness is treated[a]	All these patients still require psychological support, some may eventually require antidepressant drugs
Use diagnostic criteria that include physiological symptoms such as anorexia, fatigue, or insomnia unless fully accounted for by the medical condition	Criteria that exclude all physiological symptoms in the physically ill result in the underdiagnosis of depression[b]	False-positive diagnoses may occur. Depression is less likely when the patient is capable of appreciating humour, responds warmly to affection, and shows an active interest in life around them
Identify depression comorbid with cognitive impairment	Successful treatment may reduce disability and suffering	Diagnosis of depression in dementia is difficult with much symptom overlap, treatment response may be limited[c]

[a]Katz 1993; [b]Koenig et al. 1997b; [c]Draper 1999

Table 6.2(c) Management strategies for late-life depression—treatment

Strategy	Rationale	Caveats
Determine whether onset of depression occurred pre- or postadmission	Depressions associated with acute illnesses have a high rate of spontaneous recovery, those with onset prior to admission are more likely to require formal treatment[a]	Some depressions with onset in hospital will require antidepressants, particularly if more severe. All cases should be monitored for at least a week to determine whether formal treatment is required
Determine if patient has major depression, particularly whether psychotic or melancholic features are present	Such patients usually benefit from physical treatments, either antidepressants or ECT[b]	Patients with major depression of lesser severity may respond to non-pharmacological therapies. All patients require psychological support
Use a shorter half-life SSRI as first-choice antidepressant	In general, SSRI antidepressants are better tolerated, safer, and as effective as TCAs. Shorter half-life drugs more suited to the elderly	SSRIs may not be as effective as TCAs in severe depression and physically ill. The elderly are prone to adverse effects such as hyponatraemia, falls, and agitation
Use a non-pharmacological therapy for less severe depressions	Therapies such as CBT, IPT, and exercise may be as effective as antidepressants and avoid adverse drug effects	Only limited evidence of efficacy in physically ill elderly. Some patients are not suited for these treatments. Few therapists are available in most centres[c]
Ensure adequate postdischarge follow-up of patient	Many patients are discharged before treatment response. Adequate treatment of a depressive episode is a minimum of 6 months duration[b]	Follow-up may be provided by primary care, but there is a high risk of dropout without an assertive approach

[a]Draper 2000; [b]Chiu et al. 1999; [c]Menting et al. 1996

ECT, electroconvulsive therapy; SSRI, selective serotonin-reuptake inhibitors; TCA, tricyclic antidepressants; CBT, cognitive–behavioural therapy; IPT, interpersonal psychotherapy.

valproate are all possible treatments. The average response rate to these treatments is only approximately 50–70% (Grunze *et al.* 1999). The treatment of mania often involves a number of trials of different pharmaceutical therapies until the patient's mood state is sufficiently stable. Rare patients that have failed to respond to pharmacotherapy can be treated with ECT. A meta-analysis by Mukherjee *et al.* (1994) found that 80% of the 589 patients responded well to ECT. Prospectively, the same authors found a 60% response rate. It is worth bearing in mind that very few trials of the newer mood-stabilizing drugs (carbamazepine and sodium valproate) or the ECT studies cited by Mukherjee *et al.* (1994) have involved elderly patients. Clinical trials of a combination of antidepressants and a mood stabilizer or mood stabilizer as sole treatment, in mild cases, are also lacking.

Lithium carbonate is the most commonly used prophylaxis treatment for bipolar affective disorder in the elderly, once again very little evidence is available about its use in older people. When lithium is used as a long-term treatment, the willingness and capacity of the patient to adhere strictly to a potentially dangerous medication needs consideration. Regular blood tests and clinical assessment are a necessity.

More detailed description of the pharmacotherapy of mania can be found in Chapter 12.

References

Alexopoulos, G.S., Young, R.C., and Meyers, B.S. (1993). Geriatric depression: age of onset and dementia. *Biological Psychiatry*, **34**, 141–5.

Anderson, D.N. and Philpott, R.M. (1991). The changing pattern of referrals for psychogeriatric consultation in the general hospital: an eight-year study. *International Journal of Geriatric Psychiatry*, **6**, 801–7.

Badger, T.A. (1998). Depression, physical health impairment and service use among older adults. *Public Health Nursing*, **15**, 136–45.

Baldwin, R.C. (1999). Aetiology of late life depression. *Advances in Psychiatric Treatment*, **5**, 435–42.

Baldwin, R.C. and Jolley, D.J. (1986). The prognosis of depression in old age. *British Journal of Psychiatry* ,**149**, 574–83.

Blackburn, I.M., London, J.B., and Ashworth, C.M. (1977). A new scale for measuring mania. *Psychological Medicine*, **7**, 453–8.

Boerlin, H.L., Gitlin, M.J., Zoeliner, L.A., and Hammen, C.L. (1998). Bipolar depression and antidepressant-induced mania: a naturalistic study. *Journal of Clinical Psychiatry*, **59**, 374–9.

Broadhead, J. and Jacoby, R.J. (1990). Mania in old age—a first prospective study. *International Journal of Geriatric Psychiatry*, **5**, 215–22.

Bruce, M.L. (1997). The costs of depression in late life. *Balance (AMHCA)*, Oct/Nov, 28–30.

Burvill, P.W., Hall, W.D., Stampfer, H.G., and Emmerson, J.P. (1991). The prognosis of depression in old age. *British Journal of Psychiatry*, **158**, 64–71.

Cassidy, F., Ahearn, E., and Carroll, B.J. (1999). Elevated frequency of diabetes mellitus in hospitalized manic-depressive patients. *American Journal of Psychiatry*, **156**, 1417–20.

Chawla, M. and Lindesay, J. (1993). Polycythaemia, delirium and mania. *British Journal of Psychiatry*, **162**, 833–5.

Chiu, E., Ames, D., Draper, B., and Snowdon, J. (1999). Depressive disorders in the elderly: a review. In *Depressive disorders, WPA Series—Evidence and experience in psychiatry*, Vol. 1 (ed. M. Maj and N. Sartorius), pp. 313–63. John Wiley, Chichester.

Clark, J.E. and Clunie, F. (1996). Secondary mania occurring twice in an elderly patient following surgery carried out under local anaesthesia. *Journal of Drug Development and Clinical Practice*, **8**, 49–52.

Cole, M.G. and Bellavance, F. (1997). Depression in elderly medical inpatients: a meta-analysis of outcomes. *Canadian Medical Association Journal*, **157**, 1055–60.

Copeland, J.R.M., Dewey, M.E., Wood, N., Searle, R., Davidson, I.A., and McWilliam, C. (1987). Range of mental illness among the elderly in the community: prevalence in Liverpool using the GMS-AGECAT package. *British Journal of Psychiatry*, **150**, 815–23.

Crawford, M.J., Prince, M., Menezes, P., and Mann, A.H. (1998). The recognition and treatment of depression in older people in primary care. *International Journal of Geriatric Psychiatry*, **13**, 172–6.

Deahl, M.P. (1990). Physical illness and depression: the effects of acute physical illness on the mental state of psychiatric inpatients. *Acta Psychiatrica Scandinavica*, **81**, 83–6.

Devanand, D.P., Sano, M., Tang, M.X., Taylor, S., Gurland, B.J., Wilder, D., Stern, Y., *et al.* (1996). Depressed mood and the incidence of Alzheimer's disease in the elderly living in the community. *Archives of General Psychiatry*, **53**, 175–82.

Draper, B. (1999). The diagnosis and treatment of depression in dementia. *Psychiatric Services*, **50**, 1151–3.

Draper, B.M. (2000). The effectiveness of the treatment of depression in the physically ill elderly. *Aging and Mental Health*, **4**, 9–20.

Druss, B.G., Rohrbaugh, R.M., and Rosenheck, R.A. (1999). Depressive symptoms and health costs in older medical patients. *American Journal of Psychiatry*, **156**, 477–9.

Evans, D.L., Staab, J.P., Petitto, J.M. , Morrison, M.F., Szuba, M.P., Ward, H.E., *et al.* (1999). Depression in the medical setting: biopsychological interactions and treatment considerations. *Journal of Clinical Psychiatry.* **60** (Suppl. 4), 40–56.

Evans, M.E. (1993*a*). Development and validation of a screening test for depression in the elderly physically ill. *International Clinical Psychopharmacology*, **8**, 329–31.

Evans, M.E. (1993*b*). Depression in elderly physically ill inpatients: a 12 month prospective study. *International Journal of Geriatric Psychiatry*, **8**, 587–92.

Evans, M.E. (1995). Detection and management of depression in the elderly physically ill patient. *Human Psychopharmacology*, **10**, S235–S241.

Evans, M.E. (1996). *Development of a screening test for depression in the elderly frail or physically ill*. MD thesis, Liverpool University, UK.

Evans, M.E. and Mottram, P.G. (2000). Diagnosis of depression in elderly patients. *Advances in Psychiatric Treatment*, **6**, 49–56.

Geerlings, S.W., Beekman, A.T., Deeg, D.J., and Van Tilburg, W. (2000). Physical health and the onset and persistence of depression in older adults: an eight-wave prospective community-based study. *Psychological Medicine*, **30**, 369–80.

Georgotas, A. and McCue, R. (1989). The additional benefit of extending an antidepressant trial past seven weeks in the depressed elderly. *International Journal of Geriatric Psychiatry*, **4**, 191–5.

Grunze, H., Erfurth, A., Schafer, M., Amann, B., and Meyendorf, R. (1999). Electroconvulsive therapy in the treatment of severe mania. Case report and a state-of-art review. *Nervenarzt*, **70**, 662–7.

Hooper, S.C., Vaughan, K.J., Tennant, C.C., and Perz, J.M. (1996). Major depression and refusal of life-sustaining medical treatment in the elderly. *Medical Journal of Australia*, **165**, 416–19.

Jackson, R. and Baldwin, B. (1993). Detecting depression in elderly medically ill patients: the use of the Geriatric Depression Scale compared with medical and nursing observations. *Age and Ageing*, **22**, 349–53.

Jacoby, R.J. (1981). Depression in the elderly. *British Journal of Hospital Medicine*, **25**, 40–7.

Jorm, A.F., Henderson, A.S., Scott, R., Korten, A.E., Chritensen, H., and Machinnon, A.J (1995). Factors associated with the wish to die in elderly people. *Age and Ageing*, **24**, 389–92.

Jost, B.C. and Grossberg, G.T. (1996). The evolution of psychiatric symptoms in Alzheimer's disease: a natural history study. *Journal of the American Geriatrics Society*, **44**, 1078–81.

Katona, C.L.E. (1994). *Depression in Old Age* (pp. 65–79). Wiley, Chichester.

Katz, I.R. (1993). Drug treatment of depression in the frail elderly: discussion of the NIH Consensus Development Conference on the diagnosis and treatment of depression in late life. *Psychopharmacology Bulletin*, **29**, 101–8.

Kindermann, S.S. and Brown, G.G. (1997). Depression and memory in the elderly: a meta-analysis. *Journal of Clinical and Experimental Neuropsychology*, **19**, 625–42.

Knauper, B. and Wittchen, H.U. (1994). Diagnosing major depression in the elderly: evidence for response bias in standardized diagnostic reviews? *Journal of Psychiatric Research*, **28**, 147–64.

Koenig, H.G. and Breitner, J.C.S. (1990). Use of antidepressants in medically ill older patients. *Psychosomatics*, **31**, 22–32.

Koenig, H.G. and Kuchibhatla, M. (1998). Use of health services by hospitalized medically ill depressed elderly patients. *American Journal of Psychiatry*, **155**, 871–7.

Koenig, H.G., Goli, V., Shelp, F., Kudler, H.S., Cohen, H.J., Meador, K.G., and Blazer, D.G. (1989). Antidepressant use in elderly medical inpatients: lessons from an attempted clinical trial. *Journal General Internal Medicine*, **4**, 498–505.

Koenig, H.G., Goli, V., Shelp, F., Kudler, H.S., Cohen, H.J., and Blazer, D.G. (1992). Major depression in hospitalized medically ill older men: documentation, management, and outcome. *International Journal of Geriatric Psychiatry*, **7**, 25–34.

Koenig, H.G., George, L.K., and Meador, K.G. (1997*a*). Use of antidepressants by nonpsychiatrists in the treatment of medically ill hospitalized depressed elderly patients. *American Journal of Psychiatry*, **154**, 1369–75.

Koenig, H.G., George, L.K., Peterson, B.L., and Pieper, C.F. (1997*b*). Depression in medically ill hospitalized older adults: prevalence, characteristics, and course of symptoms according to six diagnostic schemes. *American Journal of Psychiatry*, **154**, 1376–83.

Kral, V.A. and Emery O.B. (1989). Long term follow-up of depressive pseudodementia of the aged. *Canadian Journal of Psychiatry*, **34**, 445–6.

Lipowski, Z.J. (1988). Somatisation: the concept and its clinical applications. *American Journal of Psychiatry*, **145**, 1358–68.

Lloyd, G.G. (1985). Emotional aspects of physical illness. In *Recent advances in clinical psychiatry*, **5** (ed. R. Granville-Grossman), pp. 63–85. Churchill Livingstone, London.

Menting, J.E., Honig, A., Verhey, F.R., Hartmans, M., Rozendaal, N., de Vet, H.C., *et al.* (1996). Selective serotonin reuptake inhibitors (SSRIs) in the treatment of elderly depressed patients: a qualitative analysis of the literature on their efficacy and side-effects. *International Clinical Psychopharmacology*, **11**, 165–75.

Moscowitz, H. and Burns, M.M. (1986). Cognitive performance in geriatric subjects after acute treatment with antidepressants. *Neuropsychobiology*, **15**(Suppl. 1), 38–43.

Mukherjee, S., Sackheim, H.A., and Schnur, D.B. (1994). Electroconvulsive therapy for acute manic episodes: a review of 50 years experience. *American Journal of Psychiatry*, **151**, 169–76.

Philpott, R.M. (1990). Affective disorder and physical illness in old age. *International Clinical Psychopharmacology*, **5**(Suppl. 3), 7–20.

Popkin, M.K., Callies, A.L., and Mackenzie, T.B. (1985). The outcome of antidepressant use in the medically ill. *Archives of General Psychiatry*, **42**, 1160–3.

Robinson, R.G., Boston, J.D., Starkstein, S.E., and Price, T.R. (1988). Comparisons of mania and depression after brain injury: causal factors. *American Journal of Psychiatry*, **145**, 172–8.

Rodin, G. and Voshart, K. (1986). Depression in the medically ill: an overview. *American Journal of Psychiatry*, **143**, 696–705.

Roose, S.P. and Devanand, D.P. (1999). *The interface between dementia and depression* (pp. 19–21). Martin Dunitz, London.

Shah, A. and De, T. (1998). Documented evidence of depression in medical and nursing case-notes and its implications in acutely ill geriatric inpatients. *International Psychogeriatrics*, **10**, 163–72.

Sheikh, J.I. and Yesavage, J.A. (1986). Geriatric Depression Scale (GDS): recent evidence and development of a shorter version. *Clinical Gerontologist*, **5**(1–2), 165–73.

Shulman, K. (1989). Conceptual problems in the assessment of depression in old age. *Psychiatric Journal of the University of Ottawa*, **14**, 364–71.

Shulman, K. and Post, F. (1980). Bipolar affective disorder in old age. *British Journal of Psychiatry*, **136**, 26–32.

Spitzer, R.L., Endicott, J., and Robinson, E. (1978). Research diagnostic criteria: rationale and reliability. *Archives of General Psychiatry*, **35**, 773–82.

Starkstein, S.E. and Robinson, R.G. (1989). Affective disorders and cerebral vascular disease. *British Journal of Psychiatry*, **154**, 170–82.

Strain, J.J., Lyons, J.S., Hammer, J.S., and Fahs, M. (1991). Cost offset from a psychiatric consultation-liaison intervention with elderly hip fracture patients. *American Journal of Psychiatry*, **148**, 1044–9.

Sweer, L., Martrin, D.C., Ladd, R.A., Miller, J.K., and Karpf, M. (1988). The medical evaluation of elderly patients with major depression. *Journal of Gerontology*, **3**, M53–M58.

Unutzer, J., Patrick, D.L., Simon, G., Grembowski, D., Walker, E., Rutter, C., *et al.* (1997). Depressive symptoms and the cost of health services in HMO patients aged 65 years and older. *Journal of the American Medical Association*, **19**, 169–78.

Verbosky, L.A., Franco, K.N., and Zrull, J.P. (1993). The relationship between depression and length of stay in the general hospital patient. *Journal of Clinical Psychiatry*, **54** , 177–81.

Wasserman, D. (1989). Passive euthanasia in response to attempted suicide: one form of aggressiveness by relatives. *Acta Psychiatrica Scandinavica*, **79**, 460–7.

Wragg, R.E. and Jeste, D.V. (1989). Overview of depression and psychosis in Alzheimer's disease. *American Journal of Psychiatry*, **146**, 577–87.

Young, R.C. (1997). Bipolar mood disorders in the elderly. *Psychiatric Clinics of North America*, **20**, 121–36.

Young, R.C., Moline, M., and Kleyman, F. (1997). Hormone replacement therapy and late-life mania. *American Journal of Geriatric Psychiatry*, **5**, 179–81.

7 Anxiety

Alastair J. Flint

Summary

Anxiety disorders are a heterogeneous group of conditions that fall into the following categories: phobic disorders (agoraphobia, social phobia, specific phobia), panic disorder, generalized anxiety disorder, obsessive–compulsive disorder, and post-traumatic stress disorder. This chapter reviews the clinical characteristics, risk factors, prevalence, and incidence of anxiety disorders in later life. It also discusses the relationship between anxiety and other conditions, specifically depression, dementia, delirium, and physical illness and drugs.

Introduction

Although anxiety disorders are less prevalent in the elderly than in younger adults (Flint 1994; Jorm 2000), they are still relatively common in late life. Between 5% and 10% of older people living in the community meet *Diagnostic and statistical manual* (DSM) criteria for an anxiety disorder (Uhlenhuth *et al.* 1983; Regier *et al.* 1988; Beekman *et al.* 1998). Subsyndromal symptoms of anxiety are even more prevalent. For example, Copeland *et al.* (1987*b*) found that 22% of elderly people living in Liverpool, England, had primary subsyndromal symptoms of obsessive, phobic, or generalized anxiety.

There are several reasons why it is important to diagnose and effectively treat anxiety in the elderly. First, syndromal and subsyndromal anxiety can cause distress and disability in the affected person (De Beurs *et al.* 1999; Mendlowicz and Stein 2000) and contribute to caregiver stress. Second, people with anxiety make heavy use of medical services (Kennedy and Schwab 1997; De Beurs *et al.* 1999). Thus, patients with anxiety disorders are at risk of receiving unnecessary medical investigations and inappropriate treatment for their symptoms. Third, anxiety can contribute to medical morbidity, excess disability, and mortality from physical causes (Harris and Barraclough 1998; De Beurs *et al.* 1999; Bowen *et al.* 2000). Finally, anxiety is frequently a marker of depression, a disorder that contributes to medical morbidity and mortality in its own right (NIH Consensus Development Panel 1992).

The purpose of this chapter is to review the clinical characteristics and epidemiology of anxiety disorders in the elderly, and discuss the relationship between anxiety and other psychiatric and physical conditions.

Primary anxiety disorders

Anxiety disorders are a heterogeneous group of conditions that fall into the following categories: phobic disorders, panic disorder, generalized anxiety disorder, obsessive–compulsive disorder (OCD), and post-traumatic stress disorder (PTSD). As a group, the anxiety disorders have a peak age of onset in late adolescence and early adulthood (Antony and Swinson 1996). With the exception of agoraphobia, it is unusual for a primary anxiety disorder to start for the first time in later life (Flint 1994). If an elderly person does have a primary anxiety disorder, the disorder is usually chronic, having persisted from earlier in life (Flint 1994). Late-onset anxiety usually starts in association with another condition, such as depression, physical illness, or drug toxicity or withdrawal. Throughout the adult lifespan, primary anxiety disorders are more common in women than men (Flint 1994).

Phobic disorders

A phobia is a persistent irrational fear of a situation, object, or activity that results in a compelling desire to avoid the phobic stimulus. Phobic disorders are subdivided into agoraphobia, social phobia, and specific phobia. In agoraphobia, the phobic stimulus is a situation from which there might be difficulty or embarrassment in escaping. Agoraphobic situations in the elderly are similar to those for younger individuals, and include being out of the home alone, being in an enclosed space, being in a crowd, or travelling (Lindesay 1991a). Social phobia is a fear of situations in which the individual fears humiliation or embarrassment when under the scrutiny of others (for example, public speaking, eating in public, or attending social gatherings). Specific phobia is a fear of a circumscribed stimulus such as animals, heights, or blood.

A phobic disorder can only be diagnosed if the fear is irrational (American Psychiatric Association 1994). Thus, in evaluating whether an elderly person has a phobic disorder, it is important to assess the appropriateness or reasonableness of the anxiety. For example, a diagnosis of social phobia would not apply to a man with severe Parkinson's disease who avoids eating in public because of embarrassment about the disabling effect of his tremor. Similarly, if a frail elderly woman has several falls on the street and then decides not to leave the house alone because of a realistic concern about further falls and injury, she would not meet the criteria for agoraphobia. On the other hand, a diagnosis of agoraphobia would be considered for someone who has made a good physical recovery from a myocardial infarction, yet becomes housebound because of a fear that exertion will result in a recurrence of infarction or in death.

Depending on the study, phobias are either the most common or second most common anxiety disorder among elderly people living in the community (Flint 1994). Agoraphobia appears to be more common than specific phobia or social phobia (Uhlenhuth *et al.* 1983; Lindesay 1991*a*; Manela *et al.* 1996). In the case of specific phobia, the fear is usually lifelong, having started in childhood or early adolescence (Lindesay 1991*a*; Livingston *et al.* 1997), and it is associated with little, if any, social impairment (Lindesay 1991*a*). On the other hand, many elderly people with agoraphobia report that the disorder started in later life (Lindesay 1991*a*; Livingston *et al.* 1997) and that they often experience moderate or severe social impairment as a consequence of the phobia (Lindesay 1991*a*). It has been argued that agoraphobia in younger adults is usually a conditioned response to panic attacks (Klein 1980). However, very few elderly people with agoraphobia report a current or past history of panic attacks (Lindesay 1991*a*; Burvill *et al.* 1995; Manela *et al.* 1996) and other factors appear to be associated with its onset in later life. Many cases of late-onset agoraphobia start after a sudden physical illness or some other traumatic event, such as a fall, fire, or mugging (Lindesay 1991*a*; Livingston *et al.* 1997). Burvill *et al.* (1995) found that female survivors of stroke were more likely to meet the criteria for agoraphobia compared with control subjects without stroke; in many of these cases, the agoraphobia began after the stroke. Thus, if an elderly person is reluctant to leave home after a fall or experiencing a physical illness, it is important to evaluate him or her for the presence of agoraphobia.

The apparent lack of association between agoraphobia and panic attacks in late life has important implications for management. Studies undertaken in younger adults have found that selected antidepressant medications and benzodiazepines are effective treatments for panic disorder with agoraphobia (Antony and Swinson 1996). However, there is no good evidence that pharmacotherapy is an effective treatment for agoraphobia when there is no history of panic attacks (Antony and Swinson 1996). The treatment of choice for agoraphobia without panic (that is, most cases of agoraphobia in the elderly) is exposure therapy. Family members or domiciliary services may well support elderly people with agoraphobia at home. In order for behaviour therapy to be effective, it is important to withdraw any unnecessary support since its ongoing presence will reinforce the phobic behaviour and undermine the behavioural intervention (Lindesay and Banerjee 1994).

Generalized anxiety disorder

This disorder is characterized by excessive uncontrollable worry, accompanied by motor tension (muscle tension, restlessness, fatigue) and hypervigilance (feeling keyed up or on edge, difficulty concentrating, exaggerated startle response, irritability, insomnia). The disorder is chronic; symptoms occur on most days for 6 months or more (American Psychiatric Association 1994).

Some community-based epidemiological surveys have found that generalized anxiety disorder is the most common anxiety disorder in later life, whereas others have found that it is less common than phobic disorders (Flint 1994). An important clinical point is that generalized anxiety usually does not start as a pure disorder in late life. The Epidemiologic Catchment Area study found that, when people with current major depression and panic disorder were excluded, only 3% of cases of generalized anxiety disorder began after the age of 64 years (Blazer *et al.* 1991). When generalized anxiety starts for the first time in late life, it is usually associated with a depressive illness (Lindesay *et al.* 1989; Parmelee *et al.* 1993; Manela *et al.* 1996). Thus, if an older person presents with symptoms of generalized anxiety, he or she always should be carefully evaluated for the presence of a depressive illness.

Panic disorder

Panic disorder is characterized by recurrent attacks of symptoms of panic. A panic attack is a discrete period of intense fear or discomfort, during which a number of somatic and cognitive symptoms of anxiety develop abruptly and reach a peak within 10 minutes. These symptoms include dyspnoea, chest pain, palpitations, dizziness, sweating, choking, nausea or abdominal distress, trembling or shaking, tingling, hot or cold flashes, depersonalization or derealization, fear of dying, fear of losing control, and fear of going crazy.

Epidemiological surveys consistently report a low (less than 0.5%) period prevalence of panic disorder among older people living in the community (Flint 1994). This disorder rarely starts for the first time in late life (Flint 1994). When older people do experience panic attacks, symptoms are qualitatively similar to those experienced by younger people (Sheikh *et al.* 1991). However, patients with late-onset panic attacks may have fewer symptoms and be less avoidant than younger individuals with panic disorder (Sheikh *et al.* 1991). As is the case with generalized anxiety disorder, panic disorder in late life is frequently associated with a depressive illness (Hassan and Pollard 1994; Beekman *et al.* 2000). Bona fide panic attacks can occasionally complicate medical conditions in late life (Hassan and Pollard 1994). On the other hand, symptoms of a medical disorder (for example, episodes of hypoglycaemia in someone being treated for diabetes) may, at times, be mis-diagnosed as panic attacks in an older person.

Obsessive–compulsive disorder

The essential feature of this disorder is recurrent obsessions and/or compulsions. Obsessions are ideas, thoughts, or impulses that are experienced as senseless and intrusive and persist despite attempts to suppress them. The person recognizes that the obsessions are a product of his or her own mind and not imposed from without. Compulsions are repetitive, purposeful behaviours that are performed in response to an obsession or in a stereotyped fashion, with the goal of reducing distress or preventing some dreaded event or situation. However, either the activity is not connected in a realistic way with what it is designed to prevent, or it is clearly excessive.

Preliminary data suggest that the symptomatic presentation of OCD does not differ significantly between older and younger people (Kohn *et al.* 1997). Common obsessions include contamination fears, pathological doubt, and fear of harming others (Kohn *et al.* 1997). Common compulsions are checking, counting, and washing rituals (Kohn *et al.* 1997).

As is the case with panic disorder, OCD has a low prevalence in late life (Flint 1994). Most studies report period prevalence rates of OCD of between 0% and 0.8% in community-dwelling older people (Flint 1994). OCD seldom begins in late life; most elderly people with this disorder have had symptoms for decades (Jenike 1991; Kohn *et al.* 1997).

Ruminative thoughts are common in late-life depression (Lyness *et al.* 1997) and, at times, these thoughts can take the form of obsessions. It is important to differentiate between obsessions and delusions in the depressed patient, since delusional depression has a poor response to antidepressant monotherapy (whereas depression with associated obsessions may well respond to an antidepressant alone). Patients with dementia frequently develop perseverative behaviours, such as hoarding. This type of behaviour is not considered to be a compulsion, in that it is not a purposeful behaviour that the person feels driven to perform in response to an obsession or according to rules that must be applied rigidly.

Elderly people with OCD who are admitted to hospital for medical or surgical reasons may experience a worsening of their anxiety as a result of the disruption to their routine and/or being prevented from engaging in rituals. In such a situation, psychiatric management should focus on allowing such patients to maintain as much control over themselves and their environment as possible.

Post-traumatic stress disorder

PTSD develops in persons who have been exposed to a markedly distressing event that is outside the range of normal human experience. The traumatic event is then re-experienced as recurrent and distressing recollections, dreams, and/or flashbacks. Other features of PTSD include persistent avoidance of stimuli associated with the trauma, numbing of general responsiveness (for example, feeling detached from others, restricted range of affect, diminished interest, or participation in activities), and persistent symptoms of increased arousal (for example, difficulty falling asleep, hypervigilance, exaggerated startle response, irritability). The symptoms usually begin soon after the trauma, but they can be delayed for a number of months or years.

The period prevalence and incidence of PTSD in the general elderly population is unknown. Most research into PTSD in late life has focused on people who survived the Holocaust or who were prisoners of war during World War II. Chronic symptoms of PTSD have been found in 20–50% of these individuals (Kluznik *et al.* 1986; Rosen *et al.* 1989; Speed *et al.* 1989; Kuch and Cox 1992). In these selected groups, the chronicity and intensity of symptoms were positively corre-lated with the severity of the trauma. Some studies have also found an association between the occurrence of stressful life events in old age (such as reminders of the war experience, bereavement, or a significant change in physical health) and a worsening or re-emergence of symptoms of PTSD (Kaup *et al.* 1993; Macleod 1994). These findings are particularly relevant to clinicians who are working in veterans hospitals.

Late-onset PTSD has also been found in older people who have been victims of, or witnessed, natural disasters such as earthquakes or other types of disasters such as aircraft crashes (Goenjian *et al.* 1994; Livingston *et al.* 1994). Preliminary research suggests that PTSD-like symptoms may also develop in a small proportion of people who suffer a stroke (Sembi *et al.* 1998). It is not known, however, what effect these symptoms have on recovery from the stroke.

Anxiety associated with other conditions

Depression

Throughout the life cycle there is a high level of comorbidity between anxiety and depression (Stavrakaki and Vargo 1986). In particular, symptoms of general-ized anxiety and depression are strongly associated, and there is substantial over-lap between these conditions (Piccinelli 1998). Among the elderly, major depression is present in up to 70% of people with generalized anxiety disorder (Copeland *et al.* 1987*a*; Parmelee *et al.* 1993; Manela *et al.* 1996). Significant comorbidity between generalized anxiety and depression has also been reported in patients who have suffered stroke (Starkstein *et al.* 1990) or who have Parkinson's disease (Menza *et al.* 1993). Longitudinal data suggest that when generalized anxiety and depression coexist in the elderly, the anxiety is usually symptomatic of the depression (Parmelee *et al.* 1993; Castillo *et al.* 1995; Aström 1996). For example, in a study of residents of a long-term care facility, the 1-year incidence of generalized anxiety disorder was 2.3%, and more than two-thirds of these new cases started in the context of a new or pre-existing depressive illness (Parmelee *et al.* 1993).

Anxiety that is symptomatic of depression will usually resolve with appropriate treatment of the depression (Flint and Rifat 1997*a*). Occasionally, however, symptoms of anxiety persist, despite the resolution of other depressive symptoms (Flint and Rifat 1997*a*). In such cases, there may be an increased risk of relapse or recurrence of the depression (Flint and Rifat 1997*a*). It is also important to recog-nize that anxious depression may take longer to respond to treatment compared with depression that is uncomplicated by a high level of anxiety (Flint and Rifat 1997*b*).

Dementia and delirium

The prevalence of anxiety disorders is not increased among people with dementia who are living in the community (Skoog 1993; Forsell and Winblad 1997). Subsyndromal symptoms of generalized anxiety are often present, however, in clinical populations of dementia (Wands *et al.* 1990; Ballard *et al.* 1996; Orrell and Bebbington 1996). When anxiety is present in dementia, it is frequently associated with depression (Ballard *et al.* 1994; Orrell and Bebbington 1996; Forsell and Winblad 1998). For example, in a study of elderly people with memory problems, anxiety symptoms were present in 9% of those diagnosed as dementia, 36% of those diagnosed as major depression, and 43% of those with both dementia and depression (Eisdorfer *et al.* 1981).

Agitation (purposeless motor activity) is a frequent complication of dementia. Agitation is not synonymous with anxiety. However, in some people with dementia, it may be a behavioural expression of subjective anxiety that cannot be communicated through words. The clinician should suspect anxiety as a contributor to agitation in dementia if the patient has a history of anxiety or depression (Chemerinski *et al.* 1998; Forsell and Winblad 1998), or appears to be manifesting signs of depression (for example, tearfulness, irritability, recent loss of appetite, or social withdrawal).

Although delirium in late life is often relatively 'quiet', affected individuals sometimes present with anxiety (Lindesay 1991*b*). The anxiety may be in response to hallucinations or delusions. New-onset panic attacks are uncommon in the elderly and the abrupt onset of fear or terror, especially if the patient is physically unwell and/or has pre-existing cognitive impairment, should alert the clinician to the possibility of delirium (Lindesay 1991*b*).

Medical illness and drugs

Anxiety, physical illness, and the treatment of these conditions are related in several important ways. First, a person's psychological response to having a physical illness may range from realistic worry to pathological anxiety. Examples of pathological anxiety in this situation are phobic avoidance following a myocardial infarction, stroke, or fall, and generalized anxiety complicating major depression. Second, anxiety-like symptoms may be a manifestation of underlying physical pathology (Table 7.1). In most instances, the medical condition is already known. Occasionally, however, anxiety-like symptoms may be the presenting feature of an occult physical illness (for example, hypercalcaemia, phaeochromocytoma, or thyrotoxicosis). Third, drugs used to treat medical illness may, at times, give rise to anxiety-like symptoms. Anxiety may be a side-effect of therapeutic doses of steroids or some antihypertensives, or may be a consequence of toxicity from sympathomimetics, beta-adrenergic agonists, theophylline, digoxin, or thyroxine. Anxiety-like symptoms can also result from the withdrawal of benzodiazepines, barbiturates, and

Table 7.1 Physical conditions that may cause anxiety-like symptoms

Cardiovascular
Myocardial infarction
Cardiac arrhythmia, especially paroxysmal atrial tachycardia
Congestive heart failure
Orthostatic hypotension

Respiratory
Pulmonary embolism
Pulmonary oedema
Asthma
Chronic obstructive airways disease

Endocrine
Hypo/hyperthyroidism
Hypercalcaemia
Hypoglycaemia
Phaeochromocytoma
Carcinoid syndrome

Neurological
Temporal lobe epilepsy
Demyelinating diseases
Cerebral tumours
Cerebral lupus erythematosis
Encephalopathies
Head injury
Vestibular disturbances

Drugs
Toxicity from sympathomimetics, beta-adrenergic agonists (salbutamol), theophylline, thyroxine, digoxin, amphetamines, caffeine
Withdrawal from benzodiazepines, barbiturates, antidepressants, alcohol, nicotine
Side-effects from steroids, antihypertensives, antipsychotics (akathisia)

alcohol. Clinicians should be alert to the possibility of drug or alcohol withdrawal in patients who develop symptoms of anxiety or insomnia soon after admission to hospital, or who wish to sign themselves out of hospital within the first few days of arrival. Finally, antipsychotic medication can cause akathisia, which may be mistaken for anxiety.

Conversely, anxiety can contribute to medical morbidity, disability, and mortality from physical causes. Patients with anxiety disorders have increased rates of cigarette smoking and alcohol and drug use (Coryell 1988), factors that can contribute to physical ill health and death. People with high levels of anxiety (not necessarily meeting the criteria for an anxiety disorder) are at increased risk of hypertension (Jonas *et al*. 1997; Bowen *et al*. 2000), cardiac arrhythmias (Moser and Dracup 1996; Watkins *et al*. 1999), ischaemic heart disease (Haines *et al*. 1987;

Kawachi *et al.* 1994; Bowen *et al.* 2000), and death from cardiovascular causes (Haines *et al.* 1987; Kawachi *et al.* 1994). In addition, anxiety has been associated with an increased risk of gastrointestinal and respiratory disorders (Bowen *et al.* 2000), and death from neoplasms and chronic obstructive pulmonary disease (Allgulander 1994; Harris and Barraclough 1998). Symptoms of anxiety have also been found to contribute to excess functional disability and impaired recovery in patients with cardiac disease (Sullivan *et al.* 1997) or stroke (Aström 1996; Shimoda and Robinson 1998). Benzodiazepines, frequently taken by older people with anxiety (De Beurs *et al.* 1999), can contribute to morbidity. Benzodiazepines can depress respiratory drive in people with chronic airways disease (Man *et al.* 1986), contribute to falls and fractures (Herings *et al.* 1995), and cause or exacerbate cognitive impairment (Hanlon *et al.* 1998). Finally, people with anxiety frequently consult non-psychiatric medical specialists about their symptoms (Kennedy and Schwab 1997; De Beurs *et al.* 1999). Unless the anxiety is correctly diagnosed, the patient may receive unnecessary, and potentially hazardous, medical investigations and treatment.

Conclusions

Agoraphobia and generalized anxiety account for most cases of anxiety that start for the first time in late life. Many people with late-onset agoraphobia attribute their fears to physical illness or other traumatic events such as falls. This suggests that elderly medical or surgical patients are a group of people who are vulnerable to the development of agoraphobia. Thus, agoraphobia should be enquired about in patients who are reluctant to leave home following their discharge from hospital. Most cases of late-onset generalized anxiety are associated with depression. Depression always should be sought in elderly patients with generalized anxiety, including those with general medical illness, neurological disorders, or cognitive impairment. An important practise point is that antidepressant medication, not a benzodiazepine, is the *primary* pharmacological treatment of generalized anxiety associated with depression.

References

Allgulander, C. (1994). Suicide and mortality patterns in anxiety neurosis and depressive neurosis. *Archives of General Psychiatry,* **51**, 708–12.

American Psychiatric Association. (1994). *Diagnostic and statistical manual of mental disorders,* (4th edn). American Psychiatric Association, Washington, DC.

Antony, M.M. and Swinson, R.P. (1996). *Anxiety disorders and their treatment: a critical review of the evidence-based literature*. Health Canada, Ottawa.

Aström, M. (1996). Generalized anxiety disorder in stroke patients. A 3-year longitudinal study. *Stroke, 27*, 270–5.

Ballard, C.G. Mohan, R.N.C., Patel, A., and Graham, C. (1994). Anxiety disorder in dementia. *Irish Journal of Psychological Medicine*, **11**, 108–9.

Ballard, C., Boyle, A., Bowler, C., and Lindesay, J. (1996). Anxiety disorders in dementia sufferers. *International Journal of Geriatric Psychiatry, 11*, 987–90.

Beekman, A.T.F., Bremmer, M.A., Deeg, D.J.H., van Balkom, A.J.L.M., Smit, J.H., de Beurs, E., *et al.* (1998). Anxiety disorders in later life: a report from the longitudinal aging study Amsterdam. *International Journal of Geriatric Psychiatry, 13*, 717–26.

Beekman, A.T.F., de Beurs, E., van Balkom, A.J.L.M, Deeg, D.J.H., van Dyck, R., and van Tilburg, W. (2000). Anxiety and depression in later life: co-occurrence and communality of risk factors. *American Journal of Psychiatry, 157*, 89–95.

Blazer, D., George, L.K., and Hughes, D. (1991). Generalised anxiety disorder. In *Psychiatric disorders in America: the epidemiological catchment area study* (ed. L.N. Robins and D.A. Regier), pp. 180–203. The Free Press, New York.

Bowen, R.C., Senthilselvan, A., and Barale, A. (2000). Physical illness as an outcome of chronic anxiety disorders. *Canadian Journal of Psychiatry, 45*, 459–64.

Burvill, P.W., Johnson, G.A., Jamrozik, K.D., Anderson, C.S., Stewart-Wynne, E.G. and Chakera, T.M. (1995). Anxiety disorders after stroke: results from the Perth Community Stroke Study. *British Journal of Psychiatry, 166*, 328–32.

Castillo, C.S., Schultz, S.K., and Robinson, R.G. (1995). Clinical correlates of early-onset and late-onset poststroke generalized anxiety. *American Journal of Psychiatry, 152*, 1174–9.

Chemerinski, E., Petracca, G., Manes F., Leiguarda, R., and Starkstein, S.E. (1998). Prevalence and correlates of anxiety in Alzheimer's disease. *Depression and Anxiety, 7*, 166–70.

Copeland, J.R.M., Davidson, I.A., and Dewey, M.E. (1987*a*). The prevalence and outcome of anxious depression in elderly people aged 65 and over living in the community. In *Anxious depression: assessment and treatment* (ed. G. Racagni and E. Smeraldi), pp. 43–7. Raven Press, New York.

Copeland, J.R.M., Dewey, M.E., Wood, N., Searle, R., Davidson, I.A., and McWilliam, C. (1987*b*). Range of mental illness among the elderly in the community: prevalence in Liverpool using the GMS-AGECAT package. *British Journal of Psychiatry, 150*, 815–23.

Coryell, W. (1988). Mortality of anxiety disorders. In *Handbook of anxiety,* Vol 2. *Classification, etiological factors and associated disturbances* (ed. R. Noyes, M. Roth, and G.D. Burrows), pp. 311–20. Elsevier Science Amsterdam.

De Beurs, E., Beekman, A.T.F., van Balkom, A.J.L.M., Deeg, D.J.H., van Dyck, R., and van Tilburg, W. (1999). Consequences of anxiety in older persons: its effect on disability, well-being and use of health services. *Psychological Medicine, 29*, 583–93.

Eisdorfer, C., Cohen, D., and Keckich, W. (1981). Depression and anxiety in the cognitively impaired aged. In *Anxiety: new research and changing concepts* (ed. D.F. Klein and J. Rabkin), pp. 425–30. Raven Press, New York.

Flint, A.J. (1994). Epidemiology and comorbidity of anxiety disorders in the elderly. *American Journal of Psychiatry*, **151**, 640–9.

Flint, A.J. and Rifat, S.L. (1997a). Two-year outcome of elderly patients with anxious depression. *Psychiatry Research*, **66**, 23–31.

Flint, A.J. and Rifat, S.L. (1997b). Effect of demographic and clinical variables on time to response in geriatric depression. *Depression and Anxiety*, **5**, 103–7.

Forsell, Y. and Winblad, B. (1997). Anxiety disorders in non-demented and demented elderly patients: prevalence and correlates. *Journal of Neurology, Neurosurgery and Psychiatry*, **62**, 294–5.

Forsell, Y. and Winblad, B. (1998). Feelings of anxiety and associated variables in a very elderly population. *International Journal of Geriatric Psychiatry*, **13**, 454–8.

Goenjian, A.K., Najarian, L.M., Pynoos, R.S., Steinberg, A.M., Manoukian, G., Tavosian, A., *et al*. (1994). Posttraumatic stress disorder in elderly and younger adults after the 1988 earthquake in Armenia. *American Journal of Psychiatry*, **151**, 895–901.

Haines, A.P., Imeson, J.D., and Meade, T.W. (1987). Phobic anxiety and ischaemic heart disease. *British Medical Journal*, **295**, 297–9.

Hanlon, J.T., Homer, R.D., Schmader, K.E., Fillenbaum, G.G., Lewis, I.K., and Wall, W.E. (1998). Benzodiazepine use and cognitive function among community-dwelling elderly. *Clinical Pharmacology and Therapeutics*, **6**, 684–92.

Harris, E. and Barraclough, B. (1998). Excess mortality of mental disorder. *British Journal of Psychiatry*, **173**, 11–53.

Hassan, R. and Pollard, C.A. (1994). Late-life-onset panic disorder: clinical and demographic characteristics of a patient sample. *Journal of Geriatric Psychiatry and Neurology*, **7**, 86–90.

Herings, R.M.C., Stricker, B.H.Ch., de Boer, A., Bakker, A., and Sturmans, F. (1995). Benzodiazepines and the risk of falling leading to femur fractures. *Archives of Internal Medicine*, **155**, 1801–7.

Jenike, M.A. (1991). Geriatric obsessive–compulsive disorder. *Journal of Geriatric Psychiatry and Neurology*, **4**, 34–9.

Jonas, B.S., Franks, P., and Ingram, D.D. (1997). Are symptoms of anxiety and depression risk factors for hypertension? *Archives of Family Medicine*, **6**, 43–9.

Jorm, A.F. (2000). Does old age reduce the risk of anxiety and depression? A review of epidemiological studies across the adult life span. *Psychological Medicine*, **30**, 11–22.

Kaup, B.A., Ruskin, P.E., and Nyman, G. (1993). Significant life events and PTSD in elderly World War II veterans. *American Journal of Geriatric Psychiatry*, **2**, 239–43.

Kawachi, I., Sparrow, D., Vokonas, P.S. and Weiss, S.T. (1994). Symptoms of anxiety and risk of coronary heart disease. The normative aging study. *Circulation*, **90**, 2225–9.

Kennedy, B.L. and Schwab, J.J. (1997). Utilisation of medical specialists by anxiety disorder patients. *Psychosomatics*, **38**, 109–12.

Klein, D.F. (1980). Anxiety reconceptualized. *Comprehensive Psychiatry*, **21**, 411–27.

Kluznik, J.C., Speed, N., Van Valkenburg, C., and Magraw, R. (1986). Forty-year follow-up of United States prisoners of war. *American Journal of Psychiatry*, **143**, 1443–6.

Kohn, R., Westlake, R.J., Rasmussen, S.A., Marsland, R.T., and Norman, W. H. (1997). Clinical features of obsessive–compulsive disorder in elderly patients. *American Journal of Geriatric Psychiatry*, **5**, 211–15.

Kuch, K. and Cox, B.J. (1992). Symptoms of PTSD in 124 survivors of the Holocaust. *American Journal of Psychiatry*, **149**, 337–40.

Lindesay, J. (1991*a*). Phobic disorders in the elderly. *British Journal of Psychiatry*, **159**, 531–41.

Lindesay, J. (1991*b*). Anxiety disorders in the elderly. In *Psychiatry in the elderly* (ed. R. Jacoby and C. Oppenheimer), pp. 735–57. Oxford University Press, Oxford.

Lindesay, J. and Banerjee, S. (1994). Generalized anxiety and phobic disorders. In *Functional psychiatric disorders of the elderly* (ed. E. Chiu and D. Ames), pp. 78–92. Cambridge University Press, Cambridge.

Lindesay, J., Briggs, K., and Murphy, E. (1989). The Guy's/Age Concern Survey: prevalence rates of cognitive impairment, depression and anxiety in an urban elderly community. *British Journal of Psychiatry*, **155**, 317–29.

Livingston, H.M., Livingston, M.G., and Fell, S. (1994). The Lockerbie disaster: a 3-year follow-up of elderly victims. *International Journal of Geriatric Psychiatry*, **9**, 989–94.

Livingston, G., Watkin, V., Milne, B., Manela, M.V., and Katona, C. (1997). The natural history of depression and the anxiety disorders in older people: the Islington community study. *Journal of Affective Disorders*, **46**, 255–62.

Lyness, J.M., Conwell, Y., King, D.A., Cox, C., and Caine, E. D. (1997). Ruminative thinking in older inpatients with major depression. *Journal of Affective Disorders*, **46**, 273–7.

Macleod, A.D. (1994). The reactivation of post-traumatic stress disorder in later life. *Australian and New Zealand Journal of Psychiatry*, **28**, 625–34.

Man, G.C.W., Hsu, K., and Sproule, B.J. (1986). Effect of alprazolam on exercise and dyspnea in patients with chronic obstructive pulmonary disease. *Chest*, **90**, 832–6.

Manela, M., Katona, C., and Livingston, G. (1996). How common are the anxiety disorders in old age? *International Journal of Geriatric Psychiatry*, **11**, 65–70.

Mendlowicz, M.V. and Stein, M.B. (2000). Quality of life in individuals with anxiety disorders. *American Journal of Psychiatry,* **157**, 669–82.

Menza, M.A., Robertson-Hoffman, D.E., and Bonapace, A.S. (1993). Parkinson's disease and anxiety: comorbidity with depression. *Biological Psychiatry,* **34**, 465–70.

Moser, D.K., and Dracup, K. (1996). Is anxiety early after myocardial infarction associated with subsequent ischemic and arrhythmic events? *Psychosomatic Medicine,* **58**, 395–401.

NIH Consensus Development Panel. (1992). Diagnosis and treatment of depression in late life. *Journal of the American Medical Association,* **268**, 1018–24.

Orrell, M. and Bebbington, P. (1996). Psychosocial stress and anxiety in senile dementia. *Journal of Affective Disorders,* **39**, 165–73.

Parmelee, P.A., Katz, I.R., and Lawton, M.P. (1993). Anxiety and its association with depression among institutionalized elderly. *American Journal of Geriatric Psychiatry,* **1**, 46–58.

Piccinelli, M. (1998). Comorbidity of depression and generalized anxiety: is there any distinct boundary? *Current Opinion in Psychiatry,* **11**, 57–60.

Regier, D.A., Boyd, J.H., Burke, J.D., Rae, D.S., Myers, J.K., Kramer, M., *et al.* (1988). One-month prevalence of mental disorders in the United States: based on five epidemiologic catchment area sites. *Archives of General Psychiatry,* **45**, 977–86.

Rosen, J., Fields, R.B., Hand, A.M., Falsettie, G., and Van Kammen, D.P. (1989). Concurrent posttraumatic stress disorder in psychogeriatric patients. *Journal of Geriatric Psychiatry and Neurology,* **2**, 65–9.

Sembi, S., Tarrier, N., O'Neill, P., Burns, A., and Faragher, B. (1998). Does post-traumatic stress disorder occur after stroke: a preliminary study. *International Journal of Geriatric Psychiatry,* **13**, 315–22.

Sheikh, J.I., King, R.J., and Taylor, C.B. (1991). Comparative phenomenology of early-onset versus late-onset panic attacks: a pilot study. *American Journal of Psychiatry,* **148**, 1231–3.

Shimoda, K. and Robinson, R.G. (1998). Effect of anxiety disorder on impairment and recovery from stroke. *Journal of Neuropsychiatry and Clinical Neurosciences,* **10**, 34–40.

Skoog, I. (1993). The prevalence of psychotic, depressive and anxiety syndromes in demented and non-demented 85-year-olds. *International Journal of Geriatric Psychiatry,* **8**, 247–53.

Speed, N., Engdahl, B., Schwartz, J., and Eberly, R. (1989). Posttraumatic stress disorder as a consequence of the POW experience. *Journal of Nervous and Mental Disease,* **177**, 147–53.

Starkstein, S.E., Cohen, B.S., Fedoroff, P., Parikh, R.M., Price, T.R., and Robinson, R.G. (1990). Relationship between anxiety disorders and depressive disorders in patients with cerebrovascular injury. *Archives of General Psychiatry,* **47**, 246–51.

Stavrakaki, C. and Vargo, B. (1986). The relationship of anxiety and depression: a review of the literature. *British Journal of Psychiatry,* **149**, 7–16.

Sullivan, M.D., LaCroix, A.Z., Baum, C., Grothaus, L.C., and Katon, W.J. (1997). Functional status in coronary artery disease: a one-year prospective study of the role of anxiety and depression. *American Journal of Medicine,* **103**, 348–56.

Uhlenhuth, E.H., Balter, M.B., Mellinger, G.D., Cisin, I.H., and Clinthorne, J. (1983). Symptom checklist syndromes in the general population: correlations with psychotherapeutic drug use. *Archives of General Psychiatry,* **40**, 1167–73.

Wands, K., Merskey, H., Hachinski, V.C., Fisman, M., Fox, H., and Boniferro, M. (1990). A questionnaire investigation of anxiety and depression in early dementia. *Journal of the American Geriatrics Society,* **38**, 535–8.

Watkins, L.L., Grossman, P., Krishnan, R., and Blumenthal, J.A. (1999). Anxiety reduces baroreflex cardiac control in older adults with major depression. *Psychosomatic Medicine,* **61**, 334–40.

8 Somatoform disorders in late life

Pamela S. Melding and Louise Armstrong

Summary

Of all the psychiatric disorders, the somatoform disorders seem to attract more negative attitudes from health professionals than other mental illnesses. Somatization and hypochondriasis are seen in all aspects of medical care of older people and are a challenge for the liaison psychiatrist. The phenomena can vary from transient symptoms under stress, to a lifelong coping style, to a disabling disorder. The phenomena are manifest in illness behaviour, a concept that has attracted widespread controversy as to whether it is a clinical entity or an 'idiom of distress'. The phenomena have many potential meanings for the patient–environment relationship and these are explored in this chapter. The mechanisms and phenomena of somatization are discussed as they apply to older people. In addition, the influence of gender and age, medical comorbidity, state versus trait phenomena, and definitions of illness behaviour are reviewed. The relationships of somatization phenomena to other psychiatric disorders are addressed. This chapter concludes with a brief discussion of treatment issues when somatoform psychopathology is the primary focus for treatment.

Introduction

Of all the psychiatric disorders, the somatoform disorders seem to attract more negative attitudes from health professionals than other mental illnesses. The person with hypochondriasis or somatization often seems ungrateful and they utilize considerable medical time and available resources for a relatively poor outcome. Clinical staff often resent people they believe to be hypochondriacal, and the patients can be pejoratively labelled 'crocks' (Kellner and Schneider-Braus 1988). The implicit dialogue goes something like—the patient 'fails' to do the 'right thing', which is to get better. The patient 'incorrectly' attributes a physical cause to bodily symptoms rather than making a 'true' attribution to an emotional cause; thus, the patient acquires the status of the sick-role 'illegitimately'. Note the inherent moral judgements in the discourse. Historic-ally, it was not always so.

Galen, in the second century of the Common Era, related the terms hypochondria (Greek *hupokhondriakos* = beneath the ribs) and melancholy (Greek *melankholia* = black bile) to recognizable syndromes. He thought that these disorders originated in the digestive system and somehow, through some unfathomable bowel–brain connection, caused accompanying mental symptoms of anguish and sadness. Indeed, throughout the last two millennia, hypochondria has been viewed as an admixture of the physiopathological, psychological, and sociological states of the individual. This is a view that is still consistent with a modern-day biopsychosocial approach that is particularly apposite to geriatric care.

Susan Baur (1988), taking the historical perspective in her monograph on hypochondria, wrote

> For centuries, hypochondria attracted the attention of the great doctors and philosophers who, believing the disorder to stem from a mixture of physiological imbalance and social frustration, tried every drug and therapeutic regime at their command to control this common misery. During the nineteenth century, hypo-chondria came to be associated with emotional rather than physical problems and once identified as a mental disease, quickly attracted pejorative connotations. Not only did the disorder lose its status as a yardstick by which other miseries were measured, but it was broken down into a dozen different pieces and parcelled out among the psychoses and neurosis. Hypochondria became merely a symptom of deeper troubles. (p. 2)

Baur's lamentation would seem valid. For most of our history, the single term 'hypochondria' has subsumed all the modern-day somatoform disorders. In DSM-IV (APA 1994), hypochondriasis is just one of several somatoform disorders, including somatization disorder, pain disorder, conversion disorder, body dysmorphic disorder, and somatoform disorder NOS (not otherwise specified). This review also adds somatic delusional disorder (also known as monosymptomatic hypo-chondriacal delusional psychosis), factitious disorder, and malingering. The common theme of these disorders is the presence of physical symptoms that suggest a general medical condition, not fully explained by any objective medical pathology nor by the direct effects of a substance or other mental disorder. The ICD-10 criteria are similar.

Classification systems can simultaneously be a help and a hindrance. Whilst they delineate specific criteria that can identify clinical entities, foster research, and target treatments, in real patients the boundaries between the different disorders, and even the threshold for the detection of symptoms, are often very blurred. This is particu-larly true of the somatoform spectrum, as the phenomena have multiple layers of complexity and can range in severity from mild transient symptoms to extreme disability, from being a coping style to a clinical disorder.

The core phenomenon of the somatoform spectrum is somatization. Lipowski (1988) defined somatization as:

... a tendency to *experience* and *communicate* somatic distress and symptoms unaccounted for by pathological findings, to *attribute* them to physical illness and to *seek help* for them. [our italics]

This definition highlights the interwoven socio- psycho- physiological operations that contribute in varied measure to the different presentations of somatoform disorder. Thus, using the term somatization in a generic sense, the phenomenon of somatization can be manifest as multiple physical symptoms (as in somatization disorder) or as a phobic fear of disease (as in hypochondriasis) (Schmidt 1994). There is considerable overlap of the boundaries between somatization and hypochondriasis (Leibbrand *et al*. 2000) both in the literature and in clinical life, and the terms are often confused and used interchangeably. In this review, the term 'somatization' describes the phenomena of symptom perception and attribution to physical cause, with the term 'hypochondriasis' describing somatization associated with disease conviction and or phobia.

Somatization and hypochondriasis are seen in all aspects of the medical care of older people, and somatization phenomena may be coincidental, complicating, or confounding. Blazer (1996) suggested that the psychiatric diagnoses of somatization and hypochondriasis should be de-emphasized and instead the phenomena conceptualized within a geriatric syndromal model, in keeping with the disability and rehabilitation approach of modern geriatric management. The liaison psychiatrist is likely to encounter all facets of the somatoform spectrum, from transient phenomena to clinical disorder. Consequently, this chapter addresses the following as they pertain to older people:

♦ The mechanisms and phenomena of somatization

♦ The influence of gender and age

♦ The influence of medical comorbidity

♦ The influence of ethnicity and culture

♦ State versus trait phenomena

♦ Somatization and illness behaviour

♦ Somatization as symptom of a psychiatric disorder

♦ The somatoform spectrum as medical disorders

The mechanisms and phenomena of somatization

James Pennebaker's (1982) seminal work on symptom perception theory has led to considerable interest and research on the psychological mechanisms of somatization and hypochondriasis. Briefly summarizing this large body of research, there are three key related concepts, which are: (1) the person's selective attention to physical cues (2) amplification of symptoms, and (3) cognitive appraisal and attribution of the symptoms as having a physical cause.

How bodily sensations are perceived is dependent on both the intensity of the stimulus and selective attention to bodily cues. The individual's cognitive schema and emotional state will raise or lower the threshold for detection. Boring, bland, low stimulus environments (such as experienced by many isolated elderly people or those in low-functioning nursing homes) may allow more selective attention on physical cues or, alternatively, stimulating, distracting environments with lots of activity may reduce this focus. Pennebaker (1982) considered that stimulus perception was a function of both internally and externally perceived cues. When the stimuli are perceived as an adverse state from this perceptual process, they acquire the status of symptoms (Gijsbers Van Wijk and Kolk 1997). Note that the concept of symptom perception does not assume that symptoms necessarily signify actual physical or psychological pathology.

Barsky (1992) and Barsky *et al.* (1988) postulate that symptoms, once detected by the person, are amplified and are then regarded as more noxious, adverse, intense, or ominous. The individual develops higher sensory arousal for symptoms, becomes hypervigilant and selectively attends to those symptoms that fit a preconceived explanatory hypothesis or illness belief. The person's appraisal depends on several factors that include: the relative values the person gives to health; physical appearance; physical symptoms; previous anxieties over bodily vulnerability; and aversion to ageing and dying (Barsky and Wyshak 1989,1990). These cognitions result from the person's previous illness experience, their upbringing, learned ways of perceiving and relating to the world, coping styles, and so on. The somatizing person ignores information that counters the hypothesis, and attributes the amplified symptoms to a disease or illness conceptualization rather than a physiological or emotional one. Any anxiety symptoms arising from this process may be perceived as further evidence of disorder and intensify the amplification mechanism even more.

The influence of gender and age

Pfeiffer (1977) considered that somatization was the third most common psychiatric diagnosis in the elderly after depression and paranoia, with females being most predisposed. Several authors (for example, Busse 1976; Butler 1978; Brink *et al.* 1981) have been in agreement. The assertion has persisted as a pervasive belief that old people, especially women, have more hypochondriasis and a greater tendency to somatize than younger adults. What is the evidence for this view? Is this yet another stereotype of old age, another myth?

As there is a preponderance of older women in late life, this could have some bearing on such a gender bias. The relationship of gender with somatization has been well studied, but mostly in younger subjects (Wool and Barsky 1994; Gijsbers Van Wijk and Kolk 1997), and the research suggests that women do report more physical symptoms, are more in tune with low levels of abnormality, and are more vigilant about bodily cues (Verbrugge 1989; Kroenke and Spitzer 1998). Females are socially conditioned to monitor their own physiological processes due to their reproductive cycles, and are also very practiced in monitoring health status in children and other family members. However, most research also shows that the tendency for females to report more symptoms at lower levels of acuity applies only to healthy women. In sick adults, clinical populations, or psychiatric patients, the gender difference disappears and both genders are equally likely to identify health symptoms or hypochondriacal concerns (Hernandez and Kellner 1992; Gijsbers Van Wijk and Kolk 1997).

With respect to age, and despite some contradictions, the balance of research agrees with the findings of Leventhal and Prohaska (1986) and indicates that older people seem less likely to complain about their aches and pains, tending to put these symptoms down to ageing rather than disease. Barsky *et al.* (1991) found that neither gender nor ageing was associated with an increase in hypochondriasis, despite an increase in medical illness. Furthermore, they found no difference between young and old patients on the severity of hypochondriasis. Instead, they found older patients had much higher levels of functional disability but this was due to medical comorbidity, and not to hypochondriasis.

Influence of medical comorbidity

Older people do have more illness. In late life, illness often presents in subtle ways; and even in younger adults, many physicians confidently diagnosing a somatoform disorder have been embarrassed when covert pathology is subsequently revealed (Chandler and Gerndt 1988). Such misdiagnosis is much more likely with older people. Indeed, for many older patients presenting with somatoform disorders, a physician would be able to find some explanatory pathology. Importantly, a disease state does not need to be absent for the patient to have significant and disabling somatization or hypochondriacal phenomena. History is peppered with articulate sufferers who wrote about their personal experiences of 'hypochondria', for example; diarist Dr Samuel Johnson, biographer James Boswell, writer Leo Tolstoy, and poet Sara Teasdale, all of whom were crippled, at times, by hypochondriacal concerns complicating real medical pathology (Baur 1988).

Influence of ethnicity and culture

Ethnicity, culture, and language influence how symptoms might be overtly expressed. For many cultures, a somatic construct of emotional distress is the norm. Kleinman (1982) observing patients in China considered them to have classical depressive symptoms, but noted that both doctors and patients, whilst readily admitting the emotional nature of the symptoms, preferred the diagnosis to be the more somatically ambiguous 'neurasthenia'. Farooq *et al.* (1995) compared an Asian with a Caucasian population in the United Kingdom and found that ethnicity was the main variable in determining the expression of somatic complaints. They did not find that age, gender, or social status variables related to somatic expression. In Australia,

Marmanidis *et al.* (1994), studying Greek and European Australian medical inpatients found no difference in the rate of depression or somatic complaints, but found interesting differences between the two ethnic groups in the patterns of symptom expression.

State versus trait phenomena

There is a group of patients who function perfectly well normally, but under the stress of serious medical illness, may develop state-dependent somatization phenomena. They amplify and catastrophize symptoms, with the consequence that they become more disabled than would be expected for the objective pathology. The phenomena are usually transient and would not be of sufficient severity to reach DSM diagnostic criteria. Even so, transient hypochondriacs are more likely to have a comorbid axis-1 disorder or pre-existing personality disorder, giving them fewer coping resources and less resilience to deal with medical sickness (Barsky *et al.* 1990*a,b*). As there is a greater likelihood of disease states in late life with, potentially, many more symptoms to detect, it might be expected that transient hypochondriasis would show an increase with age. In contrast, Barsky *et al.* (1991) found older people did not amplify their symptoms; nor were they any more subject to transient hypochondriasis than younger people.

For the most part, the idea that older people are more likely to have increased somatic concerns or hypochondriasis as they age does not stand up to the scrutiny of current evidence. Nevertheless, a few people develop more than transient hypochondriasis or somatic stress symptoms and progress to chronic, disabling hypochondriacal or somatoform disorders. The phenomena are much more a personal style or trait, they significantly interfere with functioning, and are objectively manifest in the person's illness behaviour.

Somatization and illness behaviour

Illness behaviour reflects the coping style of the individual. Societal expectation of normal illness behaviour is that symptoms cause the person to seek help and to co-operate with competent, technical medical help. In exchange, the person will be absolved of blame for their condition, will be cared for by others, and will be released from the normal obligations of society (Parsons 1951). These can also be powerful motivations for remaining sick. When the person amplifies the symptoms, does not appear to be motivated to get well, is non-compliant, over-dependent on care, or appears to be getting some advantage from being sick, the behaviour represents a departure from that expected. The illness and suffering state is judged to be out of proportion to the actual physical impairment caused by the disease, so-called 'abnormal illness behaviour'. It is abnormal illness behaviour that attracts most negativity from medical staff and not surprisingly this 'label' also attracts great controversy and diversity of opinion amongst commentators.

The controversy mostly concerns the idea that the phenomena inherent in illness behaviour define the *medical diagnoses* of the somatoform spectrum. Pilowsky (1978) conceptualized 'abnormal illness behaviour' as various dimensions: disease conviction (hypochondriasis), somatic focus for symptoms (somatization), denial of psychological problems and translation of psychological symptoms into somatic complaints (conversion), and affective blunting. These are also linked to the psycho-dynamic view that the person, by seeing himself or herself as a sick person, is able to deny an emotional aetiology or psychological conflict (primary gain) and may gain reinforcement for this role from the environment (secondary gain).

In contrast, Mechanic (1995), one of the original illness behaviour theorists, soundly criticizes the concept of 'abnormal' when applied to illness behaviour and the medicalization of the phenomena. He prefers to regard somatization and illness behaviour as: 'an idiom of distress shaped by culture and psychosocial factors'.

According to Mechanic (1995), it is only in modern-day societies, which are highly individualized and psychologically aware, that a somatic presentation of emotional distress is considered 'an aberration requiring re-education'. Many of today's older people have not been socialized in a psychological or emotional milieu during their lifetimes; in contrast they have been socialized into hiding emotions, and a somatic explanation for distress might be more acceptable to them.

If somatization and illness behaviour are indeed 'idioms of distress' (Mechanic 1995) for many patients, then it is important to understand how these might manifest in the older person's interaction with their environment. There are many possibilities. For example, the psychosocial processes of somatization, hypochondriasis, and illness behaviour may enable redirection of conscious focus away from emotional conflict engendered by the stress of growing old and dying. Focus on bodily symptoms may describe feelings that are poorly understood, particularly if cognition is failing. Somatization may be a way of guarding self-esteem and manipulating caregivers (Brink *et al.* 1979). Some old people, particularly if depressed, find it difficult to express distress and 'don't want to be a bother'. Somatization can be a means of communication when other channels of expression are blocked (Ford 1986). Pain and illness can justify a loss of mobility or legitimize dependency as society may be more tolerant of illness in old age, expecting frailty and infirmity. It may be more acceptable to go into a nursing home because of pain and illness than it is for loneliness. Somatization may be an adaptive way for an old person to get love and attention, particularly if institutionalized. Some political and economic systems legitimize somatic diagnoses by making accommodation subsidies more available for those with physical disorders. Lastly, it is important to remember that doctors can subtly prioritize somatic diagnoses and may actually shape illness behaviour or increase medical utilization by over-treatment (Singh *et al.* 1981)

Case study 8.1

Dr G., a longtime widower, had been a prisoner of war in Burma during World War II. Although he had witnessed several traumatic incidents during this time, he felt that he had coped well. After all, he had been a senior officer and was expected to lead and show a good example to his men. After the war he had a distinguished career as a surgeon and in his later years as a senior medical administrator. He had been a 'workaholic', and his proud boast was that he had never been sick in his life. Even after retiring, he spent considerable time working as a volunteer for various medical charities. After a small stroke he was unable to continue and he became very preoccupied about his health. Dr G. would take his blood pressure at least four times a day and would contact his doctor at least twice a week to report every symptom he feared might herald 'the big one'. He denied any depressed mood symptoms but admitted being demotivated. His daughter, a psychiatric nurse, thought he might be experiencing some delayed sadness about his deceased wife and wartime companions now that he had more to think about them. He emphatically denied this suggestion and refused to discuss these topics. Dr G. eventually decided to go into a Veteran's nursing home as he was not improving in his rehabilitation. Once there, he started to pick up and, despite his handicap, soon began organizing the residents into a social programme.

Somatization as symptom of a psychiatric disorder

Less controversial is the association of somatization with other mental disorders. The phenomena of somatic attribution (somatization) and disease phobia or conviction (hypochondriasis) occur as symptoms in a host of psychiatric problems. Several studies show a strong link between somatization phenomena and depressive symptoms (Hyer *et al*. 1987; Lipowski 1990; Kellner *et al*. 1992; Escobar *et al*. 1998; Piccinelli *et al*. 1999) and this association seems to hold true for older patients (Leventhal *et al*. 1996; Monopoli and Viccaro 1998). As depression is also significantly associated with physical disability in older adults (Lindesay *et al*. 1989), the constellation of physical illness and depression in old age complicated by hypochondriacal concerns or exaggeration of somatic symptoms would appear to be a potent mixture for inducing disability. Indeed, one of the strongest predictors for psychosocial dysfunction (Hiller *et al*. 1997) is the comorbidity of somatoform and depressive disorder. Underlying depression may not be easily recognizable as the affective disturbance may be obscured by the somatic complaints. Recognition of depression depends upon identifying symptoms other than mood state, such as loss of interest, anhedonia, or demotivation.

There are equally strong comorbid ties with anxiety disorders (Noyes *et al*. 1999). Hypochondriasis is actually defined by DSM-IV in anxiety terms, as preoccupation with a fear of having a disease. Some studies distinguish subsyndromes of hypochondriasis, such as a fear of having a disease (disease phobia) and belief of having a disease (disease conviction) (Kellner 1992). Disease conviction seems to cluster more with somatic and depressive symptoms and disease phobia with clinical anxiety, but there is considerable overlap and comorbidity between the two (Kellner

1992). Hypochondriacal symptoms can also occur in panic disorder (Barsky *et al.* 1994; Noyes *et al.* 1999) and obsessive–compulsive disorder (Schmidt 1994; Leibbrand *et al.* 2000). Some authors (reviewed by Kellner 1992) have argued that hypochondriasis is always a variant of another disorder. Others have argued that because hypochondriasis often occurs as a symptom in the course of another psychiatric disorder, it is as likely to be a secondary as much as a primary phenomenon (Pilowsky 1970).

Somatic complaints may be a feature of early cognitive impairment. There are sporadic reports, such as that by Brown (1991), of late-life somatization disorder occurring simultaneously with progressive dementia. Frisoni *et al.* (1999) studied 462 community-dwelling elderly people, and found a significant association between somatic symptoms and cognitive impairment that persisted after confounding variables were controlled.

Thus, for the liaison psychiatrist, it is important to remember that symptoms somatization and hypochondriasis do occur frequently in a range of psychiatric disorders that could be underpinning the patient's presentation. However, when the somatic preoccupation becomes central to the person's presentation and functioning it crosses the boundary to medical syndrome.

The somatoform spectrum as medical disorders

Somatoform disorders rarely appear for the first time in late life. In addition, these disorders do not preclude an associated psychiatric diagnosis or an organic substrate. Nevertheless, a diagnosis of one of the somatoform disorders is applicable for some older patients. In general, these older people will have a long history and their somatic style of functioning may be very clear.

Somatization disorder

Somatization disorder as defined by DSM-IV, is a disorder that usually starts before 30 years of age, and is characterized by multiple physical complaints in several systems. The patient is preoccupied with symptoms, is less concerned with a diagnostic label, but more in having their sickness acknowledged. Symptoms may include various pains, gastrointestinal, sexual, and pseudoneurological complaints. For DSM-IV diagnosis, there must have been at least eight different symptoms not explainable by a general medical condition at any stage in life. Escobar *et al.* (1989) argued for an abridged version of the somatization criteria because of DSM-IV's overemphasis on female reproductive system criteria. The abridged construct lowers the criteria to six separate symptoms for females and four for males from the 40 included in the Composite International Diagnostic Instrument, CIDI.

Classically, somatization disorder is a stable pattern of functioning (trait) and has a chronic relapsing lifetime course. However, a recent large international follow-up study challenges this view and indicates that 'lifetime' symptoms may improve or disappear over time (Simon and Gureje 1999), lending some weight to the idea of somatization as a state-dependent coping style.

Pain disorder

Pain disorder (formerly somatoform pain disorder) is a somatically presenting disorder where pain is the single symptom of concern. Older people have many reasons to have chronic pain problems: for example, collapsed vertebrae, hip fractures, angina, vascular insufficiency, neuropathies, and so on. In older people, a diagnosis of pain disorder, which implies that the medical condition plays a lesser role than the psychological factors, is potentially an unsafe diagnosis. The diagnosis of psychological factors affecting a general medical condition, in which both pain and psychological responses are judged to have important aetiological roles, is more appropriate.

Conversion disorders

Conversion disorders are significantly associated with dissociation phenomena and physical pathology. As dissociation phenomena tend to decrease with age (Walker *et al.* 1996) and with cognitive deficits, conversion disorder is more common in younger people, with several studies indicating mean ages of 25–35. Most studies show a preponderance of females. Conversion disorders, however, do occur in older people. Mace and Trimble (1996) and Kent *et al.* (1995) showed, in respective 10- and 4-year follow-ups of older patients with diagnosed conversion disorder, that rediagnosis of a physical disorder was less common than previously thought. In older people, the anecdotal literature reports conversion disorders presenting with neurological symptoms, such as globus hystericus, pseudoseizures, and cognitive impairments that eventually reverse (LaMancusa and Wyatt 1990; Liberini *et al.* 1993*a,b*). These accounts are rare and, whilst interesting, one should exercise great caution making such a diagnosis in the elderly with their increased prevalence of medical illness.

Hypochondriasis

Hypochondriasis (disease conviction and disease phobia) tends to start in middle age or later. It is equally common in both genders, with cardiophobia being more common in males (Hernandez and Kellner 1992). Disease conviction is an over-valued idea, often held with obsessive ruminative zeal. The patient lives with the crippling dilemma of having an intense fear of developing a disease that he or she is already convinced is present. There are very strong associations with fear of ageing and death and an overwhelming sense of body vulnerability (Barsky and Wyshak 1989). Anxious hypochondriacs often present to Accident and Emergency departments with chest pain, hyperventilation, and beliefs they are having a heart attack. Depressed older people may develop a fear of bowel cancer.

Delusional disorder, somatic type (formerly hypochondriacal delusional disorder)

In hypochondriacal delusional disorder the hypochondriacal ideas become unshakeable and hence delusional. In approximately 40% of older people with hypochondriacal delusions there is a previous history of somatization or associated depression (Opjordsmoen 1988). Delusions can be related to any bodily system.

Case study 8.2

Mr W. was admitted to the inpatient unit by a desperate general practitioner. For 2 months the patient had been ringing daily in great distress because his penis was 'rotating'. The doctor had treated him with pimozide with little effect. The patient was a bachelor with a lifelong history of social phobia. He denied any female or male liaisons, but admitted to occasionally reading 'girlie' magazines. It was after one such incident that he first experienced the 'rotation'. The sensation fluctuated during the day, being worse in the early mornings and late afternoons. He was convinced his penis would strangulate and drop off if it continued to rotate. Mr W. had marked distress and signifi-cant depressive symptoms and was not amenable to reassurance. His idea was held with delusional intensity. CT scan showed an old small infarct in the temporal lobe. Cognitive testing was suggestive of early impairment. Mr W. failed to respond to two antipsychotics and two antidepressants. As his distress persisted it was reluctantly decided that ECT should be tried. To the team's surprise, he responded well and his symptoms were virtually non-existent for the next year.

Particularly distressing are somatic delusions of socially distasteful problems such as foul body odour or delusional parasitosis. This latter disorder seems to occur mostly in people over the age of 50 (Wykoff 1987; Trabert 1995). There have been multiple anecdotes of this disorder over the past 100 years (for example, Moselhy and El-Dosoky 1996; Rasanen *et al*. 1997; Slaughter *et al*. 1998) but we do not know its true incidence. There seems to be a female preponderance. The patients mostly present to dermatologists, with a conviction that they have fleas, parasites, lice, or worms. The patients excoriate their skin trying to pick off the parasites. They bring the 'evidence' in matchboxes or jars. Indeed, the 'matchbox sign' is pathognomonic of the disorder. The matchboxes usually contain dandruff or bits of fluff but not arthropods. Some descriptions of the insects are very graphic indeed; for example, 'three-legged insects', or 'three-cornered crystals with legs' (Slaughter *et al*. 1998). Delusional parasitosis has occurred in association with several medical disorders such as dementia, alcohol, endocrine disorders, anaemia, leukaemia, hypo-vitaminosis, encephalitis, syphilis, disseminated sclerosis, asthma, arthritis, renal disease, sensory disorders, and tumours. The disorder may respond to anxiolytic and neuroleptic medications.

Somatoform disorder NOS (not otherwise specified)

This is a residual category for 'persistent somatoform presentations that do not meet the criteria for somatization disorder or other somatoform disorder' (DSM-IV). The category is something of a 'vacuum cleaner', sweeping up irritating symptoms that are out of place elsewhere and neatly putting them into a psychiatric 'tidybin', which they may not deserve. Thus, a single unexplained somatic symptom that lasts longer than 6 months and causes a decrease in functioning and or significant distress could be classified as a disorder under this category. For example, Barsky's concept of transient hypochondriasis is relegated to this category.

Factitious disorders and malingering

Although not classified with the somatoform disorders, factitious disorder with physical symptoms and malingering need to be traversed in any consideration of somatoform presentations. They should be part of the differential diagnosis of any atypical somatoform disorder to avoid unnecessary medical treatment. In clinical settings, the negative countertransference met by the 'legitimate' somatoform disorders carries underlying connotations of 'faking', and at times it can be impossible to determine where the unconscious (as in somatoform disorder) ends and the conscious (as in factitious disorder) begins. Management of the two conditions may differ little.

Factitious disorder and malingering both involve faked symptoms but differ primarily in their goals, where factitious disorder has the presumptive aim of gaining caring (and usually intervention!) from the medical profession and malingering has a more specific goal, e.g. drugs, money. The prevalence is impossible to know, as is the usual course of these illnesses or 'careers'. Information is anecdotal as this population is wary of capture. However, these disorders are seen in older people and probably not always at the end of a long career. As with the other somatoform disorders (perhaps even more so) it is important to understand the reasons for the behaviour in order to best help the individual.

Case study 8.3

Mrs S. was 67 when first seen by the liaison psychiatrist. She had a long history of asthma for which she had been admitted to hospital several times. Her asthma attack resolved within a few days in hospital but she was left with the inability to speak, the features of which were typical for conversion aphonia. Background history revealed that she had long cared for a son with antisocial personality features who was about to go to prison. Her condition resolved after reassurance that recovery was expected, with voice exercises and, probably of most importance, social work intervention to rally family and community support. She was next referred at the age of 70 after prolonged and unsuccessful rehabilitation for atypical neurological symptoms, presumptively diagnosed as multiple sclerosis. Whilst in hospital, she had become incontinent and wheelchair-bound, helped by the generous donation of an electric wheelchair. She appeared very disabled with apparent contractures of her hands, weak legs, and incontinence. A careful history-taking revealed that two important people in her life had recently died from motor neurone disease, and one suspected that her symptoms were meant to convey this disorder. To the liaison psychiatrist it appeared that her main underlying problem was dependency and loneliness. Given the extent of her disability, it seemed futile to attempt a return to full independence. A programme of physiotherapy exercises was developed in line with a 'softly softly' approach. Mrs S. improved and was discharged to a rest home (with electric wheelchair) where she appeared happy enough for a while.

Then she became depressed and made a suicide attempt by driving her electric wheel-chair out in front of traffic. She was admitted to a psychiatric hospital where she was bluntly told that she would have to walk up to her room on the next floor or sleep where she was. She walked!

Treatment

Patients with somatic attributions present to physicians, not psychiatrists, hence they present in the liaison context. Referral to a psychiatrist is usually seen in negative terms or viewed as unfair punishment perpetrated upon an innocent patient for medical failure. Sometimes the patient appears to believe that the physician has the answers to solve the problem but for some unfathomable reason is choosing to withhold. Whilst grateful to the psychiatrist for being an empathic listener, he or she appears to believe them to be therapeutically useless!

Thus, the first major obstacle in treatment is dealing with the negative transference and countertransference that the patients engender. The patients are often angry or upset and may refuse an interview. They are often unwilling to discuss emotional matters, at least until the long list of somatic problems has been heard in its entirety. A patient- and detailed-assessment process may be very therapeutic in hearing what the person and their symptoms have to say.

Once over the initial transference hurdles, it is often necessary to enter into a protracted process to engage the person on to a treatment plan. The involvement of the referring medical team is very important. A major task is in assisting the team to understand the patient's somatic concerns and to develop a conjoint therapeutic approach. The main emphasis should be to manage all the patient's problems comprehensively within a geriatric rehabilitation model (Blazer 1996) with the focus on 'care not cure' (Barsky 1993).

In the first instance, it is usually counterproductive to attempt to convince the patient that their problems are more emotional than physical. It is generally better to acknowledge the veracity of the person's somatic experience first before exploring emotional symptoms. The patient's communication is in physical terms and it is important for the liaison psychiatrist to use this frame of reference to build rapport. Symptoms should be explored and clarified carefully, as communication failure between patient and physician may have led to misinterpretation and unnecessary worry. Education on how symptoms are perceived and appraised, along the lines described by Pennebaker and Barsky, discussed earlier, may help to correct underlying misconceptions and misattributions.

Any underlying psychiatric problems, such as depression or anxiety disorders, need treating with the appropriate medication. Patients may benefit from cognitive–behavioural techniques. Simple behavioural techniques, such as deep breathing and relaxation, can assist patients with comorbid anxiety and panic to convince them that they have personal control. Occupational and physical therapists can teach very disabled older people useful strategies to enhance strength and to renew activities with confidence (Mechanic 1995). Through these activities and the physical 'hands on' approach of these therapists, trust and rapport can be developed, allowing gentle uncovering of any underlying emotional concerns whilst providing legitimate physical treatment. More formally, attention training (Papageorgiou and Wells 1998) and individual or group cognitive therapy has been suggested as potentially useful in identifying misattributions, catastrophizing thoughts, and negative schemata in older patients (Grant and Casey 1995). The process can assist in the re-education of the person towards more effective coping styles and direct expressions of emotional distress. The wider social context contributing to the patient's somatoform presentation needs to be carefully analysed and sympathetically addressed.

Finally, it is also important to provide appropriate management for physical illness substrates and to avoid overmanagement (abnormal treatment behaviour), whilst maintaining optimum care of the individual. The somatization study of Smith *et al.* (1986) showed that regular but conservative management of this condition reduced illness behaviour and healthcare costs.

In conclusion

The somatoform disorders are a challenge for the liaison psychiatrist. The phenomena of somatization and hypochondriasis have many facets and layers of complexity that can become interwoven with the individual's pathophysiology, style of functioning, and interaction with caregivers. For older adults, the phenomena need to be seen as part of a total picture. The symptoms have many potential meanings for the patient–environment relationship. Focus on somatic symptoms may be a way of getting unacknowledged and poorly understood needs met. Somatization may be a coping mechanism in adversity, but not in normal times. The phenomena may be secondary to another underlying psychiatric disorder such as anxiety or depression. Somatization may have been a lifelong trait of the person's personality or be state-dependent in late life when overwhelmed by physical illness. The phenomena may reflect legitimate concern and worry over diagnosis and investigations. Alternatively, they may truly reflect a physical disorder and be misinterpreted by clinicians as of 'psychiatric' or 'psychological' origin.

When somatization appears to be a new phenomenon, this should alert the psychiatrist that there could be real undiagnosed physical illness, significant depression, or unrecognized cognitive impairment. In older people, it is highly likely that there will be an organic substrate. By seeking to understand the phenomena in their context, rather than stigmatizing the patient's symptoms as 'not real' or deprecating a patient's need to attain the sick role as 'illegitimate', the important issues of quality of life for the older person can be addressed.

References

American Psychiatric Association (1994). *Diagnostic and statistical manual of mental disorders (DSM-IV)*. American Psychiatric Association, Washington DC.

Barsky, A.J. (1992). Amplification, somatization, and the somatoform disorders. *Psychosomatics*, **33**, 28–34.

Barsky, A.J. (1993). The diagnosis and management of hypochondriacal concerns in the elderly. *Journal of Geriatric Psychiatry*, **26**, 129–41.

Barsky, A.J. and Wyshak, G. (1989). Hypochondriasis and related health attitudes. *Psychosomatics*, **30**, 412–20.

Barsky, A.J. and Wyshak, G. (1990). Hypochondriasis and somatosensory amplification. *British Journal of Psychiatry*, **157**, 404–9.

Barsky, A.J., Goodson, J.D., Lane, R.S., and Cleary, P.D. (1988). The amplification of somatic symptoms. *Psychosomatic Medicine*, **50**, 510–19.

Barsky, A.J., Wyshak, G., and Klerman, G.L. (1990a). Transient hypochondriasis. *Archives of General Psychiatry*, **47**, 746–52.

Barsky, A.J., Wyshak, G., Klerman, G.L., and Latham, K.S. (1990b). The prevalence of hypochondriasis in medical outpatients. *Social Psychiatry and Psychiatric Epidemiology*, **25**, 89–94.

Barsky, A.J., Frank, C.B., Cleary, P.D., Wyshak, G., and Klerman, G.L. (1991). The relation between hypochondriasis and age. *American Journal of Psychiatry*, **148**, 923–8.

Barsky, A.J., Barnett, M.C., and Clary, P.D. (1994). Hypochondriasis and panic disorder. Boundary and overlap. *Archives of General Psychiatry*, **51**, 918–25.

Baur, S. (1988). *Hypochondria: woeful imaginings*. University of California Press, Berkeley, CA.

Blazer, D. (1996). Geriatric psychiatry. In *The American Psychiatric Press synopsis of psychiatry* (ed. R.E. Hales and S.C. Schaie), pp. 1307–21. American Psychiatric Press, Washington DC.

Brink, T.L., Capri, D., De Neeve, V., Janakes, C., and Oliveira, C. (1979). Hypochondriasis and paranoia: similar delusional systems in an institutionalised geriatric population. *Journal of Nervous and Mental Disease*, **167**, 226.

Brink, T.L., Janakes, C., and Martinez, N. (1981). Geriatric hypochondriasis: situational factors. *Journal of the American Geriatrics Society*, **29**, 37–9.

Brown, F.W. (1991). Somatization disorder in progressive dementia. *Psychosomatics*, **32**,463–65.

Busse, E.W. (1976). Hypochondriasis in the elderly: a reaction to social stress. *Journal of the American Geriatrics Society*, **24**, 145–9.

Butler, R.N. (1978). The doctor and the aged patient. In *The geriatric patient* (ed. W. Reichel). HP Publishing, New York.

Chandler, J.D. and Gerndt, J. (1988). Somatization, depression and medical illness in psychiatric inpatients. *Acta Psychiatrica Scandinavica*, **77**, 67–73.

Escobar, J.l., Rubrio, M., Canini, G., and Karno, M. (1989). Somatic symptom index (SSI): a new and abridged somatization construct. Prevalence and epidemiological correlates in two large community samples. *Journal of Nervous and Mental Diseases*, **177**, 140–7.

Escobar, J.I., Gara, M., Waitzkin, H., Silver, R.C., Holman, A., and Compton, W. (1998). DSM-IV hypochondriasis in primary care. *General Hospital Psychiatry*, **20**, 155–9.

Farooq, S., Gahir, M.S., Okyere, E., Sheikh, A.J., and Oyebode, F. (1995). Somatization: a transcultural study. *Journal of Psychosomatic Research*, **39**, 883–8.

Ford, C.V. (1986). The somatizing disorders. *Psychosomatics*, **27**, 327–37.

Frisoni, G.B., Fedi, V., Geroldi, C., and Trabucchi M. (1999). Cognition and the perception of physical symptoms in the community-dwelling elderly. *Behavioral Medicine*, **25**, 5–12.

Gijsbers Van Wijk, C.M.T. and Kolk, A. (1997). Sex differences in physical symptoms: the contribution of symptom perception theory. *Social Science and Medicine*, **45**, 231–46.

Grant, R.W. and Casey, D.A. (1995). Adapting cognitive behavioral therapy for the frail elderly. *International Psychogeriatrics*, **7**, 561–71.

Hernandez, J. and Kellner, R. (1992). Hypochondriacal concerns and attitudes towards illness in males and females. *International Journal of Geriatric Psychiatry*, **22**, 251–63.

Hiller, W., Rief, W., and Fichter, M.M. (1997). How disabled are patients with somatoform disorders? *General Hospital Psychiatry*, **19**, 432–8.

Hyer, L., Gouveia, I., Harrison, W.R., Warsaw, J., and Coutsouridis, D. (1987). Depression, anxiety, paranoid reactions, hypochondriasis and cognitive decline of late life in-patients. *Journal of Gerontology*, **42**, 92–4.

Kellner, R. (1992). Diagnosis and treatments of hypochondriacal syndromes. *Psychosomatics*, **33**, 278–89.

Kellner, R. and Schneider-Braus, K. (1988). Distress and attitudes in patients perceived as hypochondriacal by medical staff. *General Hospital Psychiatry*, **10**, 157–62.

Kellner, R., Hernandez, J., and Pathak, D. (1992). Hypochondriacal fears and beliefs, anxiety, and somatization. *British Journal of Psychiatry*, **160**, 525–32.

Kent, D.A., Tomasson, K., and Coryell, W. (1995). Course and outcome of conversion and somatization disorders. A four-year follow-up. *Psychosomatics*, **36**, 138–44.

Kleinman, A. (1982). Neurasthenia and depression: a study of somatization and culture in China. *Culture, Medicine and Psychiatry*. **6**, 117–90.

Kroenke, K. and Spitzer, R.L. (1998). Gender differences in the reporting of physical and somatoform symptoms. *Psychosomatic Medicine*, **60**, 150–5.

LaMancusa, J. and Wyatt, R. (1990). Recurrent conversional right hemiplegia in an elderly hospitalized patient: issues in diagnosis. *Clinical Gerontologist*, **10**, 29–33.

Leibbrand, R., Hiller, W., and Fichter, M.M. (2000). Hypochondriasis and somatization: two distinct aspects of somatoform disorders? *Journal of Clinical Psychology*, **56**, 63–72.

Leventhal, E.A. and Prohaska, T.R. (1986). Age, symptom interpretation and health behaviour. *Journal of the American Geriatrics Society*, **34**, 183–91.

Leventhal, E.A., Hansell, S., Diefenbach, M., Leventhal, H., and Glass, D.C. (1996). Negative affect and self-report of physical symptoms: two longitudinal studies of older adults. *Health Psychology*, **15**, 193–9.

Liberini, P., Faglia, L., Salvi, F., and Grant, R.P. (1993*a*). What is the incidence of conversion pseudodementia? *British Journal of Psychiatry*, **162**, 124–6.

Liberini, P., Faglia, L., Salvi, F., and Grant, R.P. (1993*b*). Cognitive impairment related to conversion disorder: a two-year follow-up study. *Journal of Nervous and Mental Disease*, **181**, 325–7.

Lindesay, J., Briggs, K., and Murphy, E. (1989). The Guy's/Age Concern Survey: prevalence rates of cognitive impairment, depression and anxiety in an urban elderly community. *British Journal of Psychiatry*, **155**, 317–29.

Lipowski, Z.J. (1988). Somatization: the concept and the clinical application. *American Journal of Psychiatry*, **145**, 1358–68.

Lipowski, Z J. (1990). Somatization and depression. *Psychosomatics*, **31**, 13–21.

Mace, C.J. and Trimble, M.R. (1996). Ten-year prognosis of conversion disorder. *British Journal of Psychiatry*, **169**, 282–8.

Marmanidis, H., Holme, G., and Hafner, R.J. (1994). Depression and somatic symptoms: a cross-cultural study. *Australian and New Zealand Journal of Psychiatry*, **28**, 274–8.

Mechanic, D. (1995). Social dimensions of illness behaviour. *Social Science in Medicine*, **41**, 1207–16.

Monopoli, J. and Vaccaro, F.J. (1998). Depression, hypochondriasis and demographic variables in a non-institutionalized elderly sample. *Clinical Gerontologist*, **19**, 75–9.

Moselhy, H. and EL-Dosoky, A.M.R. (1996). Monosymptomatic hypochondriacal psychosis: grief as a precipitant. *European Journal of Psychiatry*, **10**, 243–5.

Noyes, R., Happel, R.L., and Yagla, S.J. (1999). Correlates of hypochondriasis in a nonclinical population. *Psychosomatics*, **40**, 461–9.

Opjordsmoen, S. (1988). Hypochondriacal psychosis: a long term follow-up. *Acta Psychiatrica Scandinavica*, **77**, 587–97.

Papageorgiou, C. and Wells, A. (1998). Effects of attention training on hypochondriasis: a brief case series. *Psychological Medicine*, **28**, 193–200.

Parsons, T. (1951). Illness and the role of the physician: a sociological perspective. *American Journal of Orthopsychiatry*, **21**, 452–60.

Pennebaker, J. (1982). *The psychology of physical symptoms*. Springer, New York.

Pfeiffer, E. (1977). Psychopathology and social pathology. In *Handbook of the psychology of ageing* (ed. J.E. Birren and K.W. Schaie), pp. 650–671. Van Nostrand, New York.

Piccinelli, M., Rucci, P., Uestuen, B., and Simon, G. (1999). Typologies of anxiety, depression and somatization symptoms among primary care attenders with no formal mental disorder. *Psychological Medicine*, **29**, 677–88.

Pilowsky, I. (1970). Primary and secondary hypochondriasis. *Acta Psychiatrica Scandinavia*, **46**, 273–85.

Pilowsky, I. (1978). A general classification of abnormal illness behaviours. *British Journal Medical Psychology*, **51**, 131–7.

Rasanen, P., Erkonen, K., Isaksson U., Koho, P., Varis, R., Timonmen, M., *et al.* (1997). Delusional parasitosis in the elderly: a review and report of six cases from Northern Finland. *International Psychogeriatrics*, **9**, 459–64.

Schmidt, A.J.M. (1994). Bottlenecks in the diagnosis of hypochondriasis. *Comprehensive Psychiatry*, **35**, 306–15.

Simon, G.E. and Gureje, O. (1999). Stability of somatization disorder and somatization symptoms among primary care patients. *Archives of General Psychiatry*, **56**, 90–5.

Singh, B.S., Nunn, K., Martin, J., and Yates, J. (1981). Abnormal treatment behaviour. *British Journal of Medical Psychology*, **54**, 67–73.

Slaughter, J.R., Zanol, K., Rezvani, H., and Flax, J. (1998). Psychogenic parasitosis: a case series and literature review. *Psychosomatics*, **39**, 491–500.

Smith, G.R., Monson, R.A., and Ray, D.C. (1986). Psychiatric consultation in somatization disorder. A randomised controlled study. *New England Journal of Medicine*, **314**, 1407–13.

Trabert, W. (1995). A hundred years of delusional parasitosis. *Psychopathology*, **28**, 238–46.

Verbrugge, L.M. (1989). The twain meet: empirical explanations of sex differences in health and mortality. *Journal of Health and Social Behavior*, **30**, 282–304.

Walker, R., Gregory, J., Oakley, S. Jr, and Bloch, R. (1996). Reduction in dissociation due to ageing and cognitive deficit. *Comprehensive Psychiatry*, **37**, 31–6.

Wool, C.A. and Barsky, A.J. (1994). Do women somatize more than men? Gender differences in somatization. *Psychosomatics*, **35**, 445–52.

Wykoff, R.F. (1987). Delusions of parasitosis: a review. *Reviews of Infectious Diseases*, **9**, 433–7.

9   Psychosis and medical illness

Osvaldo P. Almeida

Summary

Delusions and hallucinations are relatively common amongst older adults treated in the general hospital. This chapter reviews the concept of psychosis, the biological and psychological mechanisms likely to be involved in its origin, the most frequent causes of psychotic symptoms in later life, and the evidence currently available on how best to manage these patients.

Introduction

Psychotic symptoms are frequent amongst older adults receiving medical care in general hospitals. These symptoms are a source of distress to both patients and medical staff, and their presence almost always triggers consultation requests to psychiatric services. Therefore, consultant psychiatrists need to be familiar with the issues involved in the assessment, diagnosis, and management of elderly psychotic patients in general medical wards. This chapter reviews the concept of psychotic symptoms, the most frequent causes of psychosis, their prevalence in later life, and the principles of assessment and management.

What is psychosis?

Psychosis is the general label used to describe a state of gross impairment in reality testing. The mechanisms that underlie the development of psychotic symptoms result in distortions of perception (e.g. illusions and hallucinations), thought content (e.g. paranoid delusions), or consciousness (e.g. delusions of influence).

Perceptual abnormalities

Karl Jaspers (1997) suggested that objects (internal or external) exist in the form of 'perceptions' (objective) or 'ideas' (subjective). Perception is the process whereby

191

information about the external and internal environment is detected through sensory organs and made available for conscious work-up. Anomalies of perception include changes in intensity (e.g. colours may seem brighter than usual with the use of morphine-like substances) and quality. Abnormal characteristics of perception include derealization (when the world is *perceived* as something strange, different from the usual), splitting of perception (e.g. when the sound and the image of someone speaking do not seem to belong together), and false perceptions. The latter describes all abnormal perceptions in which unreal objects are perceived as real, leading to the experience of illusions and hallucinations.

Illusions are defined as distortions of actual sensory perceptions. They may be due to affect (e.g. fear or depression), imagination (also called pareidolia), and decreased levels of attention. Examples of illusions include the misperception that the wire coming out of a heart monitor is a snake, or that a shadow on the wall is a threatening intruder. Illusions are considered pathological when the belief in the misperception persists despite convincing evidence to the contrary. Patients suffering from delirium are particularly prone to the development of pathological illusions secondary to the impairment of attention.

Hallucinations are perceptual experiences that are not related to external stimuli. They can occur in any sensory modality and may appear in elementary or complex forms. Elementary hallucinations are simple perceptions of sound, light, odour, etc., whereas complex hallucinations tend to be more elaborate: accusing voices, visions of dead people in the house, etc. Pseudohallucinations differ from hallucinations in two ways: they are figurative, not real, and are experienced in the subjective inner world (for example, seeing faces with the mind while keeping eyes closed or hearing voices that come from inside the head).

Distortions of thought content (delusions)

'Since time immemorial delusion has been taken as the basic characteristic of madness. To be mad was to be deluded and indeed what constitutes a delusion is one of the basic problems of psychopathology' (Jaspers 1997). Delusions manifest themselves as idiosyncratic falsified judgements about the world or oneself that lead to the development of ideas that are held with great conviction and subjective certainty. The ideas are not changed by other experiences or compelling evidence to the contrary, are impossible or highly improbable, and are not shared by other people living in the same socioeconomic environment.

Primary delusion is the name given to a delusional idea that does not arise from other psychological phenomena, such as hallucinations (for example, a patient said that when he saw the traffic lights going red he realized that an atomic bomb was about to fall on the city). Primary delusions are relatively uncommon and their presence suggests the diagnosis of schizophrenia. Secondary delusions are more frequent and represent an intellectual attempt to attribute meaning to abnormal experiences, such as primary delusions, hallucinations, or abnormal mood (for example, the patient who 'heard' a voice telling her to kill herself developed the belief that her house was bugged with microphones that had been installed by a neighbour who was trying to get rid of her). Secondary delusions are often grouped together to form a delusional system that gives support to a central delusional belief or theme. Table 9.1 lists the most frequent types of delusional ideas found in clinical practice.

Mechanisms involved in the development of psychotic symptoms

The psychological and physiological processes that underlie the development of psychotic symptoms are not well understood. A number of psychological theories have been proposed to explain the development of psychotic symptoms and, in particular, delusions. The most popular of them was introduced by Sigmund Freud in his psychoanalytical theory of psychosis. Freud (1911) suggested that delusions are the final result of repressed homosexual conflicts and that 'projection' is the psychological mechanism involved in its development: *I do not love him—I hate him, because he persecutes me* (persecutory delusion), or *I do not love her—I love him, because he loves me* (erotomanic delusion), or *I do not love him—she loves him* (delusion of infidelity). This theory has not yet received adequate empirical support.

Other theoretical models propose that delusional systems are built to make the subjective existential experience of the individual more meaningful (Fig. 9.1 see page 196). Roberts (1991), for example, investigated a sample of 17 subjects with longstanding delusional beliefs. They described a high level of perceived purpose and meaning to life in comparison to patients with chronic schizophrenia in remission. In fact, after the complete remission of psychotic symptoms, one patient described his life as meaningless and lonely. Others (for example, see Garety 1991) have proposed that patients with delusions come to conclusions at levels of probability that are too low for acceptance by normal persons. This theory suggests that delusions are a product of defective reasoning.

Chris Frith (1988, 1992) developed a model to explain the development of psychoses that brings psychopathology and neuropsychology together. He proposed the existence of an internal monitor that receives information about intended actions, which are then adjusted according to specific goals or plans in order to select the most appropriate response. In addition, the model predicts that when an action is initiated internally (i.e. with no environmental stimuli), the monitor is informed about it through a mechanism similar to the corollary discharge. For example, if a subject decides to move his arm to reach out for his cup of tea, the internal monitor will be informed that the action (i.e. movement of the arm) was initiated internally and not as a result of an external stimulus. This means that the monitor is informed, through a feedback loop, that the action that is being carried out (i.e. movement of the arm) was initiated within the limits of the individual's self. Frith (1992) has argued that if this loop is defective the subject may initiate an action and not be aware of it. In the example above, the subject may feel that his arm is being moved,

Table 9.1 Examples of the most frequent types of delusions found in clinical practice

Type of delusion	Main features	Examples
Delusions of persecution	Subjects feel pursued, tormented, persecuted by people or organizations that aim to harm, kill, undermine the reputation, or make him go mad. These symptoms are very frequent amongst patients with schizophrenia, but it can also be observed in patients with mood disorders, dementia, and other neuropsychiatric conditions.	My neighbours are trying to get rid of me. They've been pumping poisonous gases into the house.
Delusions of reference	Objects, events, and people acquire an obvious relation to the patient himself. People look at the patient in particularly meaningful ways. Odd words heard from different people are specially directed to the patient, concern his personal life, and are meant to warn or insult him. News read in the newspaper or heard on the television are specially directed at the patient. Delusions of reference are often associated with persecutory delusions. They can also be observed amongst patients with mood disorders and, less frequently, other neuropsychiatric diseases.	I went to the supermarket this morning; everybody was looking at me, they were making comments amongst themselves to indicate that nobody should get too close to me because I have a contagious disease. Last night the news was constantly making references to my health.
Grandiose delusions	Exaggerated ideas of one's importance, power, knowledge, abilities, wealth, or identity. These symptoms are typically observed amongst patients with mania. They are also frequent in dementia, particularly of frontal lobe type.	My parents came from England last century. We are the real Royal Family in England. I will now be made the Queen of Australia.
Delusions of, guilt negation, and nihilistic delusions	Exaggerated ideas about one's sin and responsibility for certain events are the main features of the delusions of guilt. In more severe cases subjects may feel that nothing, not even themselves, exist (delusions of negation). Patients with nihilist delusions feel that parts of their body are rotting away or are dead. In some cases subjects believe that they themselves are dead. These symptoms are more often associated with depression, but have also beer described amongst patients with schizophrenia and dementia.	I have ruined the life of all my family. We will now have to live in a state of total misery. Things will never get better. There is no point in taking this medication. My intestines do not exist, they've rotted away and are now dead. There is nothing inside my body, just empty and dead space

Hypochondriasis and somatic delusion	Constant concerns about one's body and physical health. Subjects are convinced that they suffer from a dreadful disease, or that a minor change of heart rate indicates an imminent heart attack. They constantly seek reassurance from doctors, but are never totally convinced that no major problems are present. In extreme forms the patient may develop somatic delusions (or hypochondriacal delusions). Delusional parasitosis (Ekbom's syndrome) is one particular type of somatic delusion. These symptoms can be observed amongst patients with psychotic depression, schizophrenia, and, less frequently, dementia.	*My liver is paralysed—I cannot digest anything I eat. I am sure it is a type of cancer that the doctors cannot see with their tests.* *My brain is being eaten by a little mouse.* *Insects are constantly walking under my skin.* *I have two little worms living inside my body: one in the vagina, the other in my rectum.*
Misidentifications	The misidentification syndromes (or symptoms) refer to delusional beliefs that other people, oneself, or the place has been substituted by impostors or replicas. The Capgras' syndrome (or symptom) is the name used to describe the belief that an imposter has replaced a person who is close to the patient. Less frequently, the patient recognizes a familiar person in others who do not show any obvious physical resemblance (Frégoli's syndrome). Other misidentifications include not recognizing oneself in the mirror and reduplicative paramnesia (when a familiar place is substituted by a replica). Capgras' symptoms are more often observed in schizophrenia, mood disorders, and dementia. The other misidentification syndromes are also relatively frequent in dementia and other neuropsychiatric disorders.	*My husband has been taken away from me. This one looks just like him, but is not him.* *Hello, how are you doing today? (looking at the mirror and not recognizing own image).*
Erotomanic delusions and delusions of infidelity	A woman with erotomanic delusions (also known as Clérambault syndrome) is convinced that a man, usually of higher socioeconomic status, is in love with her. Delusions of infidelity (also known as Othello's syndrome) are characterized by the belief that the partner is being unfaithful. The first is more frequent amongst patients with schizophrenia, whereas delusions of infidelity are more common amongst patients with alcoholism and dementia.	*When he walked passed my house I noticed that he shook his head as an indication that our love cannot yet be disclosed to the general public.* *Yes, she is having an affair. She now wants to go out every week to this club for the elderly. She denies it, but I am convinced that she meets her lover there.*

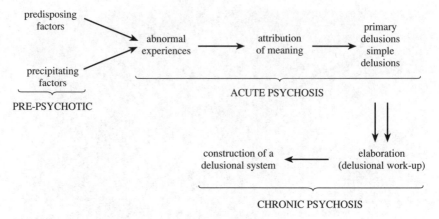

Fig. 9.1 Model of delusional formation according to Roberts (1991). Reproduced with permission of Royal College of Psychiatrists.

rather than that he is moving it (delusion of control). Similarly, one can predict that a defect in the monitoring of inner speech might be experienced as an auditory hallucination. Following this same line of thought, Frith (1992) has proposed that many psychotic symptoms can be explained as the result of a problematic initiation and monitoring of action. In addition, one can predict a number of cognitive deficits amongst psychotic patients, such as perseverative responses in tasks of attention set-shift, increased stimulus response latencies, decreased verbal fluency output, and deficits on tests of planning and working memory (see Fig. 9.2 on page 197). Such an attempt to link psychotic symptoms to cognitive deficits has received good empirical support (Frith 1992; Gold *et al.* 1992; Almeida *et al.* 1995*c*).

Sensory impairment has also been associated with the development of psychotic symptoms, particularly in the elderly. Hearing impairment, for example, has been experimentally (Zimbardo *et al.* 1981) and clinically (Almeida *et al.* 1995*a*) associated with the development of paranoid symptoms. Cooper (1976) found that the characteristics of deafness more strongly associated with psychosis were early age of onset, long duration, and profound auditory loss. Cooper and Porter (1976) suggested that these deficits might reinforce a pre-existing tendency to social isolation, withdrawal, and suspiciousness. Furthermore, it seems that auditory hallucinations are the most consistent psychopathological phenomenon associated with hearing impairment (Corbin and Eastwood 1986). Reports of a significant reduction of psychotic symptoms after the fitting of a hearing aid indicate that deafness contributes, at least as a predisposing or precipitating factor, to the development of symptoms (Almeida *et al.* 1993). Similarly, psychotic symptoms (particularly visual hallucinations) have been associated with visual impairment. In one study, for example, major ocular pathology (predominantly cataracts) was found in 30 of 54 elderly patients with psychosis (Cooper and Porter 1976).

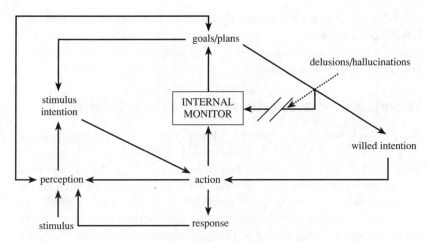

Fig. 9.2 Frith's (1988) model of the development of psychotic symptoms. The internal monitor receives information about intended actions, which are then modified according to specific goals and plans. Perception of external stimuli can be modified by goals and plans at an unconscious level, which is achieved by a signal indicating expected actions. The figure shows one possible disruption of the traffic of information within the system: goals and plans fail to reach the monitor and the subject may experience positive psychotic symptoms.
Source Frith, C.D. and Done, D.J. Towards a neuropsychology of Schizophrenia, *British Journal of Psychiatry*, 1988, 437–43. Reproduced with permission of Royal College of Psychiatrists.

Some personality traits have been associated with the later development of psychotic symptoms: quarrelsome, religious, suspicious, sensitive, unsociable, and cold-hearted (Almeida *et al.* 1992). In some patients, particularly those without hallucinations, the psychotic symptoms may be seen as an exacerbation or caricature of their deviant premorbid personality. In addition, patients with late-life psychosis are more likely to be socially isolated (Almeida *et al.* 1995*a*).

Finally, there is increasing evidence of structural and functional brain abnormalities amongst older adults with psychotic symptoms. Neuroimaging studies indicate that late-life psychosis is often associated with cerebrovascular pathology, either in the form of white matter changes or infarcts (Flint *et al.* 1991; Miller *et al.* 1992). Other signs of cerebral disease include an increased ventricle–brain ratio (Rabins *et al.* 1987; Burns *et al.* 1989) and some degree of brain atrophy (Howard *et al.* 1994, 1995). In addition, it seems that subjects with Alzheimer's disease who become psychotic have better preserved cerebral cortex than non-psychotic patients (Jacoby and Levy 1980). In fact, a neuropathological evaluation of patients with Alzheimer's disease showed that subjects with psychotic symptoms have a relatively larger number of neurons in parahippocampal areas but decreased numbers in the raphe nucleus when compared to non-psychotic patients (Förstl *et al.* 1994). Moreover, psychotic symptoms amongst patients with organic mental disorders, particularly delirium and dementia, have been associated with hypoactivity (or chemical blockade) of cholinergic systems in the brain (Gibson *et al.* 1991; Perry *et al.* 1998). This hypothesis is empirically supported by the observation that certain anticholinergic agents may produce psychotic symptoms, and by the results of recent studies reporting a beneficial effect of anticholinesterase treatment on the behavioural disturbances of patients with dementia (Morris *et al.* 1998). ᐱ

Prevalence of psychotic symptoms in later life

There is only scattered information available on the prevalence of delusions and hallucinations in later life. The Epidemiological Catchment Area (ECA) study found that 16–23% of older adults showed some form of 'organic' psychoses (Myers *et al.* 1984). Christenson and Blazer (1984) identified 40 (4%) cases of 'paranoia' amongst 997 elderly subjects living in the community. In Australia, the point prevalence of psychotic symptoms was 6% amongst the 935 subjects living in the community (approximately 10% were living in sheltered accommodation) (Henderson *et al.* 1998). Delusions and hallucinations are present in one-quarter of elderly psychiatry outpatients (Holroyd and Laurie 1999) and one-third of older adults attending day-care centres (Cohen-Mansfield *et al.* 1998). The prevalence of psychotic symptoms amongst older adults treated as inpatients in general medical wards has not yet been established.

Causes of psychotic symptoms in later life

Delusions and hallucinations in early life are almost always associated with the diagnosis of schizophrenia, mood disorder, or substance abuse or withdrawal. In later life, however, the diagnostic possibilities are much more varied (Table 9.2). A retrospective chart review of 1730 patients admitted to a psychogeriatric service in the United States indicated that dementia was the most frequent cause of psychotic symptoms in later life (40%), followed by depression (33%), delirium (7%), other medical causes (7%), bipolar disorder (5%), drug intoxication (4%), delusional disorder (2%), schizophrenia (1%), and schizoaffective disorder (1%) (Webster and Grossberg 1998). The following sections describe the main clinical features of psychosis amongst patients with dementia, delirium, mood disorders, and late-onset schizophrenia.

Dementia

Delusions and hallucinations are common in almost all types of dementia, but are particularly frequent amongst patients with Alzheimer's disease (AD), dementia with Lewy bodies (DLB), and Parkinson's disease (PD).

Estimates of the prevalence of delusions in AD range from 10 to 73% (Rao and Lyketsos 1998). These figures vary according to the setting of the study, the definition of psychotic symptoms, the period investigated, and the instruments used for the assessment of patients. The annual incidence rate of delusional beliefs has

Table 9.2 Frequent causes of psychotic symptoms

Psychiatric disorders	Metabolic and endocrine disorders	Medication
Schizophrenia (early or late onset)	Fluid and electrolyte imbalance	Anticholinergic drugs
Delusional disorder	Cardiac/hepatic/renal/respiratory failure	Dopaminergic drugs (L-dopa, agonists)
Delirium	Porphyria	Benzodiazepines
Alzheimer's disease	Cushing's disease	Antidepressants
Dementia with Lewy bodies	Thyroid disorders	Lithium
Vascular dementia	Pituitary dysfunction	Disulfiram
Frontotemporal dementia		Analgesics (narcotics)
Mood disorders (mania or depression)	_Neurological disorders_	Antituberculous drugs (isoniazid, cycloserine)
Acute psychotic reaction	Cerebrovascular disease or strokes	Anti-inflammatory drugs (indometacin, phenylbutazone)
Schizoaffective disorder	Huntington's disease	Antihypertensive agents (e.g. reserpine and methyldopa)
Factitious disorder	Parkinson's disease	Cardiac drugs (digitalis, procainamide, propranolol)
	Progressive supranuclear palsy	Idiosyncratic reaction
Infections	Brain tumours	
AIDS	Epilepsy	_Intoxication_
Encephalitis	Hydrocephalus	Alcohol
Malaria	Hypertensive encephalopathy	Barbiturates
Syphilis	Prion diseases	Hallucinogens, marijuana (LSD, amphetamines, mescaline, etc.)
Typhoid	Narcolepsy	Opiates
Neurocysticercosis	Sensory impairment	Carbon monoxide
	Multiple sclerosis	
	Brain injury	
	Subdural haematoma	
	Other	

been estimated as 2.4% (Flynn _et al._ 1991). Burns and colleagues (1990) found that 28 (16%) of 178 patients with AD living in the community displayed some type of delusional belief, particularly delusions of theft and suspicion that the patient was being watched or that the spouse was being unfaithful. Delusions of persecution, reference, jealousy, grandiosity, and somatic are also common (Burns _et al._ 1990, Deutsch _et al._ 1991; McShane _et al._ 1998).

Hallucinations, particularly of the visual type, are also relatively common amongst patients with dementia. Reported rates range from 7 to 25% for patients with AD (Burns and Levy 1992) and 23 to 72% in DLB (Ballard _et al._ 1999). The results of a recently published, prospective clinical and neuropathological study investigating the psychiatric morbidity amongst patients with dementia found that 72% of 98 patients with DLB and 16% of 92 patients with AD displayed visual hallucinations at presentation (Ballard _et al._ 1999). The authors argued that the presence of psychotic symptoms in association with parkinsonism and fluctuation of cognitive functioning is highly suggestive of DLB (McKeith *et al.* 1996). The diagnosis of DLB is of clinical significance, as these patients may develop severe adverse reactions to the use of typical antipsychotics (McKeith *et al.* 1992, 1995).

Psychotic symptoms have also been associated with the development of aggressive behaviour. Lyketsos *et al.* (1999) described that aggressive patients were 3.8 times more likely to be deluded and 3.2 times more likely to experience hallucinations than non-aggressive patients. In addition, a 4-year cohort study showed that patients who had delusions or hallucinations at baseline were more likely to become physically aggressive or hyperactive during the follow-up period (McShane *et al.* 1998).

Parkinson's disease, with or without dementia, has also been associated with the development of psychotic symptoms in later life. Aarsland and colleagues (1999) have recently described the prevalence and clinical correlates of psychotic symptoms in 235 patients with PD living in nine Norwegian towns. Of these, 23 (9.8%) had hallucinations with insight retained, and 14 (6.0%) had psychosis with hallucinations or delusions during the week prior to assessment. Some 32 subjects (13.6%) reported having experienced clear psychotic symptoms at some point after the clinical diagnosis of PD was made. Patients with psychotic symptoms or hallucinations were older, had higher depressive and lower cognitive scores, and a more severe illness according to the Unified Parkinson's Disease Rating Scale. Surprisingly, there was no difference between patients with and without psychotic symptoms with regard to the dose of levodopa received. The authors (Aarsland *et al.* 1999) concluded that levodopa treatment and the widespread brain changes that characterize severe PD may interact to render patients more vulnerable to the development of psychotic symptoms (see also Wolters 1996).

Delirium

Delirium is a disorder characterized by an impairment of consciousness and reduced ability to direct, sustain, or shift attention. This diagnosis is present in 10–25% of older adults on hospital admission, although rates can be even higher in intensive care or surgical units (see Chapter 10). Early recognition of delirium is important, as morbidity and mortality may increase if the condition is not quickly reversed.

Webster and Grossberg (1998) reported that 11 (6.6%) of the 166 patients admitted to a psychogeriatric unit due to the presence of psychotic symptoms had delirium. Similarly, Holroyd and Laurie (1999) found that 6 (12.2%) out of 49 psychotic patients referred to a geriatric outpatient mental health service met criteria for the diagnosis of delirium. However, the exact prevalence of psychotic symptoms amongst older adults with delirium admitted to general medical wards has not yet been established.

The clinical presentation of delirium in later life is extremely variable. For some patients the most prominent features may be the sudden development of illusions, hallucinations, fleeting delusions, or agitated behaviour. Ross and colleagues (1991) found that these symptoms were present in approximately one-third of their 58 patients meeting criteria for the diagnosis of delirium in a general hospital. They also described that psychotic symptoms were more likely to be associated with psycho-motor agitation. In such cases, the consultant psychiatrist may be able to assist the consulting medical practitioner in clarifying the diagnosis of delirium and organiz-ing appropriate investigations and management plans for the patient.

Mood disorders

Depression is frequent amongst older adults admitted to general hospitals due to conditions such as cardiovascular disease, cancer, stroke, and Parkinson's disease (see Chapter 6). An as yet unknown proportion of patients will develop delusions and hallucinations during the course of their depressive illness. Data from psycho-geriatric services suggest that 28–50% of older adults with depression report the presence of delusions and hallucinations (Soares and Gershon 1997; Webster and Grossberg 1998). In addition, Henderson and colleagues (1998) found that depres-sion was one of the most robust predictors of psychosis amongst older adults living in the community (a small fraction was living in nursing homes). They also described that 9.7% of all older adults with psychotic symptoms met criteria for the diagnosis of a depressive disorder according to ICD-10. Clinical reports suggest that the most frequent delusional themes amongst these patients are somatic and persecutory. Less often, subjects may report delusions of guilt, sin, poverty, jealousy, or nihilism (Ruegg *et al.* 1988).

Older adults with psychotic depression seem to differ from non-psychotic patients in some respects. Simpson and colleagues (1999), for example, investigated the clinical features of 99 patients with depression enrolled consecutively from two psychogeriatric services in the UK. The 18 patients with psychotic symptoms had worse physical health, worse performance on tests of executive functioning and mental processing, increased number of brain lesions on MRI scan, and poorer response to antidepressant treatment. In addition, Flint and Rifat (1998*a*) have shown that subjects with psychotic depression who recover after treatment were more likely to relapse (9 out of 19) than non-psychotic patients (10 out of 68) during a 2-year follow-up.

Schizophrenia and delusional disorder in later life

The incidence and prevalence of schizophrenia and delusional disorders of later life (also known as 'late paraphrenia or late-life schizophrenia-like psychosis') are still uncertain, as basic epidemiological data are sparse and difficult to interpret (differ-ent studies tend to use different diagnostic and age cut-off criteria). Most epidemio-logical surveys of the condition have retrospectively examined the rate of patients admitted to mental hospitals, but there are a few case-register evaluations and community surveys that provide an overall idea of the frequency of such conditions. Late-life psychosis seems to represent approximately 10% of the elderly population of psychiatric hospitals. The reported prevalence of the disorder among the elderly living in the community ranges from 0.1 to 1.7% (Henderson and Kay 1997), and its incidence has been estimated to be between 10–26/100 000 per year. On average, only 1.5% of those who receive the diagnosis of schizophrenia have the onset of illness after 60 years of age, in contrast to 23% and 16% of patients with other paranoid states and reactive psychoses, respectively. Schizophrenia and delusional disorder with onset in later life are more frequent amongst women, and people who have sensory impairment or are socially isolated (Almeida *et al*. 1995*a*).

A wide range of delusional activity has been observed amongst these patients, including delusions of persecution, reference, misidentification, delusions of control, hypochondriasis, grandiosity, and sexual and religious delusions. Persecutory delusions have been found in 80–90% of patients (Almeida *et al*. 1995*a*), and auditory hallucinations in up to 75% of cases (Almeida *et al*. 1995*b*). Visual, olfactory, tactile, and somatic hallucinations are less common, but not rare. Other frequent symptoms include the first-rank symptoms of Schneider (FRS), present in 35–64% of patients, and a variety of depressive features, found in 42–60% of subjects (Almeida *et al*. 1995*b*). Thought disorder and negative symptoms are uncommon (Almeida *et al*. 1995*b*).

A specific type of delusional disorder that is reasonably frequent among older adults in the general hospital is monosymptomatic hypochondriasis. Hypochondriacal ideas can be divided into primary and secondary (i.e. associated with depression, schizophrenia, dementia, etc.). Primary hypochondriasis is often associated with longstanding hypochondriacal traits and can, in later life, develop into a full-flown delusional disorder (with the subjective experience of disease conviction—see Table 9.1). Hypochondriasis is also covered in Chapter 8.

Management of psychosis in later life

Managing elderly subjects with psychotic symptoms is a complex task. First, it is important to ensure that patients receive a thorough clinical assessment leading up to the correct diagnosis of the underlying condition. Second, all current medical disorders and medications should be clarified before new drugs are prescribed—older adults are more likely to experience adverse drug reactions and some interactions between medication may be particularly harmful (e.g. urinary retention when two drugs with anticholinergic properties are use concomitantly). Finally, treatment is unlikely to succeed if the clinician fails to establish good rapport and build a trusting relationship with the patient, who is often guarded, suspicious, and has limited insight into his or her mental state (Almeida *et al*. 1996).

Treatment will depend on the causes leading up to the development of psychotic symptoms, although the use of antipsychotic medication should be considered as an option in the treatment of most patients. Table 9.3 summarizes the issues physicians should be aware of before prescribing antipsychotic drugs to older adults.

Table 9.3 Issues to be considered when prescribing antipsychotic medication for older adults

	Effects associated with ageing	Consequence of the use of antipsychotic drugs
Pharmacokinetics	Decrease in gastric acidity Decrease in splanchnic blood flow Decrease in lean body mass Decreased clearance Decline in function of CYP3A Decline in function of CYP1A No age-related changes in CYP2D6	Increased biological availability of medication. Note that perphenazine, thioridazine and risperidone are metabolized by CYP2D6. Olanzapine and clozapine are metabolized by CYP3A4.
Extrapyramidal side-effects	Increased sensitivity to development of parkinsonism, acathisia, and TD	Whenever possible, avoid the use of typical antipsychotic medication. Risperidone in daily doses higher than 2 mg (or less) may also produce significant EPS. The risk of TD increases with increasing daily dose. Approximately half of the elderly exposed to antipsychotic medication will develop TD during the following 36 months.[a]
Falls	Orthostatic hypotension Impaired mobility Decreased reflexes Increased risk of fractures Cognitive decline	Orthostatic hypotension is a common side-effect of antipsychotic medication, particularly low-potency antipsychotics such as thioridazine and chlorpromazine. Clozapine is also associated with an increased risk of postural hypotension.[b]
Osteoporosis	Increased bone catabolism	The use of typical antipsychotic medication and risperidone is associated with elevation in the levels of prolactin. Prolactin decreases the levels of gonadal hormones and, as a consequence, may lead to decreased bone mineral density and osteoporosis.
Cognition	Mild decline in some cognitive abilities Increased risk of dementia	The anticholinergic effect of antipsychotic drugs may contribute to deterioration in cognitive functioning. This is particularly important for patients with delirium and dementia. It is still unclear whether atypical antipsychotic medication interferes with cognitive functioning.

Table 9.3 Issues to be considered when prescribing antipsychotic medication for older adults (cont.)

	Effects associated with ageing	Consequence of the use of antipsychotic drugs
Constipation, urinary retention, and others	Increased susceptibility to the effects of anticholinergic drugs	Low-potency antipsychotic drugs have clinically significant anticholinergic properties and may increase the risk of constipation, dry mouth, and urinary retention.
Weight gain	Increase in the proportion of fat tissue	Low-potency antipsychotic drugs such as chlorpromazine are associated with significant weight gain. The use of atypical drugs such as clozapine, olanzapine, quetiapine, and risperidone may also lead to weight gain.[d] Beware of the interaction between obesity and the risk of cardiovascular diseases and diabetes.
Heart functioning	Increased risk of heart-related problems	Antipsychotic agents (including atypical) may produce postural hypotension, tachycardia, conduction disturbances, arrhythmia, and ventricular fibrillation. Patients on calcium-channel blockers or diuretics may be at an increased risk of potassium and magnesium depletion—this may predispose even further to the risk of QT prolongation and arrhythmia.[e]
Ocular	Increased risk of cataract, macular degeneration, glaucoma	Typical antipsychotic drugs may produce corneal, conjunctival, and retinal pigmentation—this side-effect is more often associated with the use of thioridazine. The anticholinergic properties of some agents may cause difficulties with visual accommodation and worsen the clinical symptoms of previously existing glaucoma. Quetiapine may produce lens opacities.[e]
Sexual functioning	Increase in time to become sexually aroused Increase in time to reach orgasm Ageing-associated genitourinary changes	Antipsychotic medication may decrease sexual interest and pleasure. Thioridazine, fluphenazine, and trifluoperazine have been associated with female anorgasmia. Agents with alpha-adrenergic activity (cf. chlorpromazine and thioridazine) may produce sexual dysfunction and ejaculatory impairment.[e]

[a]Woerner et al. 1998; [b]Verhaeverbeke and Mets 1997; [c]Halbreich et al. 1995; [d]McManus et al. 1999; [e]Maixner et al. 1999. TD, tardive dyskinesia; EPS, extrapyramidal side-effects.

Managing psychotic patients in general medical wards

Patients with psychotic symptoms are usually avoided by other patients and staff and often labelled as 'mad' and 'weird'—this contributes to increasing their isolation and suspiciousness. Unfortunately, the development of 'plots' to get rid of patients do not only take place in their imagination—consultation requests are frequently used to persuade the psychiatrist to take responsibility for the care of psychotic patients and move them to psychiatric wards. Hence, supporting and educating staff working with these patients is an essential part of the consultation process. It is worth remembering that these patients have been placed in an unfamiliar environment and have, to some extent, lost control over their lives. For this reason, it is important that patients regain some control over the situation by actively getting involved in the decisions about investigations and therapies that may be introduced. This involvement is the first step to ensure long-term compliance with treatment (psychiatric or otherwise) and to reduce the threat associated with hospitalization.

Most older adults who experience psychotic symptoms can be managed in general medical wards. However, patients should be transferred to more secure environments when safety issues arise (e.g. aggressive behaviour towards self/others or inappropriate intrusive activities such as the manipulation of the medical equipment used by other patients).

There are few placebo-controlled studies looking at the efficacy and safety profile of antipsychotic medication for the treatment of delusions and hallucinations in later life. They can be generally divided into two groups: management of behavioural problems in dementia; and treatment of late-onset schizophrenia.

Use of antipsychotic medication in patients with dementia

Thioridazine is one of the most widely prescribed antipsychotic drugs for the management of behavioural problems in dementia. A recent meta-analysis by Kirchner et al. (1998) concluded that there is no clear evidence that thioridazine use improves general measures of behaviour, although they did find that the drug reduces anxiety when compared to placebo. Surprisingly, thioridazine had no obvious effect on delusions and hallucinations. In addition, recent concerns over its cardiac safety further limits its utility.

Haloperidol is another drug often used in clinical practice for the treatment of behavioural problems in subjects with dementia. Devanand and colleagues (1998) reported its efficacy for the treatment of 'psychosis and disruptive behaviours' in a 6-week, double-blind, placebo-controlled clinical trial of 60 outpatients with AD (there were 11 dropouts). Subjects were randomly allocated to receive either placebo or treatment with haloperidol in low dose (0.5–0.75 mg per day) or standard dose (2–3 mg per day). They reported a 25% improvement on the psychotic subscale of the BPRS (brief psychiatric rating scale) in 12/20 patients receiving the standard dose of haloperidol—6/20 patients receiving low doses of haloperidol and 5/20 given a placebo also improved. The authors claimed that haloperidol in doses of 2–3 mg/day had a favourable therapeutic profile, although these results are rather difficult to generalize. First, the study was limited to outpatients, possibly with mild dementia. Second, the duration of the trial was short and the long-term impact of the use of the medication unclear. Third a reduction of 25% on the psychotic subscore of the BPRS is unlikely to be of great clinical significance.

It seems, therefore, that there is little data available at the moment to support the use of traditional antipsychotic medication for the treatment of psychotic symptoms in dementia. On the other hand, there is compelling evidence that the use of these drugs is associated with high rates of tardive dyskinesia (Woerner et al. 1998; Jeste et al. 1999), increased cognitive decline, and lower survival rate (McShane et al. 1997).

The poor efficacy and safety profile of neuroleptics has encouraged the study of the new atypical drugs for the treatment of behavioural problems and psychosis in dementia. Clozapine, the prototype of atypical antipsychotic drugs, has not been used extensively in dementia—the drug produces intense anticholinergic effects and requires regular blood tests. In contrast, numerous case reports have suggested that risperidone may decrease behavioural disturbances and psychotic symptoms in dementia. A retrospective analyses of 41 patients treated with risperidone (2 mg/day on average) showed that 9/15 patients with hallucinations and 7/13 subjects with delusions experienced full remission of symptoms with treatment (the average length of treatment was 4 months) (Irizarry et al. 1999). A more systematic investigation of the efficacy of risperidone to treat behavioural disturbances in dementia was recently reported by Katz and colleagues (1999). The results of this 12-week, double-blind, placebo-controlled trial of 625 patients with AD, vascular dementia, or both showed that doses between 1 and 2 mg/day, but not 0.5 mg, reduced psychotic scores significantly. However, higher doses were also associated with increased rates of extrapyramidal signs, sedation, and oedema when compared to placebo.

The use of olanzapine for the treatment of psychotic symptoms in dementia has not yet been investigated systematically. Few reports suggest that the drug may be useful in the management of psychotic symptoms in patients with Parkinson's disease (Wolters et al. 1996). A recent open-label, 8-week study of olanzapine for the treatment of 21 patients with Parkinson's disease and psychotic symptoms showed that 80% of them were rated as much or very much improved at the end of the trial (Aarsland et al. 1999). They also noted that treatment did not produce a decline on Mini Mental State Examination (MMSE) scores or worsening of parkinsonian symptoms. The results of this and other studies (Tollefson et al. 1997) suggest that olanzapine use is safe and less likely to produce extrapyramidal side-effects than typical antipsychotic drugs.

Table 9.4 summarizes the recommended doses for the prescription of anti-psychotic medication in later life.

Table 9.4 Recommended doses of common antipsychotic drugs used in later life

Drug	Starting dose (mg)	Maintenance dose (mg)	Comments of safety
Haloperidol	0.25–0.5	1–3	High incidence of EPS, including TD
Thioridazine	10–25	50–100	Should be avoided in patients with dementia—poor efficacy, cognitive decline, sedation, and EPS
Clozapine	6.25–12.5	50–100	Should be avoided in later life—intense anticholinergic properties and need for regular blood tests
Risperidone	0.25–0.5	1–3	Doses higher than 2 mg/day are associated with a high incidence of EPS
Olanzapine	1–5	5–10	Sedation, dizziness, and weight gain are the most frequent side-effects

Use of antipsychotic medication in patients with late-onset schizophrenia

Maixner and colleagues (1999) have recently reviewed the controlled trials of antipsychotic drugs in later life. They found that fluphenazine, haloperidol, loxapine, trifluoperazine, and thioridazine were all associated with a moderate response to treatment, particularly of symptoms such as suspiciousness, delusions, hallucinations, agitation, and anxiety. However, they also noted that the use of these drugs was associated with postural hypotension, extrapyramidal symptoms (EPS), unsteadiness, falls, and drowsiness. The results of an open-label study reported by Howard and Levy (1992) suggested that treatment with 'depot' medication may help in the management of patients with late-onset schizophrenia—its use was associated with good compliance and positive treatment outcome.

There are only limited data available to date on the use of atypical antipsychotic drugs for the treatment of patients with late-onset schizophrenia or delusional disorder. Recently, Madhussodanan and colleagues (1999) investigated the efficacy and safety of risperidone in a sample of 103 elderly inpatients with schizophrenia or schizoaffective disorder in a 12-week, open-label study. At the end of the trial, 36 patients were much or very much improved according to the Clinical Global Impression Scale. Dizziness, EPS side-effects, somnolence, agitation, and falls were frequent adverse events. At the time of writing, there were no published data from double-blind, placebo-controlled trials of atypical antipsychotic medication for the treatment of late-onset schizophrenia.

Use of antipsychotic medication in patients with other mental disorders associated with psychosis

Clinicians managing elderly patients with delirium often use antipsychotic medication to control agitation and psychotic symptoms. Surprisingly, however, there is only scarce empirical evidence to support this type of treatment. Breitbart and colleagues (1997) investigated the effects of haloperidol, chlorpromazine, and lorazepam for the treatment of delirium in a sample of 30 adult patients with AIDS. They found that both haloperidol and chlorpromazine use were associated with significant improvement of symptoms as measured by the Delirium Rating Scale. Patients receiving lorazepam deteriorated. Another small, open-label study compared the effects of olanzapine and haloperidol in the treatment of 22 older adults (mean age = 64 years) with delirium (Sipahimalani and Masand 1998). Of the 11 patients treated with olanzapine (mean dose = 8.2 mg), 5 showed significant improvement on the Delirium Rating Scale, compared with 6/11 of those treated with haloperidol (mean dose = 5.1 mg). In addition, the authors reported that five patients in the haloperidol treatment group developed significant side-effects. There is certainly a need for large, double-blind, controlled clinical trials on how best to manage psychosis and behavioural disorders in elderly inpatients with delirium.

Antipsychotic medication is also used in the treatment of patients with psychotic depression, almost always in association with an antidepressant (see Chapter 12).

Alternative treatment strategies

The treatment of delusions and hallucinations does not always involve the use of antipsychotic medication. A recent review showed that some adult patients improve with cognitive–behavioural treatment, although controlled trial evaluations are still few in number (Norman and Townsend 1999). For the elderly, the situation is much worse—there has been no systematic evaluation to date of the effect of psychological therapies on delusions and hallucinations arising in later life.

Other psychotropic drugs have also been tried for patients with AD presenting delusions and hallucinations. Morris and colleagues (1998) reported that the behaviour of patients receiving metrifonate (a cholinesterase inhibitor) improved significantly after 26 weeks of treatment. In addition, they found that hallucinations (as measured by the Neuropsychiatric Inventory) were particularly responsive to this form of treatment. A similar study (Bodick et al. 1997) designed to investigate the effect of xanomeline (a selective muscarinic receptor agonist) on cognitive function and behavioural symptoms in AD described a significant reduction of delusions and hallucinations amongst patients who completed treatment with 225 mg/day of the drug. A note of caution: 49 of the 87 subjects randomized to this dose of xanomeline had to discontinue treatment due to side-effects.

Electroconvulsive therapy (ECT) is another form of treatment that has been used to manage psychotic patients (Tharyan 1999), particularly if the symptoms are part of a depressive disorder (i.e. psychotic depression). Flint and Rifat (1998*b*) compared, in an open-label study, the response to treatment of 8 elderly patients treated with nortriptyline and perphenazine with 17 subjects treated with ECT. ECT was associated with a higher frequency of response than pharmacotherapy (15/17 vs 2/8). ECT has also been used in Parkinson's disease, schizophrenia, and mania, although there is only scarce data available to support its use for the treatment of patients with these disorders.

Discharge recommendations

The long-term management of patients with psychotic symptoms will depend on the cause of their illness. None the less, some general principles apply:

+ Patients and carers should be advised as to the nature of the condition and the importance of ensuring compliance with treatment. The use of depot medication can be considered for subjects with schizophrenia and a prior history of poor compliance.

+ General practitioners should be advised as to the nature of the psychotic symptoms, diagnoses, and potential benefits and risks associated with the use of antipsychotic medication.

+ Follow-up with mental health services should be organized for subjects who remain actively psychotic, particularly when the diagnosis of schizophrenia, mood disorder, or dementia is present.

In conclusion

Delusions and hallucinations are relatively frequent in later life and their presence often indicates the existence of an organic mental disorder (such as dementia, delirium, or medication-induced psychosis), depression, schizophrenia, or delusional disorder. Clinical trials and case series suggest that antipsychotic medication can be used to control psychotic symptoms, regardless of aetiology. The newer atypical antipsychotic agents may be particularly appropriate for the treatment of older adults, as they do not seem to produce high rates of EPS or tardive dyskinesia. However, clinicians should remember that although antipsychotic drugs produce symptomatic relief, they do not treat the underlying cause of symptoms. For this reason, the appropriate management of psychosis should always include the education of carers and psychosocial support of patients.

Acknowledgements

I am grateful to Felicity Roche for proof-reading this paper and Cheryl Ackoy for organizing the list of references.

References

Aarsland, D., Larsen, J.P., Lim, N.G., and Tandberg, E. (1999). Olanzapine for psychosis in patients with Parkinson's disease with and without dementia. *Journal of Neuropsychiatry and Clinical Neurosciences*, **11**, 392–4.

Almeida, O.P., Howard, R., Förstl, H., and Levy, R. (1992). Late paraphrenia: a review. *International Journal of Geriatric Psychiatry*, **7**, 543–8.

Almeida, O.P., Howard, R., Förstl, H., and David, A. (1993). Unilateral auditory hallucinations. *British Journal of Psychiatry*, **162**, 262–4.

Almeida, O.P., Howard, R., Levy, R., and David, A. (1995*a*). Psychotic states arising in late life—the role of risk factors. *British Journal of Psychiatry*, **166**, 215–28.

Almeida, O.P., Howard, R., Levy, R., and David, A. (1995*b*). Psychotic states arising in late life—psychopathology and nosology. *British Journal of Psychiatry*, **166**, 205–14.

Almeida, O.P., Howard, R., Levy, R., David, A., Morris, R., and Sahakian, B.J. (1995*c*). Cognitive features of psychotic states arising in late life (late paraphrenia). *Psychological Medicine*, **25**, 685–98.

Almeida, O.P., Levy, R., Howard, R., and David, A. (1996). Insight and paranoid disorders in late life (late paraphrenia). *International Journal of Geriatric Psychiatry*, **11**, 653–8.

Ballard, C., Holmes, C., McKeith, I., Neill, D., O'Brien, J., Cairns, N., *et al.* (1999). Psychiatric morbidity in dementia with Lewy bodies: a prospective clinical and neuropathological comparative study with Alzheimer's disease. *American Journal of Psychiatry*, **156**, 1039–45.

Bodick, N.C., Offen, W.W., Levey, A.I., Cutler, N.R., Gauthier, S.G., Satlin, A., *et al.* (1997). Effects of xanomeline, a selective muscarinic receptor agonist, on cognitive function and behavioural symptoms in Alzheimer disease. *Archives of Neurology*, **54**, 465–73.

Breitbart, W., Marotta, R., Platt, M.M., Weisman, H., Derevenco, M., Grau, C., *et al.* (1997). Double-blind trial of haloperidol, chlorpromazine, and lorazepam in the treatment of delirium in hospitalized AIDS patients. *American Journal of Psychiatry*, **153**, 231–7.

Burns, A. and Levy, R. (1992). *Clinical diversity in late onset Alzheimer's disease*. Oxford University Press, London.

Burns, A., Carrick, J., Ames, D., Naguib, M., and Levy, R. (1989). The cerebral cortical appearance in late paraphrenia. *International Journal of Geriatric Psychiatry*, **4**, 31–4.

Burns, A., Jacoby, R., and Levy, R. (1990). Psychiatric phenomena in Alzheimer's disease. *British Journal of Psychiatry*, **157**, 72–6.

Christenson, R. and Blazer, D. (1984). Epidemiology of persecutory ideation in an elderly population in the community. *American Journal of Psychiatry*, **141**, 1088–91.

Cohen-Mansfield, J., Taylor, L., and Werner, P. (1998). Delusions and hallucinations in an adult day care population. *American Journal of Geriatric Psychiatry*, **6**, 104–21.

Cooper, A.F. (1976). Deafness and psychiatric illness. *British Journal of Psychiatry*, **129**, 216–26.

Cooper, A.F. and Porter, R. (1976). Visual acuity and ocular pathology in the paranoid and affective psychoses of later life. *Journal of Psychosomatic Research*, **20**, 107–14.

Corbin, S.L. and Eastwood, M.R. (1986). Sensory deficits and mental disorders of old age: causal or coincidental associations? *Psychological Medicine*, **16**, 251–6.

Deutsch, L.H., Bylsma, F.H., Rovner, B.W., Steele, C., and Folstein, M.F. (1991). Psychosis and physical aggression in probable AD. *American Journal of Psychiatry*, **198**, 1159–63.

Devanand, D.P., Marder, K., Michaels, K.S., Sackeim, H.A., Bell, K., Sullivan, M.A., *et al.* (1998). A randomized, placebo-controlled dose-comparison trial of haloperidol for psychosis and disruptive behaviors in Alzheimer's disease. *American Journal of Psychiatry*, **155**, 1512–20.

Flint, A.J. and Rifat, S.L. (1998*a*). Two-year outcome of psychotic depression in late life. *American Journal of Psychiatry*, **155**, 178–83.

Flint, A.J. and Rifat, S.L. (1998*b*). The treatment of psychotic depression in later life: a comparison of pharmacotherapy and ECT. *International Journal of Geriatric Psychiatry*, **13**, 23–8.

Flint, A.J., Rifat, S.L., and Eastwood, M.R. (1991). Late-onset paranoia: distinct from paraphrenia? *International Journal of Geriatric Psychiatry*, **6**, 103–9.

Flynn, F.G., Cummings, J.L., and Goinbar, T. (1991). Delusions in dementia syndromes: investigation of behavioural and neuropsychological conditions. *Journal of Neuropsychiatry and Clinical Neurosciences*, **3**, 364–70.

Förstl, H., Burns, A., Levy, R., and Cairns N. (1994). Neuropathological correlates of psychotic phenomena in confirmed Alzheimer's disease. *British Journal of Psychiatry*, **165**, 53–9.

Freud, S. (1911). Psychoanalytic notes upon an autobiographic account of cases of paranoia (Schreber). In *The standard edition of the complete psychological works* (1958), 12, pp. 1–82. Hogarth Press, London.

Frith, C.D. (1992). *The cognitive neuropsychology of schizophrenia*. Lawrence Erlbaum, Hove/Hillsdale.

Frith, C.D. and Done, D.J. (1988). Towards a neuropsychology of schizophrenia. *British Journal of Psychiatry*, **153**, 437–43.

Garety, P. (1991). Reasoning and delusions. *British Journal of Psychiatry*, **159**(Suppl. 14), 14–18.

Gibson, G.E., Blass, J.P., Huang, H.M., and Freeman, G.B. (1991). The cellular basis of delirium and its relevance to age-related disorders including Alzheimer's disease. *International Psychogeriatrics*, **3**, 373–95.

Gold, J.M., Goldberg, T.E., and Weinberger, D.R. (1992). Prefrontal function and schizophrenic symptoms. *Neuropsychiatry, Neuropsychology and Behavioral Neurology*, **5**, 253–61.

Halbreich, U., Rojansky, N., Palter, S., Hreshchyshyn, M., Kreeger, J., Bakhai, Y., *et al.* (1995). Decreased bone mineral density in medicated psychiatric patients. *Psychosomatic Medicine*, **57**, 485–91.

Henderson, A.S. and Kay, D.W.K. (1997). The epidemiology of functional psychoses of late onset. *European Archives of Psychiatry and Clinical Neurosciences*, **247**, 176–89.

Henderson, A.S., Koerten, A.E., Levinos, C., Jorm, A.F., Christensen, H., Jacomb, P.A., *et al.* (1998). Psychotic symptoms in the elderly: a prospective study in a population sample. *International Journal of Geriatric Psychiatry*, **13**, 484–92.

Holroyd, S. and Laurie, S. (1999). Correlates of psychotic symptoms among elderly outpatients. *International Journal of Geriatric Psychiatry*, **14**, 379–84.

Howard, R. and Levy, R. (1992). Which factors affect treatment response in late paraphrenia? *International Journal of Geriatric Psychiatry*, **7**, 667–72.

Howard, R., Almeida, O., Levy, R., Graves, P., and Graves, M. (1994). Quantitative magnetic resonance imaging volumetry of the brain, third and lateral ventricles in late paraphrenia distinguishes delusional disorder from late-onset schizophrenia. *British Journal of Psychiatry*, **165**, 474–80.

Howard, R., Mellers, J., Petty, R., Bonner, D., Menon, R., Almeida, O., *et al.* (1995). Magnetic resonance imaging volumetric measurements of the superior temporal gyrus, hippocampus, parahippocampal gyrus, frontal and temporal lobes in late paraphrenia. . *Psychological Medicine*, **25**, 495–503.

Irizarry, M.C., Ghaemi, S.N., Lee-Cherry, E.R, Gomez-Isla, T., Binetti, G., Hyman, B.T., *et al.* (1999). Risperidone treatment of behavioral disturbances in outpatients with dementia. *Journal of Neuropsychiatry and Clinical Neurosciences*, **11**, 336–42.

Jacoby, R. and Levy, R. (1980). Computed tomography in the elderly. 2. Senile dementia: diagnosis and functional impairment. *British Journal of Psychiatry*, **136**, 256–69.

Jaspers, K. (1997). *General psychopathology*, Vol. 1. Johns Hopkins, Baltimore, MD.

Jeste, D.V., Rockwell, E., Harris, M.J., Lohr, J.B., and Lacro, J. (1999). Conventional vs. newer antipsychotics in elderly patients. *American Journal of Geriatric Psychiatry*, **7**, 70–6.

Katz, I.R., Jeste, D.V., Mintzer, J.E., Clyde, C., Napolitano, J., and Brecher, M. (1999). Comparison of risperidone and placebo for psychosis and behavioural disturbances associated with dementia: a randomised, double-blind trial. *Journal of Clinical Psychiatry*, **60**, 107–15.

Kirchner, V., Kelly, C.A., and Harvery, R.J. (1998). A systematic review of the evidence for the safety and efficacy of thioridazine in dementia. The Cochrane Database of Systematic Reviews **4**.

Lyketsos, C.G., Steele, C., Galik, E., Rosenblatt, A., Steinberg, M., Warren, A., *et al.* (1999). Physical aggression in dementia patients and its relationship to depression. *American Journal of Psychiatry*, **156**, 66–71.

McKeith, I.G., Fairbairn, A., Perry, R., Thompson, P., and Perry, E. (1992). Neuroleptic sensitivity in patients with senile dementia of Lewy body type. *British Medical Journal*, **305**, 673–8.

McKeith, I.G., Ballard, C.G., and Harrison, R.W.S. (1995). Neuroleptic sensitivity to risperidone in Lewy body dementia. *Lancet*, **346**, 699.

McKeith, I.G., Galasko, D., Kosaka, K., Perry, E.K., Dickson, D.W., Hansen, L.A. *et al.* (1996). Consensus guidelines for the clinical and pathologic diagnosis of dementia with Lewy bodies (DLB): report of the consortium on DLB international workshop. *Neurology*, **47**, 1113–24.

McManus, D.Q., Arvanitis, L.A., and Kowalcyk, B.B. (1999). Quetiapine, a novel antipsychotic: experience in elderly patients with psychotic disorders. Seroquel Trial 48 Study Group. *Journal of Clinical Psychiatry*, **60**, 292–8.

McShane, R., Keene, J., Gedling, K., Fairburn, C., Jacoby, R., and Hope, T. (1997). Do neuroleptic drugs hasten cognitive decline in dementia? Prospective study with necropsy follow up. *British Medical Journal*, **314**, 266–70.

McShane, R., Keene, J., Fairburn, C., Jacoby, R., and Hope, T. (1998). Psychiatric symptoms in patients with dementia predict the later development of behavioural abnormalities. *Psychological Medicine*, **28**, 1119–27.

Madhussodanan, S., Brecher, M., Brenner, R., Kasckow, J., Kunik, M., Negrón, A.E., *et al.* (1999). Risperidone in the treatment of elderly patients with psychotic disorders. *American Journal of Geriatric Psychiatry*, **7**, 132–8.

Maixner, S.M., Mellow, A.M., and Tandon, R. (1999). The efficacy, safety, and tolerability of antipsychotics in the elderly. *Journal of Clinical Psychiatry*, **60**(Suppl. 8), 29–41.

Miller, B.L., Lesser, I.M., Mena, I., Villanueva-Meyer, J., Hill-Gutierrez, E., Boone, K., *et al.* (1992). Regional cerebral blood flow in late-life-onset psychosis. *Neuropsychiatry, Neuropsychology, and Behavioral Neurology*, **5**, 132–7.

Morris, J.C., Cyrus, P.A., Orazem, J., Mas, J., Bieber, F., Ruzicka, B.B., *et al.* (1998). Metrifonate benefits cognitive behavioral, and global function in patients with Alzheimer's disease. *Neurology*, **50**, 1222–30.

Myers, J.K., Weissman, M.M., and Tischler, G. (1984). Six-month prevalence of psychiatric disorders in three communities. *Archives of General Psychiatry*, **41**, 959–70.

Norman, R.M.G. and Townsend, L.A. (1999). Cognitive-behavioural therapy for psychosis: a status report. *Canadian Journal of Psychiatry*, **44**, 245–2.

Perry, E., Ballard, C., Spurden, D., Cheng, A., Johnson, M., McKeith, I., *et al.* (1998). Cholinergic systems in the human brain: psychopharmacology and psychosis. *Alzheimer's Disease Review*, **3**, 117–24.

Rabins, P., Pearlson, G., Jayaram, G., Steele, C., and Tune, L. (1987). Increased ventricle-to-brain ratio in late-onset schizophrenia. *American Journal of Psychiatry*, **142**, 557–9.

Rao, V. and Lyketsos, C.G. (1998). Delusions in Alzheimer's disease: a review. *Journal of Neuropsychiatry and Clinical Neurosciences*, **10**, 373–82.

Roberts, G. (1991). Delusional belief systems and meaning in life: a preferred reality? *British Journal of Psychiatry*, **159**(Suppl. 14) 19–28.

Ross, C.A., Peyser, C.E., Shapiro, I., and Folstein, M.F. (1991). Delirium: phenomenologic and etiologic subtypes. *International Psychogeriatrics*, **3**, 135–47.

Ruegg, R.G., Zisook, S., and Swerdlow, N.R. (1988). Depression in the aged: an overview. *The Psychiatric Clinics of North America*, **11**, 83–99.

Simpson, S., Baldwin, R.C., Jackson, A, and Burns, A. (1999). The differentiation of the DSM-III-R psychotic depression in later life from nonpsychotic depression: comparisons of brain changes measured by multispectral analysis of magnetic resonance brain images, neuropsychological findings, and clinical features. *Biological Psychiatry*, **45**, 193–204.

Sipahimalani, A. and Masand, P.S. (1998). Olanzapine in the treatment of delirium. *Psychosomatics*, **39**, 422–30.

Soares, J.C. and Gershon, S. (1997). Therapeutic targets in late-life psychoses: review of concepts and critical issues. *Schizophrenia Research*, **27**, 227–39.

Tharyan, P. (1999). Electroconvulsive therapy for schizophrenia. The Cochrane Database of Systematic Reviews 2.

Tollefson, G.D., Beasley, C.M. Jr, Tamura, R.N., Tran, P.V., and Potvin, J.H. (1997). Blind, controlled, long-term study of the comparative incidence of treatment-emergent tardive dyskinesia with olanzapine or haloperidol. *American Journal of Psychiatry*, **154**, 1248–54.

Verhaeverbeke, I. and Mets, T. (1997). Drug-induced orthostatic hypotension in the elderly: avoiding its onset. *Drug Safety*, **17**, 105–18.

Webster, J. and Grossberg, G.T. (1998). Late-life onset of psychotic symptoms. *American Journal of Geriatric Psychiatry*, **6**, 196–202.

Woerner, M.G., Alvir, J.M.J., Saltz, B.L., Lieberman, J.A., and Kane, J.M. (1998). Prospective study of tardive dyskinesia in the elderly: rates and risk factors. *American Journal of Psychiatry*, **155**, 1521–8.

Wolters, E.C., Jansen, E.N.H., Tuynman-Qua, H.G., and Bergmans, P.L.M. (1996). Olanzapine in the treatment of dopaminomimetic psychosis in patients with Parkinson's disease. *Neurology*, **47**, 1085–7.

Zimbardo, P.G., Anderson, S.M., and Kabat, L.G. (1981). Induced hearing deficit generates experimental paranoia. *Science*, **212,** 1529–31.

10 Organic mental disorders

David G. Taylor and Ajit K. Shah

Summary

This chapter aims to give an overview of the principal organic mental disorders encountered in old age psychiatry consultation liaison settings. A brief overview is given of those aspects of the diagnostic process having particular relevance to organic mental disorders. Individual disorders are then covered, including delirium, dementia, amnestic disorder, and other disorders. The dementia section places special emphasis on the three most common conditions of old age, namely dementia of the Alzheimer's type (DAT), vascular dementia (VaD), and dementia with Lewy bodies (DLB). Emerging pharmacotherapeutic interventions for DAT in the form of cholinesterase-inhibitor therapy are reviewed. Finally, a number of other conditions are considered, including aphasia, apraxia, agnosia, executive disorder, and personality change. Case studies occur throughout the text, to illustrate commonly encountered liaison consultation scenarios.

Organic mental disorders of varied aetiologies are commonly referred to old age psychiatry liaison services. Some are due to neurological disorders, whilst others are due to systemic general medical conditions or the effects of ingested substances such as medications, drugs of abuse, or toxins. They are subclassified according to the predominant clinical features. The International Classification of Diseases, 10th edition (ICD-10) (WHO 1992) and the Diagnostic and Statistical Manual of Mental Disorders, 4th edition (DSM-IV) (APA 1994) have broadly equivalent categories.

The diagnostic process

The assessment and diagnostic process is discussed in detail in Chapter 5. Points of particular relevance for patients suspected of having organic mental disorders are discussed below.

History of presenting complaint

Patients with organic mental disorders are often unable to give a clear history of the presenting complaint. It is therefore essential to acquire a collateral history from other informants such as spouses, relatives, friends, neighbours, wardens, nursing-home staff, social workers, general practitioners, and the hospital medical team. It is particularly important to obtain a longitudinal history of the clinical features noted prior to admission, as this is useful for differentiating disorders. The inpatient nursing staff is a most valuable source of information on the patients' current clinical features.

Past psychiatric history

Review of the previous psychiatric history will provide useful information. A previous diagnosis of delirium due to a specific general medical condition may assist with understanding the nature and cause of subsequent episodes. A previous history of depression may be a risk factor for the subsequent development of dementia of the Alzheimer's type (DAT) (Broe *et al.* 1990) or may herald its onset. Patients with Huntington's disease may present with clinical features mimicking several mental disorders (Folstein 1989).

Past and current medical history

Review of the medical case-notes may reveal general medical conditions important in the diagnosis of organic mental disorders. A wide range of general medical conditions and ingested substances can result in the development of delirium (Lipowski 1990). Certain pre-existing general medical conditions may help clarify the aetiology of dementia; for example: head injury and DAT (Mortimer *et al.* 1985); atherosclerosis and vascular dementia (VaD) (Meyer *et al.* 1988); parkinsonism and dementia with Lewy bodies (DLB) (McKeith *et al.* 1996); motor neurone disease and frontotemporal dementia (FTD) (Snowden *et al.* 1996); chorea and Huntington's dementia (Lipe *et al.* 1993); ataxia and prion dementia (Yamada *et al.* 1999).

Family history

In some families, dementia is associated with specific genetic defects (McGuffin and Martin 1999). Huntington's disease is inherited as an autosomal dominant trait (Conneally *et al.* 1985). Some prion diseases show heritability due to polymorphic variability of the prion protein (PrP) gene on chromosome 20 (Berr *et al.* 1998). The amyloid precursor protein (APP) gene on chromosome 21 (Goate *et al.* 1991), and the presenilin 1 and 2 genes on chromosomes 14 and 1, respectively (Sherrington *et al.* 1995; Hutton and Hardy 1997), directly cause early-onset DAT. Only a few families (1–2%) with these genetic patterns have been identified. On chromosome 19 is a gene that codes for the isoforms of apolipoprotein E, a lipid transporter protein that is essential for the integrity of neuronal cell walls. Homozygosity for the ApoEε4 allele increases the risk for developing DAT (Roses and Saunders 1997). Recent work also suggests that possession of the ApoEε4 phenotype also increases the risk of developing DLB (Lamb *et al.* 1998).

Although the issue of genetic counselling in the liaison context is uncommon, well-read or Internet-familiar patients and families are increasingly assertive in seeking information and advice on the genetic risk to family members.

Personal history

Enquiry about birth, infancy, childhood, and adolescence may reveal evidence of a learning disability. The life expectancy of intellectually handicapped patients is increasing and they have a higher prevalence of dementia than the general population (Patel *et al.* 1993). Poor educational attainment may be a risk factor for the development of dementia (Frataglioni *et al.* 1991). Higher education endows an individual with greater cognitive reserve, and intelligent people who develop dementia are commonly observed to mask their symptoms in the early stages (Cummings *et al.* 1998).

Some occupations are associated with risk factors for organic mental disorders, for example repeated head injury in professional boxers (dementia pugilistica and possibly DAT) (Roberts *et al.* 1990). A history of occupational exposure to toxins (such as mercury, lead, or manganese) increases the risk for some organic disorders (Verity 1993). Some occupations such as medicine are associated with higher than average rates of substance abuse.

Substance-use history

It is important to ascertain a detailed history of both prescribed and non-prescribed medications. Some drugs individually, and others in combination, can have adverse consequences on cognitive and non-cognitive mental functioning (Mehta 2000). Many drugs have anticholinergic properties, which can precipitate delirium in some patients (Tune and Bylsma 1991).

Alcohol can cause organic mental disorders both directly (for example, alcohol withdrawal delirium) and indirectly (for example, dementia due to vitamin B_{12} and folate deficiency). Cigarette smoking is a risk factor for cerebrovascular disease and thus VaD.

Cognitive status examination

A detailed cognitive examination is essential in organic mental disorders. A hierarchical approach is essential. Assessment of consciousness comes first, as impairment in this domain may confound the subsequent cognitive assessment. Language follows, as aphasia in clear consciousness may confound the assessment of memory, praxis, gnosis, and executive function. These last four domains may be assessed in any order. Fluctuating cognition in disorders such as delirium may result in a normal cognitive examination if the patient is assessed during a lucid interval, and a grossly abnormal one at other times. A detailed chronological collateral history is helpful to clarify the diagnosis.

Physical examination

The physical examination may provide clues about aetiology (for example, goitre), risk factors (for example, hypertension), and sequelae (for example, dehydration and malnutrition due to self-neglect). The psychiatrist may be required to perform a focused physical examination, and any previously undetected abnormal findings should be reported back to the referring team.

Disability assessment

The disability assessment should consider both premorbid and current functional ability to allow identification of any decline. It also allows identification of coping strategies utilized by patients and their professional and family carers. Information on physical, psychological (presence or absence of distress), social, self-care activities of daily living (ADL), and instrumental ADL disabilities can be ascertained from the medical and nursing case-notes, discussion with the nursing staff, occupational therapists, physiotherapists, and social workers. Busy nursing staff may have insufficient time to assist a slow patient to function optimally, or may inadvertently provide too much assistance. An assessment by an occupational therapist may give a more accurate picture, particularly if it is done in the patient's home.

Screening investigations for organic mental disorders are listed in Table 10.1

Table 10.1 Screening investigations for organic mental disorders

Routine:	
Full blood count	Thyroid function tests
C-reactive protein	Serum glucose
Erythrocyte sedimentation rate	Syphilis serology
Vitamin B_{12} and folate	Midstream urine and culture
Urea and electrolytes	Electrocardiogram
Liver function tests	Chest radiograph
Calcium	CT scan of the brain
Sometimes indicated:	
Electroencephalogram	MRI brain scan
Lumbar puncture	Functional neuroimaging: SPECT/PET

CT, computed tomography; MRI, magnetic resonance imaging; SPECT, single-photon emission tomography; PET, positron emission tomography.

Specific organic mental disorders

Delirium

Epidemiology

Between 15% and 50% of acutely medically ill geriatric inpatients have delirium (Johnston *et al.* 1987; MacDonald *et al.* 1989; Ramsey *et al.* 1991; Levkoff *et al.* 1992; Kolbeinsson and Jonsson 1993). The incidence rises substantially after admission, and the prevalence is generally greater on surgical as opposed to general medical wards (Bucht *et al.* 1999). Up to 25% of referrals to geriatric psychiatry liaison services have delirium (Scott *et al.* 1988; Wrigley and Loane 1991; Collinson and Benbow 1998; Baheerathan and Shah 1999). It is often associated with diagnostic difficulties (Treloar and MacDonald 1997*a,b*).

Aetiology

Almost any general medical condition can result in delirium. The commonest causes include myocardial infarction, cerebrovascular accident, metastatic spread of cancer, chest infection, urinary tract infections, and alcohol withdrawal. A large number of prescribed and non-prescribed drugs can also produce delirium (Ford and Folks 1985; Larson *et al.* 1987; Katzman *et al.* 1988; Katz *et al.* 1991; De and Shah 1998). The common categories and some examples of medications that can cause the disorder are listed in Table 10.2. The aetiology of delirium is best understood as an interaction of predisposing vulnerability factors and precipitating cerebral toxic/injury factors. Very often, there are multiple contributing causes rather than a single one. In contrast, it is not uncommon that no 'clear ' cause can be found, and this does not invalidate the diagnosis.

The list is not exhaustive and any drug with sedative side-effects may be aetiologically implicated. Benzodiazepines and drugs with anticholinergic properties are particularly important (Tune and Bylsma 1991). Individual drugs may not have sufficient anticholinergic properties to produce symptoms, but the additive effect of several drugs may do so (Tune and Bylsma 1991). The altered pharmacodynamics and pharmacokinetics in the elderly means they are particularly susceptible to these effects (De and Shah 1998).

Diagnosis

Diagnostic criteria for delirium (DSM-IV 1994) are listed in Table 10.3.

A useful clinical distinction can be made between hyperactive and hypoactive states. In hyperactive states, for example in alcohol withdrawal, the patient may be at risk of harm to self or others due to extreme agitation. Delirium due to medical illnesses such as hepatic encephalopathy can produce hypoactive states, with the consequence that the diagnosis is likely to be missed. In patients with cognitive impairment, slowness, vague speech, poor attention, and incoherent speech may be

Table 10.2 Common medications that cause delirium in the elderly

Class of medication	Common examples
Analgesics–narcotic and non-narcotic	Buprenorphine, codeine, dextropropoxyphene, dextromoramide, nefopam, morphine, pethidine, tramadol
Antiarrythmics	Digoxin, propranolol, procainamide, quinidine, sotalol, verapamil
Anticonvulsants	Carbamazepine, phenytoin, valproate
Antidepressant drugs, particularly tricyclics	Amitriptyline, clomipramine, doxepin, nortriptyline
Antihistamines	Dexchlorpheniramine, pheniramine, promethazine
Antihypertensives, particularly β-blockers	Captopril, clonidine, enalapril, oxprenolol, metoprolol, quinapril
Antiparkinsonian drugs, particularly anticholinergics	Benztropine, bromocryptine, L-dopa, phencyclidine, selegiline
Antispasmodics	Dicycloverine (dicyclomine), hyoscine, oxybutynin, probanthine
Benzodiazepines	Bromazepam, diazepam, clonazepam, lorazepam, oxazepam, triazolam
Cyclopegics and mydriatics	Atropine, homatropine, hyoscine, tropicamide
Cytotoxics	Cyclophosphamide, chlorambucil, tamoxifen
Histamine H_2-receptor antagonists	Cimetidine, famotidine, ranitidine
Lithium	Lithium carbonate
Neuroleptics, particularly phenothiazines	Chlorpromazine, trifluoperazine, thioridazine, haloperidol
Sedatives	Chlomethiazole (chlormethiazole), hydroxyzine
Steroids	Hydrocortisone, prednisone

observed, along with episodes of hyperactivity (Treloar and MacDonald 1997a,b). Screening with instruments such as the Confusion Assessment Method (CAM) can allow general physicians and surgeons to identify possible cases of delirium within a few minutes (Inouye et al. 1990).

Non-cognitive features often associated with delirium include agitation, aggres-

Table 10.3 Diagnostic criteria for delirium[a]

A Disturbance of consciousness (i.e. reduced clarity of awareness of the environment) with reduced ability to focus, sustain, or shift attention.
B A change in cognition (such as memory deficit, disorientation, language disturbance) or the development of a perceptual disturbance that is not better accounted for by a pre-existing, established, or evolving dementia.
C The disturbance develops over a short period (usually hours to days) and tends to fluctuate during the course of the day.
D There is evidence from the history, physical examination, or laboratory findings that the disturbance is caused by the direct physiological consequences of a general medical condition or substance. If substance-related, the symptoms in Criteria A and B developed during substance intoxication or during or shortly after substance withdrawal.
Note: A diagnosis of 'substance intoxication delirium' or 'substance withdrawal delirium' should be made instead of a diagnosis of 'substance intoxication' or 'substance withdrawal' only when the cognitive symptoms are in excess of those usually associated with the intoxication or withdrawal syndrome, and when the symptoms are sufficiently severe to warrant independent clinical attention.

[a]Taken from DSM-IV 1994 with permission of the American Psychiatric Association.

sion, wandering, delusions, and perceptual disturbances such as misidentifications, illusions, and hallucinations. These features often pose management challenges that lead to requests for psychiatric consultation.

The sequelae of delirium are various, and mainly depend on the underlying general medical condition. For example, a delirious patient with raised intracranial pressure or alcohol withdrawal may make a full recovery or be left with varying degrees of brain damage. These could include dementia, amnestic disorder, personality change, psychotic disorder, and depressive disorder (Taylor and Lewis 1993).

The importance of diagnosing delirium is reinforced in the demonstration that it acts as a predictor of adverse outcome, independent of the patient's general medical status (Inouye *et al.* 1998).

Case study 10.1

Mr AB., aged 77 years, was assessed on a general medical ward where he had been admitted following a stroke. Later in the admission he developed disruptive and aggressive behaviour that was characterized by extreme agitation with the (correct) belief that he was being kept in hospital against his wishes. He had several episodes of altered consciousness, lack of awareness of the immediate external environment, and inability to focus or sustain attention. When lucid, he was co-operative with nursing and medical interventions and pleasant in his interactions.

The clinical diagnosis of delirium was made, and a full medical review revealed a urinary tract infection. The referring team was advised on reassurance techniques and antibiotics were prescribed. Regular visits from the patient's daughters were encouraged to assist with orientation. The behaviour disturbance settled after these interventions were implemented.

Management

Junior doctors working in inpatient wards and emergency rooms often seek advice on the management of behaviour disturbance associated with delirium. If an accurate diagnosis is made and appropriate treatment implemented, early intervention may avoid a full-blown crisis. Any potentially reversible cause(s) should be identified and treated. Medications implicated in the aetiology, for example anticholinergics or benzodiazepines, should be stopped, if possible. Visual and auditory deficits may require correction (Shah and Ames 1994; De and Shah 1998). Adequate analgesia will be required for pain. Dehydration needs to be rectified.

Calming strategies are helpful (Shah and Ames 1994; De and Shah 1998). Disturbed patients should be approached gently and calmly from the front. Communication should be clear and unambiguous. The judicious use of touch and non-threatening postures may help. Meticulous attention should be paid to nutrition, fluid balance, skin care, and mobilization. Ideally, patients with delirium should be nursed in a well-lit room with changes of staff or nursing environment kept to a minimum. Staff should be easily identifiable. Family and friends can be very helpful by staying with the patient and providing familiar objects from home. Simple strategies such as orientating cues (clocks, calendars, and signs); sensory aids (night lights); and the provision of a quiet and relaxing night environment will also assist.

Sometimes, if patients are very disturbed they may require sedation with psycho-active medication (Alexopoulos *et al.* 1998). Haloperidol is the drug of choice as it has the least anticholinergic, cardiovascular, and sedative side-effects of the neuro-leptics. The efficacy of other medications for behavioural disturbance in delirium is modest at best. Most have potent side-effects (Risse and Barnes 1986; Sunderland and Silver 1988) and can increase cognitive impairment because of anticholinergic side-effects. Newer neuroleptics, such as risperidone, olanzapine, quetiapine, and amisulpiride have not been adequately investigated in delirium (Goldberg and Goldberg 1997; Katz *et al.* 1999).

Medications should be used sparingly in elderly patients, due to age-related alterations in pharmacokinetics and pharmacodynamics and the potential for polypharmacy to cause drug–drug interactions. Whenever possible, oral medication should be used. Small doses should be prescribed initially, with gradual increments in dosage, if necessary, whilst carefully monitoring for side-effects. Oral haloperidol given in increments of 0.25–0.5 mg titrated with the mental state to total doses of 0.5–2 mg per day is effective in mild to moderate cases. Rarely should it be neces-sary to exceed these doses. In severe agitation, haloperidol 1–2 mg intramuscularly immediately, then 1–2 mg intramuscularly an hour later may be necessary. In emergency situations (such as when patients are in immediate danger of causing harm to themselves or others), midazolam 2.5–5 mg intramuscularly or diazepam (as diazemuls) 2.5–5 mg intravenously (IV) and/or droperidol 2.5–5 mg IV, may be necessary. In all such cases, close cardiorespiratory (including pulse oximetry) and neurological observation is mandatory due to the heavy sedation that might occur. As it may be necessary to continue prescribing these drugs for a few days, the doses need to be continually monitored and kept as low as possible. Several of these drugs have long half-lives and their effect can be cumulative in older people. If given for prolonged periods, they can make delirium worse. Use of a nurse 'sitter' may be a better option than heavy doses of tranquillizers. Carefully applied physical restraints are occasionally justified for short periods, but require regular monitoring to prevent injuries and allow review of their effectiveness.

Patients with alcohol withdrawal delirium (delirium tremens) will require treatment for potential withdrawal seizures, detoxification, and sedation. Oral diazepam 2.5–5 mg several times a day is given as needed for 7–10 days. High-potency multi-vitamin replacement is essential (for example, IV injections three times a day for 3–4 days, followed by oral therapy for at least 6 months). Appropriate fluid and electrolyte replacement must also be given (Chick 1989).

Delirium can appear very alarming. An explanation of the diagnosis, management plan, and possible sequelae should be provided to the relatives and medical team. During lucid periods, the patient can be appraised of the diagnosis. Specific issues that should be addressed include the nature and cause of the delirium and its likely implications. In addition, the associated behavioural disturbance, role of medication, possible management strategies, and need for further psychiatric assessment or follow-up can be discussed. Both relatives and staff in medical settings may need an opportunity to ventilate their feelings. Despite the best efforts of the medical team, there will be situations where behaviour disturbance does not improve and admission to an old age psychiatry unit may be indicated.

Prognosis

Delirium is a medical emergency and is associated with increased morbidity, including failure to regain full premorbid cognitive capacity and increased length of inpatient stay (Kolbeinsson and Jonsson 1993). Delirium may persist for several weeks, despite rectification of the underlying causes. There is a significantly increased mortality (Ramsey et al. 1991; Kolbeinsson and Jonsson 1993), with mortality rates from 18% to 37% (Lipowski 1990). However most cases, if adequately treated, are reversible (Taylor and Lewis 1993).

Dementia

Epidemiology

Up to 62% of acute (Ramsay et al. 1991; Ames and Tuckwell 1994) and 94% of continuing-care (Hodkinson et al. 1988; Harrison et al. 1990; Shah et al. 1992) inpatients over the age of 65 years have dementia. Moreover, up to 44% of patients referred to old age psychiatry liaison services have dementia (Scott *et al.* 1988; Wrigley and Loane 1991; Collinson and Benbow 1998; Baheerathan and Shah 1999).

Aetiology

The three most common types of dementia seen in liaison old age psychiatry settings are: dementia of the Alzheimer type (DAT), vascular dementia (VaD), and dementia with Lewy bodies (DLBT). Combinations of these conditions may also occur. Other primary degenerative disorders such as frontal lobe dementia (FTD), Huntington's dementia, and prion dementia have a younger average age of onset, often present to neurologists, and are therefore less common in liaison old age psychiatry settings

Diagnosis

All types of dementia share the DSM-IV criteria listed in Table 10.4.

Specific diagnostic features characterize the different types of dementia. For example in DAT, which is the most common disorder (60% of dementias), the course is characterized by the insidious onset and gradual decline of memory and other cognitive functions. Numerous behavioural and psychological symptoms of dementia (BPSD) may also be present, including behavioural disturbance, depressed mood, and psychotic features (delusions and/or hallucinations).

Vascular dementia VaD (10–15% of dementias) is a heterogeneous category, most frequently caused by cerebral infarction (usually multiple) or white-matter ischaemia (leucoaraiosis). Risk factors such as hypertension, hypercholesterolaemia, ischaemic heart disease, smoking, and diabetes should alert the clinician to the possibility of VaD. In multi-infarct dementia a natural history of sudden onset and step-wise deterioration in cognition is classically described. 'Patchiness' of cognitive deficits may help to distinguish VaD from the characteristic pattern of

Table 10.4 DSM-IV diagnostic criteria for dementia[a]

A The development of multiple cognitive deficits manifested by both:
1. memory impairment (impaired ability to learn new information or to recall previously learned information)
2. one (or more) of the following cognitive disturbances: aphasia, apraxia, agnosia, disturbance in executive functioning.
B The cognitive deficits cause significant impairment in social or occupational functioning and represent a significant decline from a previous level of function.
C There is evidence of an organic aetiological disorder.
D The deficits do not occur exclusively in the course of a delirium.

[a]Taken from DSM-IV 1994 with permission of the American Psychiatric Association.

deficits seen in DAT. There may be clinical evidence of focal neurological signs and symptoms, such as exaggeration of deep tendon reflexes, extensor plantar response, pseudobulbar palsy, gait abnormalities, and weakness of an extremity. In VaD, computed tomographic (CT) scanning may show evidence of infarction and/or ischaemia. If clinical suspicion of cerebrovascular disease is not be confirmed on CT, magnetic resonance imaging (MRI) should be considered, as this technique provides better resolution of vascular brain lesions.

Specific diagnostic criteria for DLB, which makes up 12–15% dementias, have been identified by McKeith *et al.* (1996) and are listed in Table 10.5. This condition is associated with widespread cortical Lewy neurites (visible on anti-alpha-synuclein immunohistochemistry) and Lewy bodies (visible on both anti-alpha-synuclein and anti-ubiquitin immunohistochemistry). A recent report (McKeith *et al.* 1999) has upheld the current diagnostic criteria, but also points to the frequency of depressive features and REM sleep behaviour disorder in the condition. One of the most characteristic features is fluctuating cognition with pronounced variations in conscious alertness and attention, similar to that seen in delirium. This can cause difficulties in the differential diagnosis of the two conditions (see Table 10.6). Although spontaneous parkinsonism (motor rigidity, tremor, bradykinesia) is common in DLB, a formal diagnosis of Parkinson's disease coexists in only 33 per cent of DLB patients at the point of diagnosis (McKeith *et al.* 1996).

It is envisioned that acetylcholinesterase inhibitor therapy will have significant

Table 10.5 Diagnostic criteria for dementia with Lewy bodies

A	The central feature required for a diagnosis of DLB is progressive cognitive decline of sufficient magnitude to interfere with normal social or occupational function. Prominent or persistent memory impairment may not necessarily occur in the early stages, but it is usually evident with progression. Deficits on tests of attention and of frontosubcortical skills and visuospatial ability may be especially prominent.
B	Two of the following core features are essential for a diagnosis of probable DLB, and one is essential for possible DLB: – fluctuating cognition with pronounced variations in attention and alertness; – recurrent visual hallucinations that are typically well formed and detailed; – spontaneous motor features of parkinsonism.
C	Features supportive of the diagnosis are: transient loss of consciousness; syncope; repeated falls; systematized delusions; hallucinations in other modalities; neuroleptic sensitivity; depression; REM sleep behaviour disorder.
D	A diagnosis of DLB is less likely in the presence of: stroke disease, evident as focal neurological signs or on brain imaging evidence, on physical examination and investigation of any physical illness, or other brain disorder sufficient to account for the clinical picture.

*From McKeith *et al.* 1996, 1999 with permission to adapt granted by *Neurology*.

Table 10.6 Differential diagnosis between DLB and delirium

	DLB	Delirium
History	Gradual deterioration, may be step-wise	May have history of decline or none
Onset	Gradual	Sudden
Physiological or pathological cause	None found	Infection, drugs, metabolic cause, etc.
Alertness	Fluctuating	Fluctuating
Cognition	Fluctuating	Fluctuating
Attention	Unable to sustain	Variable
Perceptual phenomena	Complex visual and auditory hallucinations	Misperceptions of actual stimuli
Psychotic phenomena	Well-formed delusions	Secondary delusions
Syncope	Common	Not common
Visuospatial distortion and falls	Common	Common
Response to neuroleptics	Very poor, may have marked parkinsonian side-effects	Good response

benefits in the treatment of the cognitive impairment, behavioural disturbance, and psychotic features of DLB (McKeith *et al.* 2000). Conventional neuroleptics are poorly tolerated and are likely to result in marked extrapyramidal symptoms. The atypical neuroleptic olanzapine can be poorly tolerated in patients with DLB and should be used with caution (Walker *et al.* 1999). Therefore, the use of quetiapine, given in the minimum possible dose, is recommended when an antipsychotic is essential.

Case study 10.2

Mr C., aged 68 years, was admitted to a general medical ward because of repeated falls. He had been noted to be behaving oddly, and was referred for an old age psychiatry liaison consultation. From his wife, the psychiatrist obtained a collateral history of 1 year of progressive cognitive decline, manifested by intermittent loss of attention, difficulties in organizing tasks such as domestic bill payment, and getting lost in his local neighbourhood. He was intermittently 'confused' on the ward, and often spoke about groups of children and animals he could see gathered around his bed. The patient had developed the belief that the staff was trying to poison him and consequently had acted aggressively towards his perceived assassins, requiring forcible restraint. Neurological examination revealed some parkinsonian features. Investigations (including a CT scan of brain) failed to reveal an identifiable general medical condition to account for his mental state changes. Cognitive assessment revealed executive dysfunction, apraxia, agnosia, and mild amnesia. A clinical diagnosis of dementia with Lewy bodies was made.

Parkinsonism is associated with dementia in 10 to 80% of all cases (Brown and Marsden 1984). This may be due to Lewy body disease, cerebrovascular disease, or advanced Alzheimer's disease. Dementia may also occur rarely in idiopathic Parkinson's disease. Numerous less common conditions, such as progressive supranuclear palsy, multiple system atrophy, and corticobasal degeneration can also present with the combination of dementia and parkinsonism (Harding 1993).

Subcortical dementia is characterized by bradyphrenia, as elicited by timed cognitive tests (Fleminger 1991). Amnesia and executive dysfunction predominate, with a relative lack of aphasia, apraxia, and agnosia. Parkinsonism is common, and other movement disorders may be present such as dystonia, dyskinesia, or ataxia. Many different pathologies may be implicated, such as cerebrovascular disease (including Binswangers disease), Parkinson's disease, Huntington's disease, and multiple sclerosis.

Frontotemporal lobar degeneration (FTLD) describes a group of disorders that includes FTD, progressive non-fluent aphasia, and semantic dementia (Robert *et al.* 1999). They constitute 15% of all dementias, and usually present in patients under 65 years of age. Approximately 50% of patients have a positive family history. Histologically, two main types are identified, characterized by either prominent microvacuolar change without specific histological features (frontal lobe degeneration-type), or severe astrocytic gliosis with or without ballooned cells and inclusion bodies (Pick-type). Clinical features of FTD include loss of personal and social awareness, personal neglect, disinhibition, apathy, mental rigidity and inflexibility, motor and verbal perseveration, stereotyped behaviour, utilization behaviour, hyperorality, and impairment in speech (Lund and Manchester Groups 1994; Snowden *et al.* 1996). Autopsy studies have shown that some patients with FTD are misdiagnosed as having other forms of dementia during life (Litvan *et al.* 1997). The use of instruments such as the BEHAVE-AD (Reisberg *et al.* 1987) or the Executive Interview to measure neuropsychiatric symptoms may help to distinguish these conditions from each other (Royall *et al.* 1993; Mendez *et al.* 1998). The FTLDs, together with their differential diagnoses, are reviewed in detail by Snowden, Neary, and Mann, in their monograph, *Fronto-temporal lobar degeneration: Frontotemporal dementia, progressive aphasia and semantic dementia* (1996).

The clinical presentations of frontal lobe lesions vary depending upon the main site of pathology. A correlation has been demonstrated between lesions of the dorsolateral prefrontal cortex, giving rise to avolitional or attentional deficit states, and lesions of the orbitofrontal cortex, giving rise to behavioural change. The former may be described as 'executive disorder' (or 'catatonic disorder' when abulia is marked), whilst the latter may be described as 'personality change' (Table 10.7). the cardinal features of executive disorder include:

- impaired ability to plan, organize, and sequence information, and thus perform purposeful activities;
- impaired ability to abstract information, leading to impaired reasoning ability and faulty judgement;
- impaired ability to shift attention; perseveration;
- loss of volition, aspontaneity, self-neglect;
- stereotypies, echolalia, echopraxia;
- affective change, blunted or incongruous (facetious);
- perceptual inability to process simultaneous sensory inputs;

Table 10.7 Diagnostic criteria for personality change due to a general medical condition[a]

A	A persistent personality disturbance that represents a change from the individual's previous characteristic personality pattern.
B	There is evidence from the history, physical examination, or laboratory findings that the disturbance is the direct physiological consequence of a general medical condition.
C	The disturbance is not better accounted for by another mental disorder (for example, a manic episode).
D	The disturbance does not occur exclusively during the course of a delirium and does not meet the criteria for a dementia.
E	The disturbance causes clinically significant distress or impairment in social, occupational, or other important areas of functioning.

Specify type:
- labile type: if the predominant feature is affective lability
- disinhibited type: if the predominant feature is poor impulse control as evidenced by sexual indiscretions, etc.
- aggressive type: if the predominant feature is aggressive behaviour
- paranoid type: if the predominant feature is suspiciousness or paranoid ideation
- other type: if the predominant feature is not one of the above, for example personality change associated with a seizure disorder
- combined type: if more than one feature predominates in the clinical picture.

Unspecified type:
Coding note: include the name of the general medical condition on Axis I, for example personality change due to
temporal lobe epilepsy; also code the general medical condition on Axis III.

[a]Taken from DSM-IV 1994 with permission of the American Psychiatric Association.

- lack of insight;
- relative preservation of memory;
- relative preservation of praxis and gnosis.

Frontal lobe dysfunction may occur as a result of either frontal lobe lesions or diaschisis. The latter term refers to functional impairment in one brain region occurring as a result of a structural lesion in another neurally connected region. Thus, diaschisis in the neural network connecting the frontal lobes, the hippocampus, the basal ganglia, and the thalamus can account for an executive disorder due to caudate nucleus infarction or Huntington's disease (Petty *et al.* 1996).

The treatment of executive disorder and personality change presents considerable challenges, and often competency or placement issues are prominent if poor insight and faulty judgement are evident. The likelihood of avoiding long-term institutionalization is principally dependent on the treatability or otherwise of the underlying general medical condition. The possibility of potentially reversible dementias including normal pressure hydrocephalus, brain tumours, subdural haematomas, cerebral infections, endocrine disorders, and vitamin deficiency states should always be considered.

Management

Patients with dementia may be referred because of diagnostic difficulties, non-cognitive features, discharge advice, and determination of mental competency. Meticulous assessment should enable accurate diagnosis and formulation of a management plan, both of which should be communicated to the patient, the relatives, or significant others and the members of the referring team.

Investigations

Neuroimaging can often assist in the diagnosis of dementia. Sometimes, techniques such as a CT can be diagnostic (for example, normal pressure hydrocephalus or frontal meningiomas). The demonstration of generalized atrophy and ventricular dilatation on CT, in the absence of additional findings, is of positive clinical and diagnostic value as it helps to limit the number of conditions from which the patient might be suffering. In such cases, serial scans or a rotated view of the medial temporal lobe and hippocampus may further aid in the diagnosis of DAT (Smith and Jobst 1996). With the emergence of several new anti-Alzheimer's drugs, the role of neuroimaging has increased currency, as information to assist in accurate diagnosis is often needed.

MRI provides better resolution than CT. However, availability and cost factors often preclude its use in routine clinical practice as a first-line investigation. Thus, it is usually undertaken when CT is inconclusive, such as when findings do not match clinical features, or when brainstem imaging is particularly important.

Single-photon emission computed tomography (SPECT) (Rodriguez *et al.* 1999), positron emission tomography (PET) (Berent *et al.* 1999), and functional MRI

(Small *et al.* 1999) represent major advances in the neurophysiological investigation of organic mental disorders. PET and functional MRI are strictly limited in availability, whilst SPECT scanning is still not routinely available in many hospitals.

Characteristic patterns of brain function have been demonstrated with SPECT for many of the dementias, such as parietotemporal hypoperfusion in DAT and frontotemporal hypofunction in FTD. If SPECT is performed in addition to CT scanning, the diagnostic accuracy for Alzheimer's disease is further improved (Jobst *et al.* 1998). In liaison settings, SPECT is most likely to be available for unusual cases where further data are needed to establish the diagnosis. Functional imaging (such as SPECT) should only ever be used in association with structural imaging (such as CT) because of diaschisis–functional abnormalities resulting in one brain region as a result of structural pathology in another.

The electroencephalogram (EEG) has a limited place in liaison old age psychiatry. Epileptic seizures can occur in dementia, and whilst epilepsy is a clinical diagnosis, nevertheless EEG confirmation can improve and enhance clinical management. A characteristic triphasic or partial triphasic pattern is sometimes observed in Creutzfeldt–Jakob disease (Brenner 1990). More sophisticated EEG techniques, including sphenoidal leads (for temporal lobe epilepsy), telemetry, and sleep EEGs are sometimes indicated.

Treatment

If mild to moderate DAT is diagnosed, treatment with neurocholinesterase inhibitors such as donepezil 10 mg per day (Rogers *et al.* 1998), rivastigmine up to 12 mg per day (Rosler *et al.* 1999), or galantamine up to 24 mg per day (Raskind *et al.* 2000) should be considered. The cost of these drugs is not inconsiderable, and the treatment population is potentially huge (up to half a million patients in the UK alone). Thus, many countries have proposed or adopted stringent prescribing criteria using an evidence-based approach that generally excludes patients with serious medical illnesses (Harvey 1999). This in turn reduces the likelihood that these drugs will be prescribed in liaison settings.

The BPSD of dementia include disorders of behaviour, mood, thought content, perception, and personality (Shah and Allen 1999; Foli and Shah 2000). For some patients the personality change is an exaggeration of premorbid traits, disinhibited by executive dysfunction, but not all personality change can be attributed to the disease process.

Challenging behaviours can often be reduced by psychosocial interventions alone. A behavioural analysis demonstrates the uniqueness of the behaviour for that individual (Stokes 1986). Monitoring, through keeping a record of the frequency, duration, and type of Antecedent events, Behaviour, and the Consequences following the behaviour (ABC approach), provides this information (Stokes 1986). The aim is to change the behaviour by altering the antecedent stimuli or consequent events (Hussian 1984; Stokes 1986). Thus, depressed mood may be identified with understimulation, or paranoia with contact with unfamiliar people, or aggression with a misinterpreted situation. More detail on the non-pharmacological management of BPSD is given in Chapters 11 and 14.

Case study 10.3

Mrs C., an 87-year old widow, had DAT of moderate severity and was in a long-stay ward. She had several challenging behaviours including screaming and hitting out at caregivers. The nursing staff found her extremely difficult to look after. An ABC behaviour chart was implemented over a 5-day period. Analysing the chart, it was noted that the only time Mrs C. did not exhibit any challenging behaviour was on Thursday evenings when she behaved impeccably. The only identifiable difference was the presence of a certain part-time staff nurse who only worked Thursday evenings and regularly nursed the patient on that shift. Other staff members on the same shift invoked the usual reaction. The nurse involved always wore a pink apron over her uniform and this was the only factor that seemed different. All the nursing staff involved with Mrs C. started wearing pink aprons with a complete resolution of the challenging behaviour. No clear reason for this association was established.

There is a paucity of convincing evidence for effective pharmacological interventions in BPSD. Also, many of these features may remit spontaneously. Thus, Ballard and O'Brien (1999) recommend that, unless symptoms are extremely distressing, BPSD should be monitored for at least 1 month before starting pharmacological treatment.

Psychotic features may require treatment with neuroleptics if they are distressing, disabling, or lead to a risk of self-harm, self-neglect, or harm to others. Doses of more than 3 mg per day of haloperidol are associated with high rates of unacceptable extrapyramidal side-effects (Devanand *et al.* 1998). Neuroleptics with a relatively high 5-HT$_2$/D$_2$ receptor-blocking ratio (such as risperidone, olanzapine, and quetiapine) have fewer extrapyramidal side-effects than older neuroleptics. Quetiapine 25 mg twice a day titrated to 75 mg twice a day is often an effective dose. Non-neurological side-effects may be less marked with relatively D-specific medications such as sulpiride (for example 200 mg twice daily) and amisulpiride (for example, 100 mg twice daily). Recently, large, double-blind, controlled studies have shown that risperidone is as effective as haloperidol in treating psychotic features in dementia and is better tolerated (Burns and Craig 1998; Katz *et al.* 1999).

It may be necessary to treat depression with an antidepressant. Modern antidepressants, including selective serotonin-reuptake inhibitors (SSRIs), have fewer side-effects and have efficacy for depressive features in dementia (Katona *et al.* 1998). Short half-life SSRIs, such as citalopram 10–20 mg per day or sertraline 25–100 mg per day, are recommended.

Patients with VaD may be given low-dose aspirin prophylaxis, provided there are no contraindications, but as yet there is no clear evidence of efficacy. Attention should be paid to the optimal control of coexistent hypertension (including avoidance of intermittent hypotension), hypercholesterolaemia, cardiac disease, and diabetes mellitus.

Assessment of disability status is an important part of the management plan and crucial to decision-making on future accommodation and support needs. Problems are best identified via an occupational therapy and/or physiotherapy home visit. The appropriate management of the finances of mentally incapacitated patients may require legal guardianship (see Chapters 15 and 16). Relatives should be given advice on voluntary organizations such as the Alzheimer's Disease and Related Disorders Society (ADARDS) or a local Alzheimer's Association, which will often provide a range of useful services.

Professional community services tailored to the individual's needs should be organized before discharge to minimize the risk of readmission. Services required may include day-centre care, assistance with self-care, housework, home-delivered meals, shopping, personal finance activities, medication supervision, communication aids (e.g. large-key phone pads, scan alarms), and transport needs.

Prognosis

In many cases dementia is unrecognized for several years due to its insidious onset and slow progress in the early stages (Reisberg *et al.* 1996). By the time a formal diagnosis is made, the mortality rate for late-onset DAT is 9% at 6 months, rising to 35% at 2 years (Christie and Wood 1990). Even in a medical setting, dementia is poorly recognized and treated and can contribute to increases in length of stay in hospital (Johnston *et al.* 1987; Ramsay *et al.* 1991), delirium (Taylor and Lewis 1993), and mortality (Shah *et al.* 1993).

Case study 10.4

Mrs C. was a 78-year-old woman with one son who was a doctor. He had no inkling that his mother had any problems until his father died suddenly of a heart attack. At first, he put down his mother's incoherence and disorganization after the funeral to a grief reaction. A month later he discovered she had lost a considerable amount of weight, was incontinent of faeces, and was ungroomed. He realized to his horror that his mother was suffering from marked cognitive impairment. He also recognized that he had never questioned his father's helpful tendency towards his wife, nor his habit of finishing her sentences and taking over tasks. When Mrs C. was admitted for assessment he was most embarrassed to learn that the dementia was well advanced and that she needed to be placed in a nursing home.

Amnestic disorder

Epidemiology and aetiology

The prevalence of amnestic disorder in liaison settings is unclear. It is most frequently associated with chronic alcohol abuse and head injury. There is evidence in North America of a declining association with alcohol abuse and an increasing association with head injury (Kaplan and Sadock 1998).

Clinical features

DSM-IV criteria for amnestic disorder are listed in Table 10.8. Strong reciprocal connections between the medial temporal lobe and the dorsolateral prefrontal cortex probably underlie the frequent coexistence of amnesia and executive dysfunction. However, in amnestic disorder the executive dysfunction is not prominent relative to the amnesia.

Alcohol abuse is common in the elderly (Luttrell *et al.* 1997), particularly in liaison settings (Scott *et al.* 1988; Wrigley and Loane 1991; Swanwick *et al.* 1994; Ticehurst 1994; Collinson and Benbow 1998). A variety of syndromes may present. Many amnestic patients have a previous history of alcohol withdrawal delirium (delirium tremens or Wernicke's encephalopathy). In Wernicke's encephalopathy there are distinctive features such as a staggering gait, ocular palsy, nystagmus, and peripheral neuropathy. It should be noted, however, that such features are not invariably present. The disorder is partially or totally reversible if identified early and appropriately treated with thiamine (Cutting 1978). Wernicke's encephalopathy can cause a persisting amnestic disorder (Korsakoff's syndrome) after the delirium has cleared, if inadequately treated. The memory disturbance is particularly marked in the ability to learn new information. Less distinctively, an alcohol-induced

Table 10.8 Diagnostic criteria for amnestic disorder

A The development of memory impairment as manifested by impairment in the ability to learn new information or the inability to recall previously learned information.

B The memory disturbance causes significant impairment in social or occupational functioning and represents a significant decline from a previous level of functioning.

C The memory disturbance does not occur exclusively during the course of a delirium or a dementia (and in cases of substance-related disorder, persists beyond the usual duration of substance intoxication or withdrawal).

D There is evidence from the history, physical examination, or laboratory findings that the disturbance is the direct physiological consequence of a general medical condition (including physical trauma) or, in substance-related cases, is aetiologically related to the persisting effects of substance use (for example, a drug of abuse, a medication).

Specify if:
– transient: if memory impairment lasts for 1 month or less
– chronic: if memory impairment lasts for more than 1 month.

Coding note: include the name of the general medical condition on Axis I, for example amnestic disorder due to head
trauma; also code the general medical condition on Axis III.

Taken from DSM-IV 1994 with permission of the American Psychiatric Association.

persisting dementia can occur without a clear history of delirium tremens/ Wernicke's encephalopathy. The patient presents with cognitive impairment on a background of prolonged, heavy drinking over many years and without other cause for the impairment being apparent (Beresford 1993).

Management

The liaison psychiatrist may be asked to advise on several aspects of alcohol-related cognitive disorders, including the management of acute behavioural disturbance, specific treatment of delirium or dementia, or suitability for an abstinence programme. In alcohol-induced persisting amnestic disorder, there is an association between the development of irreversible cognitive and neurological disability and delay in diagnosis. The principal reason for this is delay in treatment with thiamine (Cutting 1978). Parenteral thiamine should be given immediately, followed by oral thiamine and other multivitamin preparations for at least 6 months.

Patients presenting with delirium tremens or Wernicke–Korsakoff's syndrome may also suffer from clinically significant alcohol-related complications of other organ systems, and these may require assessment and treatment from a range of specialties. Cognitive impairment may modify and reduce the urge to drink alcohol. Formal treatment may be needed where the urge to drink alcohol continues; this may need long-term follow-up and rehabilitation, and requires liaison between old age psychiatry and substance misuse services.

Other cognitive disorders

These include aphasias, apraxias, and agnosias (for definitions see Table 10.9). They can be caused by circumscribed lesions of the brain in association with disorders such as cerebrovascular accidents and cerebral neoplasms, or by focal cerebral lobar atrophy. Epidemiological data for these disorders in liaison settings are absent.

Aphasic disorder

Aphasia is caused by lesions of Broca's area in the dominant frontal lobe or Wernicke's area in the dominant temporal lobe. Broca's aphasia is an expressive aphasia and may occur after a stroke in the dorsolateral area of the prefrontal cortex. A similar type of aphasia, progressive non-fluent aphasia, is due to a focal lobar degeneration. It is one of the FTLDs and is often familial. The extent of clinical impairment is usually associated with the extent of the lesion. Speech is reduced in quantity, non-fluent, and ungrammatical, with phonemic paraphrasias and impaired word retrieval. (Snowden *et al.* 1996). In Broca's aphasia and progressive non-fluent aphasia, patients often become distressed and frustrated at their inability to correctly

Table 10. 9 Miscellaneous disorders of cognition

	Definition
Agnosia	Lack of ability to perceive or recognize sensory stimuli at a cortical level.
Aphasia	Impaired or absent comprehension of/or communication by speech, writing, or signs, due to dysfunction of brain centres in the dominant hemisphere.
Apraxia	1. Partial or complete incapacity to execute purposeful movements, despite preservation of muscular power, sensibility, and coordination. 2. The proper use of an object can not be carried out, although the object can be named and its uses described.
Dyscalculia	Difficulty in performing mathematical calculations at a cortical level.
Dysgraphia	Difficulty in writing at a cortical level.
Executive	Impairment of central co-ordinating and processing of mental tasks.
Disorder	Associated with dysfunction of frontal–subcortical–thalamic neural networks.

formulate words for verbal communication. If it can be demonstrated that the patient's comprehension for the spoken or written word is intact, then psycho-therapeutic support may help the patient come to terms with the disability. Although treatment is difficult, a speech therapy assessment should be sought. An active treatment and rehabilitation programme may result in improved verbal (spoken and written) and non-verbal communication (Greener *et al.* 1998).

Comprehension impairment involves lesions of Wernicke' area in the temporal lobe. A range of language disturbances may be found in an individual patient, including disturbance of comprehension, expression, naming, repetition, reading, and writing. It is sometimes assumed that a condition with expressive impairment must represent an 'expressive aphasia' (i.e. Broca's aphasia). However, the expressive abnormality of a 'comprehension aphasia' (i.e. Wernicke's aphasia), includes increased quantity of speech with fluent breakdown of phonetic, syntactical, and semantic components, sometimes resulting in 'word salad'. It is often less intelligible than the expressive abnormality of an 'expression aphasia' (Benson and Geschwind 1971).

Semantic dementia (Snowden *et al.* 1989), the third variant of FTLD, is a rare disorder of the (dominant) temporal lobe characterized by a loss of meaning and significance to words, whilst speech is fluent and syntactically normal. Some words may be used idiosyncratically or there may be excessive use of generic terms such as 'water' for all forms of fluid. There may be an associated visual agnosia. Episodic, day-to-day, autobiographical memory is preserved, along with visuospatial and calculation skills, allowing a fair degree of independence. Often the relatives report a 'memory failure', which when investigated closely is due to the patient's inability to recognize word meanings, faces, or objects. Structural imaging with CT or MRI may show temporal lobe atrophy, whilst functional techniques such as SPECT and PET localize the impairment to the dominant lobe (Hodges *et al.* 1992).

Apraxic and agnostic disorders

Isolated apraxias and agnosias can occur independently, but frequently occur together. This reflects their neuroanatomical relationship. An agnosia may be conceptualized as the sensory component, and an apraxia as the motor component, of a higher order reflex loop. They most frequently occur in relation to circum-scribed lesions of the posterior cortex, classically the parietal lobe. Thus, they are frequently seen in patients with stroke, and can lead to considerable difficulties in rehabilitation if the patient exhibits a lack of concern about the hemiparesis (Denes *et al.* 1982). Ideomotor apraxia refers to the inability to carry out a requested movement properly, such as waving goodbye (Geschwind and Damasio 1985). In ideational apraxia, the patient is unable to carry out sequential tasks, such as the three-stage command in the Mini-Mental State Examination (Folstein *et al.* 1975). Constructional apraxia refers to the inability to perform visuospatial tasks such as copying intersecting pentagrams (Folstein *et al.* 1975). A vast number of agnosias are described, including the failure to recognize facial characteristics in prosopagnosia, external space in topographical agnosia, and internal body schema in autotopagnosia. These conditions are comprehensively reviewed by Frederiks (1985).

Case study 10.5

Mr E.F., aged 73 years, was admitted to a general medical ward because of haemat-emesis. Following transfusion his general condition improved, but he was then referred as an emergency to the old age psychiatry liaison service after having sexually assaulted a female member of staff. Collateral history revealed that he was a previously devout Muslim gentleman of good character in whom, premorbidly, such behaviour would be unthinkable. There was a 2-year history of intrafamilial relationship problems and a history of alcohol abuse, despite the prohibition of his religion. Mental state examination revealed intact conscious awareness of the immediate external environment with marked attentional impairment. There was a delayed response time to all questions and marked impairment on tests of reverse counting, reverse spelling, clockface drawing, verbal fluency, and similarities/differences. Mild amnesia and apraxia were noted, which were judged to be secondary to the patient's marked attentional deficit. A diagnosis was made of personality change due to a general medical condition, and supportive advice given to the general medical team on how to manage the patient's behaviour whilst awaiting the results of CT brain scan. This revealed a large subcortical infarct of the white matter underlying the left frontal lobe. The patient required admission to a continuing-care unit.

Conclusions

Organic mental disorders represent some of the most frequent conditions leading to referral to psychogeriatric liaison services. Delirium represents a medical emergency and thus requires an urgent response. Patients with dementia may be referred for a wide range of reasons, including behavioural difficulties and determination of mental competency with regard to treatment and discharge placement. Optimum management of all conditions is facilitated by close working with patients, relatives, carers, and all members of the referring team.

References

Alexopoulos, G.S., Silver, J.M., Kahn, D.A., Frances, A., and Carpenter, D. (1998). Treatment of agitation in older persons with dementia. The Expert Consensus Guidelines Series. *Postgraduate Medicine*, Special Report, April.

American Psychiatric Association (1994). *Diagnostic and statistical manual of mental disorders (DSM-IV)*, 4th edn. American Psychiatric Association, Washington DC.

Ames, D. and Tuckwell, V. (1994). Psychiatric disorders among elderly patients in a general hospital. *Medical Journal of Australia*, **160**, 671–5.

Baheerathan, M. and Shah, A.K. (1999). The impact of two changes in service delivery on a geriatric psychiatry liaison service. *International Journal of Geriatric Psychiatry*, **14**, 767–75.

Ballard, C. and O'Brien, J. (1999). Treating behavioural and psychological signs in Alzheimer's disease. *British Medical Journal*, **319**, 38–39.

Benson, D.F. and Geschwind, N. (1971). Aphasia and related cortical disturbances. In *Clinical neurology* (ed. A.B. Baker and L.H. Baker), pp. 77–98. Harper and Row, New York.

Berent, S., Giordani, B., Foster, N., Minoshima, S., Lajiness-O'Neill, R., Koeppe, R., *et al.* (1999). Neuropsychological function and cerebral glucose utilisation in isolated memory impairment and Alzheimer's disease. *Journal of Psychiatric Research*, **33**, 7–16.

Beresford, T.P. (1993). Alcoholism and the elderly. *International Review of Psychiatry*, **5**, 477–83.

Berr, C., Richard, F., Dufouil, C., Amant, C., Alpervitch, A., and Amouyel, P. (1998). Polymorphism of the prion protein is associated with cognitive impairment in the elderly: the EVA study. *Neurology*, **51**, 734–7.

Brenner, R.P. (1990). Periodic EEG patterns: classification, clinical correlation and pathophysiology. *Journal of Clinical Neurophysiology*, **7**, 249–67.

Broe, G.A., Henderson, A.S., Creasey, H., McCusker, E., Korten, A.E., Jorm, A.F., *et al.* (1990). A case-control study of Alzheimer's disease in Australia. *Neurology*, **40**, 1698–707.

Brown, R.G. and Marsden, C.D. (1984). How common is dementia in Parkinson's disease? *Lancet*, **2**, 1262–5.

Bucht, G., Gustafson, Y., and Sandberg, O. (1999). Epidemiology of delirium. *Dementia and Geriatric Cognitive Disorders*, **10**, 315–18.

Burns, A. and Craig, S. (1998). Neuroleptics in the treatment of Alzheimer's disease. *Neurobiology of Ageing*, **19** (Suppl. 4), 450.

Chick, J. (1989). Delirium tremens. *British Medical Journal*, **298**, 3–4.

Christie, A.B. and Wood, E.R.M. (1990). Further change in the pattern of mental illness in the elderly. *British Journal of Psychiatry*, **157**, 228–31.

Collinson, Y. and Benbow, S.M. (1998). The role of an old age consultation liaison nurse. *International Journal of Geriatric Psychiatry*, **13**, 159–63.

Conneally, P.M., Gusella, J.F., and Wexler, N.S. (1985). Huntington's disease: linkage with G8 on chromosome 4 and its consequences. *Progress in Clinical and Biological Research*, **177**, 53–60.

Cummings, J.L., Vinters, H.V., Cole, G.M., and Khachaturian, Z.S. (1998). Alzheimer's disease: etiologies, pathophysiology, cognitive reserve, and treatment opportunities. *Neurology*, **1**(Suppl. 1), S2–S17.

Cutting, J. (1978). The relationship between Korsakoff's syndrome and 'alcoholic dementia'. *British Journal of Psychiatry*, **132**, 240–51.

De, T. and Shah, A.K. (1998). Dementia: behavioural problems can be managed effectively. *Geriatric Medicine*, **28**, 60–4.

Denes, G., Semenza, C., Stoppa, E., and Lis, A. (1982). Unilateral spatial neglect and recovery from hemiplegia. *Brain*, **105**, 543.

Devanand, D.P., Marder, K., Michaels, K.S., Sackeim, H.A., Bell, K., Sullivan, M.A., *et al.* (1998). A randomized, placebo-controlled dose-comparison trial of haloperidol for psychosis and disruptive behaviors in Alzheimer's disease. *American Journal of Psychiatry*, **55**, 1512–20.

Fleminger, S. (1991). Subcortical dementia–defining a clinical syndrome. In *Neurobiology and psychiatry* (ed. R. Kerwin), pp. 137–54. Cambridge University Press, Cambridge.

Foli, S. and Shah, A.K. (2000). Measurement of disturbed behaviour, non-cognitive features and quality of life. In *Dementia* (ed. J. O'Brien, D. Ames, and A. Burns), pp. 87–100. Chapman and Hall, London.

Folstein, M.F., Folstein, S.E., and McHugh, P.R. (1975). Mini-mental state: a practical method for grading the cognitive state of patients for the clinician. *Journal of Psychiatric Research*, **12**, 189–98.

Folstein, S.E. (1989). *Huntington's disease: a disorder of families*. Johns Hopkins University Press, Baltimore, MD.

Ford, C.V. and Folks, D.G. (1985). Psychiatric disorders in geriatric medical and surgical patients. *Southern Medical Journal*, **78**, 397–402.

Frataglioni, L., Grut, M., Forsell, Y., Viitanen, M., Grafstrom, M., Holmen, K., *et al.* (1991). Prevalence of Alzheimer's disease and other dementias in an elderly urban population: relationship with sex and education. *Neurology*, **41**, 1886–92.

Frederiks, J.A.M. (1985). Disorders of the body schema. In *Handbook of clinical neurology, Revised series*, Vol. 1, *Clinical neuropsychology* (ed. J.A.M. Frederiks), pp. 373–93. Elsevier Science, Amsterdam.

Geschwind, N. and Damasio, A.R. (1985). Apraxia. In *Handbook of clinical neurology, Revised series*, Vol. 1, *Clinical neuropsychology* (ed. J.A.M. Frederiks), pp. 423–32. Elsevier Science, Amsterdam.

Goate, A., Chartier Harlin, M.C., Mullan, M., Brown, J., Crawford, F., Fidani, L., *et al.* (1991). Segregation of a missense mutation in the amyloid precursor protein gene with familial Alzheimer's disease. *Nature*, **349**, 704–6.

Goldberg, R.J. and Goldberg, J. (1997). Risperidone for treating dementia related disturbed behaviour in nursing home residents: a clinical experience. *International Psychogeriatrics*, **9**, 65–8.

Greener, J., Enderby, P., Whurr, R., and Grant, A. (1998). Treatment for aphasia following stroke: evidence for effectiveness. *International Journal of Language and Communicative Disorders*, **33**(Suppl.), 158–61.

Harding, A.E. (1993). Movement disorders. In *Brain's diseases of the nervous system* (ed. J. Walton), 393–425. Oxford Medical, Oxford.

Harrison, R., Savla, N., and Kafetz, K. (1990). Dementia, depression and physical disability in a London Borough: a survey of elderly people in and out of residential care and implications for future care. *Age and Ageing*, **19**, 97–103.

Harvey, R. (1999). A review and commentary on a sample of 15 UK guidelines for drug treatment of Alzheimer's disease. *International Journal of Geriatric Psychiatry*, **14**, 249–56.

Hodges, J.R., Patterson, K., Oxbury, S., and Funnell, E. (1992). Semantic dementia. Progressive fluent aphasia with temporal lobe atrophy. *Brain*, **115**, 1783–806.

Hodkinson, E., McCafferty, F.G., Scott, J.N., and Stout, R.W. (1988). Disability and dependency in elderly people in residential and hospital care. *Age and Ageing*, **17**, 147–54.

Hussian, R.A. (1984). Behavioral geriatrics. *Progress in Behavior Modification*, **16**, 159–83.

Hutton, M. and Hardy, J. (1997). The presenilins and Alzheimer's disease. *Human Molecular Genetics*, **6**, 1639–46.

Inouye, S.K., van Dyck, C.H., Alessi, C.A., Balkin, S., Siegal, A.P., and Horwitz, R.I. (1990). Clarifying confusion: the Confusion Assessment Method. *Annals of Internal Medicine*, **113**, 941–8.

Inouye, S.K., Rushing, J.T., Foreman, M.D., Palmer, R.M., and Pompei, P. (1998). Does delirium contribute to poor hospital outcomes? A three-site epidemiologic study. *Journal of General Internal Medicine*, **13**, 234–42.

Jobst, K.A., Barnetson, L.P., and Shepstone, B.J. (1998). Accurate prediction of histologically confirmed Alzheimer's disease and the differential diagnosis of dementia: the use of NINCDS-ADRDA and DSM-III-R criteria, SPECT, X-ray CT, and Apo E4 in medial temporal lobe dementias. Oxford Project to Investigate Memory and Aging. *International Psychogeriatrics*, **10**, 271–302.

Johnston, M., Wakeling, A., Graham, N., and Stokes, F. (1987). Cognitive impairment, emotional disorder and length of stay of elderly patients in a district general hospital. *British Journal of Medical Psychology*, **60**, 133–9.

Kaplan, H.I. and Sadock, B.J. (1998). Amnestic disorders. In *Synopsis of psychiatry* (8th edn), (eds. Kaplan, H.I. and Sadock, B.J.), pp. 345–50. Williams and Wilkins, Baltimore, MD.

Katona, C.L.E., Hunter, B.N., and Bray, J. (1998). A double blind comparison of the efficacy of paroxetine and imipramine in the treatment of depression in dementia. *International Journal of Geriatric Psychiatry*, **13**, 100–8.

Katz, I.R., Parmelee, P., and Brubaker, K. (1991). Toxic and metabolic encephalopathies in long-term care patients. *International Psychogeriatrics*, **3**, 337–47.

Katz, I.R., Jeste, D., Mintzer, J.E., Clyde, C., Napolitano, J., and Brecher, M. (1999). Comparison of risperidone and placebo for psychosis and behavioural disturbances associated with dementia: a randomised double blind trial. *Journal of Clinical Psychiatry*, **60**, 107–15.

Katzman, R., Lasker, R., and Bernstein, N. (1988). Advances in the diagnosis of dementia: accuracy of diagnosis and consequences of misdiagnosis of disorders causing dementia. *Aging and the Brain*, **32**, 17–62.

Kolbeinsson, H. and Jonsson, A. (1993). Delirium and dementia in acute medical admissions of elderly patients in Iceland. *Acta Psychiatrica Scandinavica*, **87**, 123–7.

Lamb, H., Christie, J., Singleton, A.B., Leake, A., Perry, R.H., Ince, P.G., *et al.* (1998). Apolipoprotein E and alpha-1 antichymotrypsin polymorphism genotyping in Alzheimer's disease and in dementia with Lewy bodies. Distinctions between diseases. *Neurology*, **50**, 388–91.

Larson, E.B., Kukall, W.A., Buchner, D., and Reifler, B.V. (1987). Adverse drug reactions associated with global cognitive impairment in elderly patients. *Annals of Internal Medicine*, **107**, 169–73.

Levkoff, S., Evans, D., Liptzin, B., Cleary, P., Lipsitz, L., Wetle, T., *et al.* (1992). Delirium, the occurrence and persistence of symptoms among elderly hospitalised patients. *Archives of Internal Medicine*, **152**, 334–40.

Lipe, H., Schultz, A., and Bird, T.D. (1993). Risk factors for suicide in Huntington's disease: a retrospective case controlled study. *American Journal of Medical Genetics*, **48**, 231–3.

Lipowski, Z.J. (1990). *Delirium: acute confusional states*. Oxford University Press, Oxford.

Litvan, I., Agid, Y., Sastrj, N., Jankovic, J., Wenning, G.K., Goetz, C.G., *et al.* (1997). What are the obstacles for an accurate clinical diagnosis of Pick's disease? A clinicopathologic study. *Neurology*, **49**, 62–9.

Lund and Manchester Groups (1994). Clinical and neuropathological criteria for frontotemporal dementia. *Journal of Neurology, Neurosurgery and Psychiatry*, **57**, 416–18.

Luttrell, S., Watkin, V., Livingston, G., Walker, Z., D'Ath, P., Patel, P., *et al.* (1997). Screening for alcohol misuse in older people. *International Journal of Geriatric Psychiatry*, **12**, 1151–4.

MacDonald, A., Simpson, A., and Jenkins, D. (1989). Delirium in the elderly: a review and suggestions for a research programme. *International Journal of Geriatric Psychiatry*, **4**, 311–19.

McGuffin, P. and Martin, N. (1999). Behaviour and genes. *British Medical Journal*, **319**, 37–40.

McKeith, I.G., Galasko, D., Kosaka, K., Perry, E.K., Dickson, D.W., Hansen, L.A., *et al.* (1996). Clinical and pathological diagnosis of dementia with Lewy bodies: report of the CLBD international workshop. *Neurology*, **47**, 1113–24.

McKeith, I.G., Perry, E.K., and Perry, R.H. (1999). Report of the second dementia with Lewy body international workshop: diagnosis and treatment. *Neurology*, **53**, 902–5.

McKeith, I.G., Grace, J.B., Walker, Z., Byrne, E.J., Wilkinson, D., Stevens, T., *et al.* (2000). Rivastigmine in the treatment of dementia with Lewy bodies: preliminary findings from an open trial. *International Journal of Geriatric Psychiatry*, **15**, 387–92.

Mehta, D.K. (ed.) (2000). *The British national formulary* (39th edn). British Medical Association and the Royal Pharmaceutical Society of Great Britain, London.

Mendez, M.F., Perryman, K.M., Miller, B.L., and Cummings, J.L. (1998). Behavioral differences between frontotemporal dementia and Alzheimer's disease: a comparison on the BEHAVE-AD rating scale. *International Psychogeriatrics*, **10**, 155–62.

Meyer, J.S., McClintic, K.L., Rogers, R.L., Sims, P., and Mortel, K.F. (1988). Aetiological considerations and risk factors for multi-infarct dementia. *Journal of Neurology, Neurosurgery and Psychiatry*, **51**, 1489–97.

Mortimer, J.A., French, L.R., Hutton, J.T., and Schuman, L.M. (1985). Head trauma as a risk factor for Alzheimer's disease. *Neurology*, **35**, 264–7.

Patel, P., Goldberg, D., and Moss, S. (1993). Psychiatric morbidity in older people with moderate and severe learning disability (mental retardation). Part II: The prevalence study. *British Journal of Psychiatry*, **163**, 481–91.

Petty, R.G., Bonner, D., Mouratoglou, V., and Silverman, M. (1996). Acute frontal lobe syndrome and dyscontrol associated with bilateral caudate nucleus infarctions. *British Journal of Psychiatry*, **168**, 237–40.

Ramsay, R., Wright, P., Katz, A., Bielawska, C., and Katona, C. (1991). The detection of psychiatric morbidity and its effect on outcome in acute elderly medical admissions. *International Journal of Geriatric Psychiatry*, **6**, 861–6.

Raskind, M.A., Peskind, E.R., Wessel, T., and Yuan, W. (2000). Galantamine in AD: a 6-month randomized, placebo-controlled trial with a 6-month extension. The Galantamine USA-1 Study Group. *Neurology*, **54**, 2261–8.

Reisberg, B., Borenstein, J., Salob, S.P., Ferris, S.H., Franssen, E.H., and Georgotas, A. (1987). Behavioral symptoms in Alzheimer's disease: phenomenology and treatment. *Journal of Clinical Psychiatry*, **48**(Suppl.), 9–15.

Reisberg, B., Ferris, S.H., Franssen, E.H., Shulman, E., Monteiro, I., Sclan, S.G., *et al*. (1996). Mortality and temporal course of probable Alzheimer's disease: a 5-year prospective study. *International Psychogeriatrics*, **8**, 291–311.

Risse, S.C. and Barnes, R.I. (1986). Pharmacologic treatment of agitation associated with dementia. *Journal of the American Geriatrics Society*, **34**, 368–76.

Robert, P.H., Lafont, V., Snowden, J.S., and Lebert, F. (1999). Diagnostic criteria for fronto-temporal lobar degeneration. *Encephale*, **25**, 612–21.

Roberts, G.W., Allsop, D., and Bruton, C. (1990). The occult aftermath of boxing. *Journal of Neurology, Neurosurgery and Psychiatry*, **53**, 373–8.

Rodriguez, G., Nobili, F., Copello, F., Vitali, P., Gianelli, M.V., Taddei, G., *et al*. (1999). 99mTc-HMPAO regional cerebral blood flow and quantitative electroencephalography in Alzheimer's disease: a correlative study. *Journal of Nuclear Medicine*, **40**, 373–8.

Rogers, S.L., Doody, R.S., Mohs, R.C., and Friedhoff, L.T. (1998). Donepezil improves cognition and global function in Alzheimer's disease: a 15-week, double-blind, placebo controlled study. *Archives of Internal Medicine*, **158**, 1021–31.

Roses, A.D. and Saunders, A.M. (1997). Apolipoprotein E genotyping as a diagnostic adjunct for Alzheimer's Disease. *International Psychogeriatrics*, **9**(Suppl. 1), 277–88.

Rosler, M., Anand, R., Cicin-Sain, A., Gautheir, S., Agid, Y., Dal-Bianco, P., *et al*. (1999). Efficacy and safety of rivastigmine in patients with Alzheimer's disease: international randomised controlled trial. *British Medical Journal*, **318**, 633–8.

Royall, D.R., Mahurin, R.K., and Gray, K.F. (1993). Bedside assessment of executive cognitive impairment: the executive interview. *Journal of the American Geriatrics Society*, **40**, 1221–26.

Scott, J., Fairbairn, A., and Woodhouse, K. (1988). Referrals to a psychogeriatric consultation-liaison service. *International Journal of Geriatric Psychiatry*, **3**, 131–5.

Shah, A.K. and Allen, H. (1999). Is improvement possible in the measurement of behaviour disturbance? *International Journal of Geriatric Psychiatry*, **14**, 512–19.

Shah, A.K. and Ames, D. (1994). Behavioural problems in patients with dementia. *Modern Medicine*, **5**, 67–72.

Shah, A., Phongsathorn, V., George, C., Bielawska, C., and Katona, C. (1992). Psychiatric morbidity among continuing care geriatric inpatients. *International Journal of Geriatric Psychiatry*, **7**, 517–25.

Shah, A.K., Phongsathorn, V., George, C., Bielawski, C., and Katona, C. (1993). Does psychiatric morbidity predict mortality in continuing care geriatric inpatients? *International Journal of Geriatric Psychiatry*, **8**, 255–9.

Sherrington, R., Rogaev, E.L., Liang, Y., Rogaeva, E.A., Levesque, G., Ikeda, M., *et al.* (1995). Cloning of a gene bearing mis-sense mutations in early onset familial Alzheimer's disease. *Nature*, **375**, 754–60.

Small, S.A., Perera, G.M., DeLapaz, R., Mayeux, R., and Stern, Y. (1999). Differential regional dysfunction of the hippocampal formation among elderly with memory decline and Alzheimer's disease. *Annals of Neurology*, **45**, 466–72.

Smith, A.D. and Jobst, K.A. (1996). Use of structural imaging to study the progression of Alzheimer's disease. *British Medical Bulletin*, **52**, 575–86.

Snowden, J.S., Goulding, P.J., and Neary, D. (1989). Semantic dementia: a form of circumscribed atrophy. *Behavioural Neurology*, **2**, 167–82.

Snowden, J.S., Neary, D., and Mann, D.M.A. (1996). Lobar atrophy and motor neurone disease. In *Fronto-temporal lobar degeneration: fronto-temporal dementia, progressive aphasia and semantic dementia*, pp. 59–72. Churchill Livingstone, New York.

Stokes, G. (1986). *Screaming and shouting*. Winslow Press, Bicester, Oxfordfordshire.

Sunderland, T. and Silver, M.A. (1988). Neuroleptics in the treatment of dementia. *International Journal of Geriatric Psychiatry*, **3**, 784–90.

Swanwick, G.R.J., Lee, H., Clare, A.W., and Lawlor, B. (1994). Consultation-liaison psychiatry: a comparison of two service models for geriatric patients. *International Journal of Geriatric Psychiatry*, **9**, 495–9.

Taylor, D. and Lewis, S. (1993). Delirium. *Journal of Neurology, Neurosurgery and Psychiatry*, **56**, 742–51.

Ticehurst, S. (1994). Substance use and abuse. In *Functional psychiatric disorders of the elderly* (ed. E. Chiu and D. Ames), pp. 269–84. Cambridge University Press, Cambridge.

Treloar, A. and MacDonald, A. (1997*a*). Outcome of delirium diagnosed by DSM-III-R, ICD-10 and CAMDEX and derivation of the reversible cognitive dysfunction scale among acute geriatric inpatients. *International Journal of Geriatric Psychiatry*, **12**, 609–13.

Treloar, A. and MacDonald, A. (1997*b*). Clinical features of reversible cognitive dysfunction—are they the same as accepted definitions of delirium? *International Journal of Geriatric Psychiatry*, **12**, 614–18.

Tune, L.E. and Bylsma, F.W. (1991). Benzodiazepine-induced and anticholinergic-induced delirium in the elderly. *International Psychogeriatrics*, **3**, 397–408.

Verity, M.A. (1993). Environmental neurotoxicity of chemicals and radiation. *Current Opinions in Neurology and Neurosurgery*, **6**, 397–408.

Walker, Z., Grace, J., Overshot, R., Satarasinghe, S., Swan, A., Katona, C.L., *et al.* (1999). Olanzapine in dementia with Lewy bodies: a clinical study. *International Journal of Geriatric Psychiatry*, **14**, 459–66.

World Health Organization (1992). *The international classification of diseases classification of mental and behavioural disorders, 10th edn (ICD-10): diagnostic criteria for research*. World Health Organization, Geneva.

Wrigley, M. and Loane, R. (1991). Consultation-liaison referrals to the North Dublin old age psychiatry service. *Irish Medical Journal*, **84**, 89–91.

Yamada, M., Itoh, Y., Inaba, A., Wada, Y., Takashima, M., Satoh, S., *et al.* (1999). An inherited prion disease with a PrP P 105L mutation: clinicopathologic and PrP heterogeneity. *Neurology*, **53**, 181–8.

11 Specific patients and problems

Ajit Shah and David Ames

Summary

A range of special patients and problems are encountered in liaison geriatric psychiatry settings. Some examples include patients labelled as 'difficult to like', 'undesirable', and 'bed blockers'. These patients may have specific problems, such as behaviour disturbance, suicidal ideation, poor compliance with treatment, refusal to eat, mental incapacity, squalor, neuropsychiatric complications of prescribed and non-prescribed drugs, and alcohol misuse. Case studies are used to illustrate some typical cases.

Introduction

Liaison geriatric psychiatry occurs at the interface between geriatric psychiatry and almost all other hospital specialties involving older people. Consequently, a wide and challenging range of patients and problems are encountered. These include patients with behaviour disturbance, suicidal ideation, poor compliance with treatment, refusal to eat, mental incapacity, squalor syndrome, neuropsychiatric complications of prescribed and non-prescribed drugs, and alcohol misuse. Staff members, individually or collectively, from all these specialties and disciplines may label such patients as 'difficult to like' and 'undesirable'. Anecdotally, in a recent liaison study, about a third of patients were estimated to fit this description (Baheerathan and Shah 1999). As epidemiological and clinical data are sparse, the true incidence of patients thus described is unknown.

'Difficult to like patients' and 'undesirable patients'

Pejorative labelling such as ' difficult to like' or 'undesirable patients' may be influenced by factors related to the patient, the clinical setting, and the doctor (Ewing 1965; Anonymous 1969; Papper 1969; Weiner 1993; Short 1994). Patient characteristics include the illness, previous experience, premorbid personality, clinical presentation, and social circumstances. Factors related to the clinical setting include delay in transportation (e.g. the ambulance service), long waiting lists for appointments, long waiting delays in outpatient and casualty departments, missing medical case-notes and investigations, and the timing of the assessment (working or duty hours). Factors related to doctors include tiredness and fatigue, previous knowledge of the patient, previous experience, clinical and research interests, personal bias and prejudice, and conflict within the multidisciplinary team. Patients labelled as 'undesirable' have been further classified into several separate, but overlapping, categories of undesirability (Papper 1969). These are as follows:

- socially undesirable;
- attitudinally undesirable;
- undesirable on physical grounds;
- circumstantially undesirable;
- distraction undesirability.

Socially undesirable patients include people with eccentricities (e.g. hoarding, strange eating behaviours, unusual sleep habits, poor hygiene), socially maligned conditions (e.g. substance abuse, sexually transmitted diseases, mental illness), those with communication difficulties (e.g. deaf, poor command of local language, rambling historians, uneducated), non-compliant patients (e.g. refusing food, medication, consent), and the elderly (Anonymous 1969; Papper 1969; Short 1994). The elderly mentally ill may find themselves in double or multiple jeopardy, not only from their mental illness or age but also from bias as a result of the socially undesirable consequences (Norman 1985; Rait *et al*. 1996).

Case study 11.1

Mrs G.S, a 70-year-old Indian lady, was admitted with poorly controlled diabetes. Her vision was reduced, she was deaf without a hearing aid, and spoke no English. This resulted in staff feeling that she was deliberately non-compliant with treatment and that she had an underlying mental illness. Luckily the psychiatrist spoke the patient's mother tongue. After acquiring her hearing aid from her home, the psychiatrist was able to establish two points: (1) she did not have a mental illness and (2) she had great deal of difficulty in understanding the instructions of the nursing staff because of her deafness and poor English. Simple explanation of this to the staff was sufficient to improve her management.

There are two basic groups of patients who are regarded as undesirable due to their attitudes towards the clinical staff. First, those who are perceived as ungrateful, critical, or complaining, and second, those who ask too many questions, make staff feel inadequate, or know too much (Ewing 1965; Anonymous 1969; Papper 1969; Weiner 1993; Short 1994). The doctor may be disconcerted by the assertiveness of such patients. Doctor–patient relationships often get strained when medical negligence is alleged or actually occurs (Short 1994). Some patients may exploit potentially different views offered by the referring specialist and the liaison geriatric psychiatrists, and so complicate management issues.

Case study 11.2

Miss D.K, a 76-year-old single female, was admitted for the management of her urinary tract infection. From the outset, although compliant with her specific treatment, she was highly critical of the health service, long casualty waiting time, shortage of nursing staff on the ward, aesthetic quality of the ward environment, and ward meals. During the admission she began to complain about the specific care offered by the nursing and medical staff, and started to write formal letters of complaint about various issues and specific individuals. These complaints were then investigated in accordance with the complaints procedure. Both medical and nursing staff found all of this very time-consuming and stressful. They wondered if the patient had a mental illness and referred the patient to the geriatric liaison psychiatry team. Formal psychiatric evaluation did not reveal a mental illness. Nevertheless, irrespective of the accuracy of her complaints, the staff felt attacked and victimized by the patient and needed considerable support, which the geriatric psychiatry liaison team was able to offer.

A group of patients who have several large volumes of case-notes, are seen by doctors from several specialties, and have had numerous special investigations are labelled as 'fat file', 'fat envelope' or 'heart sink' (O'Dowd 1988; Short 1994). How do patients acquire such a pejorative label? Patients who fail to respond to treatment may earn this label due to clinical staff projecting their therapeutic impotency and regarding the patients as 'deliberately' not wanting to get better. Patients thought to feign symptoms, to malinger, or have Munchausen's syndrome could also be included in this category (Shah 1990; Short 1994).

Other patients, who may be labelled as 'bed blockers', are those who are considered clinically fit for discharge but who cannot leave the hospital for a variety of reasons. Up to 40% of referrals to liaison geriatric psychiatry services may be for advice on placement into supervised or sheltered care (Scott *et al.* 1988; Wrigley and Loane 1991; Baheerathan and Shah 1999), even when up to 10% of these individuals are free of mental illness (Wrigley and Loane 1991). Such patients may need to wait until a comprehensive care package is provided to enable them to return to their own home or until long-term residential care is organized. Delays in accessing sources of funding, whether from the patient, health service, or social service, often contributes to the delay in discharge.

Undesirability can take various forms. Circumstantial undesirability is associated with a state of affairs that are beyond the patient's control (Papper 1969; Short 1994). One example is an internal dispute between various members of the multi-disciplinary team or across different specialties. Another potentially difficult circumstance is where there is controversy between psychiatrists and referring specialists about the precise management advice offered by either party. Distraction undesirability occurs when there is reduced interest in a specific patient because of idiosyncratic research and clinical interests (Papper 1969; Short 1994).

Patients with these pejorative labels are likely to be referred to liaison geriatric psychiatry services. The liaison psychiatrist needs to make sure such patients are properly assessed for psychiatric or psychological morbidity and are treated adequately according to the usual management principles of geriatric psychiatry. The liaison team needs to identify the circumstances that led to deprecatory labelling. A behavioural analysis can be used to assist the referring team's understanding and knowledge of the patient and the clinical difficulties they are encountering. By educating the staff, the liaison psychiatrist hopes to increase their understanding and knowledge base in order to improve management for the individual patient. The psychotherapeutic training and skills of the liaison psychiatrist can be very useful in such complex clinical systems.

The behaviourally disturbed patient

The non-cognitive features of dementia include disorders of behaviour, personality, mood, perception and thought content, and functional disability (Shah and Allen 1999; Foli and Shah 2000) have been categorized as 'behavioural and psychological symptoms of dementia' (BPSD) by the International Psychogeriatric Association (Finkel 1996). The broad features of BPSD can be extended to cover all psychiatric disorders encountered in liaison geriatric psychiatry settings.

Epidemiology

Over a third of all geriatric patients with dementia and behaviour disturbance admitted to a psychiatry unit have untreated significant medical illness (O'Connor 1987), illustrating the importance of medical illness in behaviour disturbance. Up to 25% of liaison referrals are for behaviour disturbance (Scott *et al.* 1988; Wrigley and Loane 1991; Swanwick *et al.* 1994; Baheerathan and Shah 1999). Common behavioural problems observed in medical settings are listed in Table 11.1, although epidemiological data on the true incidence are sparse (Shah 1999, 2000).

Patients showing aggressive behaviour, sexual disinhibition, or intimidation, cause the most anxiety, fear, and concern among general hospital staff. Possibly up to 40% of medically ill, elderly inpatients have aggressive behaviours (Anderson 1970; Hallberg *et al.* 1993). Aggressive behaviour includes shouting, threatening behaviour, excessive vocal activity, and physical aggression. Verbal aggression is most common, but only a small number of patients are repeatedly physically aggressive. This challenging behaviour can lead to distress, psychological disorders, and physical injury in the victims (Shah 1999). Sexual disinhibition may take several forms, including suggestive remarks, removal of clothing, masturbation in public, physical sexual contact, and sexual assaults including rape. Some behaviour may be misinterpreted by referrers or perceived as aberrant, and it is wise to carefully analyse the behaviour to make sure that it is abnormal or inappropriate.

Table 11.1 Examples of common forms of behaviour disturbances

Aggressive behaviour
  including irritability and verbal aggression

Activity disturbance
  including pottering, checking, pacing, and wandering

Eating behaviour
  including changes in food preference and eating inedible items

Disturbances of diurnal rhythm
  including sundowning and alterations in sleep–wake cycle

Sexual behaviour
  including self-exposure and attempted fondling

Miscellaneous behaviours
  including screaming, and hoarding and moving objects from one part of the ward
  to another

Case study 11.3

Mr V.G, a 75-year-old man, with a history of chronic mild schizophrenia, resident in a long-stay geriatric unit was referred to the geriatric liaison psychiatry team because of 'sexual disinhibition and inappropriate behaviour'. He had made friends with a newly admitted female patient. One evening whilst attempting intercourse with his new friend in his own room, he had been interrupted by a junior nurse delivering his supper tray. He had become very angry at the interruption and the nurse complained to her supervisor who initiated the referral. Having established that the patient did not have current psychiatric symptoms and that his partner was both willing and competent to consent, the psychiatrist facilitated a well-received staff forum on sexuality in elderly people. The nursing staff subsequently took care to knock on the doors of their long-term residents before entering uninvited.

Although epidemiological data are lacking, anecdotally, aggression and sexual disinhibition are relatively common, whereas other problem behaviours are less prevalent. Not only do these groups of patients acquire a reputation for socially undesirable behaviour but, even after their behaviour improves, the label of undesirability may remain and nursing homes may be reluctant to admit them, resulting in inappropriate long-term psychiatric hospitalization (Shah 1992).

What causes behavioural disturbances?

The pathological disease process may primarily cause behaviour disturbances. They can also stem from affective and psychotic symptoms in psychosis, delirium, dementia, or other psychiatric disorders. For example, persecutory delusions may lead to overt aggression because the patient fears harm to him or herself. Perhaps more commonly, behaviour disturbance may be secondary to cognitive changes, for example when a patient with dementia becomes anxious and agitated or when cognitive deficits are exposed during interview. Other factors that contribute to behaviour disturbance include sensory impairment, visuospatial dysfunction, intercurrent medical illnesses, pain, noise, and change of environment or personnel in the environment (Shah and Ames 1994; De and Shah 1998; Shah 1999). Dementia sufferers with delirium may suddenly present with new behavioural problems. Sensory impairment may exacerbate cognitive impairment, affective or psychotic symptoms. As these patients have difficulty in adjusting to change, exposure to a new environment and personnel in hospital may actually induce behavioural problems. Challenging behaviours may result from disinhibition or exaggeration of the premorbid personality traits. For example, a previously quiet and introverted patient may suddenly display out of character, sexually disinhibited behaviour.

Treatment

Treatment strategies will need to be directed at the patient, but it should also involve relatives and the staff on medical wards. Any potentially reversible causes of delirium, dementia, and other psychiatric disorders should be identified and treated. Treatment of intercurrent medical illnesses such as constipation, urine infection, and chest infection is likely to reduce acute confusion and behaviour disturbance. Visual or auditory deficits should be corrected, if possible, by the appropriate use of glasses, hearing aids, and the removal of ear wax (Shah and Ames 1994; De and Shah 1998).

Many drugs can cause delirium and may worsen the cognitive impairment of dementia (Ford and Folks 1985). Psychotropics, antiparkinsonian drugs, digoxin, steroids, anticholinergics, and opiate analgesics are particularly important (see Table 10.2 in Chapter 10). Careful consideration should be given to discontinuing these drugs, particularly if the indications for their use are no longer present.

Simple calming strategies are helpful (Shah and Ames 1994; De and Shah 1998) since early identification and intervention may avoid a full-blown crisis. Disturbed patients should be approached gently and calmly from the front. Communication should be clear and unambiguous. The judicious use of touch and non-threatening postures may also help. As studies are difficult to conduct in medical inpatients because of frailty, medical illnesses, emergent nature of symptoms, and multiple medications, the efficacy of various psychotropic drugs to treat behaviour disturbance is unclear (Risse and Barnes 1986; Schneider *et al.* 1990).

A meta-analysis of seven double-blind, placebo-controlled and parallel-group studies of neuroleptics and placebo showed neuroleptics to be modestly effective (Schneider *et al.* 1990), but it is unclear whether they reduce behaviour disturbance or simply sedate the patient. Most of these drugs have potent side-effects (Risse and Barnes 1986; Sunderland and Silver 1988) and because of their anticholinergic properties can increase the cognitive impairment. Newer neuroleptics like risperidone, olanzapine, quetiapine, and amisulpiride may have fewer side-effects and evidence of their efficacy in methodologically improved studies is emerging (Goldberg and Goldberg 1997; Katz *et al*. 1999). Oversedation is a common side-effect of clomethiazole (chlormethiazole), diazepam, oxazepam, and chlordiaze-poxide. Moreover, paradoxical rage reaction and disinhibition have also been reported with diazepam and chlordiazepoxide (Risse and Barnes 1986). There is also increasing evidence of the efficacy of anticonvulsants like carbamazepine in the treatment of patients with aggressive behaviour disturbances (Tariot *et al*. 1998).

If these drugs are prescribed, small doses should be used with careful monitoring of side-effects and gradual increments in dosage. The drug dose to achieve efficacy and the duration of treatment is unclear. Until further evidence emerges, dosages should be reduced as soon as possible after achieving efficacy.

A simple explanation of the diagnosis, management plan, and possible sequelae should be provided to the patient, relatives, and staff. Specific issues that should be addressed include the diagnosis of mental illness and its likely implications; causes of behaviour problems; possible management strategies; the role of medication, if any; and the proposed psychiatric follow-up. Both relatives and staff in medical settings may need an opportunity to ventilate their feelings.

Staff in medical units need regular support, training, and ongoing continuing professional development to tackle behaviour disturbance. Such liaison programmes can be clinically effective and cost-effective (Baheerathan and Shah 1999). Joint medical and psychiatric beds are useful for the management of medically ill patients with behaviour disturbance, since patients have ready access to multidisciplinary staff trained in psychiatry and medicine. However, such units are rare, as shown by a recent UK survey where these were only available in 5% of services (Wattis *et al*. 1999). Data on the clinical and cost-effectiveness of such provision is also lacking.

The unclean patient

Physical illnesses are common among patients with a syndrome variously labelled as Diogenes' syndrome (Clark *et al*. 1975), senile squalor syndrome, squalor syndrome (Shah 1995*a*), senile breakdown (MacMillan and Shaw 1966), and senile recluse. Many of these patients are encountered in liaison settings. The clinical features include extreme-self neglect, domestic filth, social withdrawal, apathy, a tendency to hoard rubbish, lack of shame (Cybulska and Rucinski 1986) and insight (Halliday *et al*. 2000).

Case study 11.4

Mrs A.J. was a 74-year widowed lady who was admitted to a geriatric medical ward following a severe fall and wound infection. She had been known to social services for several years as she had a history of living in squalid conditions in her own home. However, their previous offers of help had been consistently rejected and she was resistant to the idea of having her home cleaned or the hoarded material disposed. The patient had diminished vision secondary to diabetic retinopathy. Mrs A.J. couldn't understand why the social services and medical team were making such a fuss about her living at home as she considered herself a good housekeeper. After a detailed multidisciplinary assessment it was clarified that she had no clear mental illness.

Published studies have examined differing patient samples, including those known to geriatricians, general practitioners, social workers, and the clergy (MacMillan and Shaw 1966). Some are referred to geriatric medical services (Clark *et al.* 1975; Roe 1977), others to geriatric psychiatry services (Wrigley and Cooney 1992; Shaw and Shah 1996) or community health centres (Snowdon 1987).

The annual incidence has been estimated as 0.5 per 1000 population over the age of 60 years (MacMillan and Shaw 1966). The prevalence in liaison settings is unclear as only biased samples have been studied. The gender ratio is equal in some studies (Clark *et al.* 1975; Shaw and Shah 1996), and in favour of women in others (MacMillan and Shaw 1966; Snowdon 1987). The vast majority of squalor subjects live alone (MacMillan and Shaw 1966; Clark *et al.* 1975; Wrigley and Cooney 1996). Although most patients are known to the community authorities, they tend to decline offers of help (Shah 1995*a*). Many own properties, have substantial financial reserves, and come from all social classes (MacMillan and Shaw 1966; Clark *et al.* 1975; Shah 1992).

Sensory impairments, including deafness and particularly blindness in up to one-third of cases, make it more difficult to pick up sensory cues regarding the squalor (MacMillan and Shaw 1966; Shah 1992; Wrigley and Cooney 1992). About 50% of such people have psychiatric illness in the following order of frequency: dementia, schizophrenia, alcohol misuse, and manic-depressive illness (MacMillan and Shaw 1966; Anonymous 1975; Snowdon 1987; Shah 1992; Wrigley and Cooney 1992; Shaw and Shah 1996). A significant proportion may have unrecognized psychiatric illness in the form of frontal lobe dysfunction (Orrell *et al.* 1989; Shah 1992).

A study looking at subjective ratings of an index patient's personality from informants, including relatives, showed that quarrelsome, domineering, or independent traits were prominent (MacMillan and Shaw 1966). Other studies have found no significant personality abnormality (Clark *et al.* 1975) or have labelled these individuals as eccentric (Snowdon 1987).

The final common pathway in the development of this syndrome may be frontal lobe dysfunction, although systematic intellectual testing has not been undertaken in any study (Shah 1995*a*). Many features of frontal lobe dysfunction, including disinhibition, lack of concern, apathy, and the lack of initiative and spontaneity, overlap the syndrome's cardinal features (Shah 1992; Orrell *et al.* 1989). If this is coupled with concomitant sensory impairment, the patient can be oblivious to the squalid conditions in which they live. Death of a relative living with the patient may act as the precipitator of squalor syndrome. However, it is more likely that the deceased relative would have kept the house and the patient clean. Upon the relative's death, squalor is likely to worsen and come to the attention of the authorities.

Hospital admission may result in a rapid deterioration in the patient's condition and the development of apathy (Macmillan and Shaw 1966). However, admission may be necessary for severely physically ill patients (Clark *et al*. 1975). There is a mortality of up to 50% during the index admission due to physical disorders, including carcinoma, bronchopneumonia, heart disease, gangrene, and cerebrovascular disease (MacMillan and Shaw 1966; Clark *et al*. 1975; Roe 1977). A model of day care has been suggested (MacMillan and Shaw 1966) that allows the development of social networks and an improvement in emotional and physical well-being.

Once admitted as an inpatient or as a day patient, good nursing care is paramount. Orem's self-care nursing model where individuals are treated holistically with biological, psychological, and social approaches, has been suggested (Moore 1989). Patients retain personal responsibility for self-care, and nursing interventions are avoided unless the patient is unable to achieve a balance between their self-care abilities and demands placed upon them.

This syndrome elegantly illustrates the complex relationship between geriatric psychiatry and geriatric medicine and the need to work together. Many survivors (40%) find their way to more dependent settings including residential homes, nursing homes, and continuing-care geriatric and geriatric psychiatry beds (MacMillan and Shaw 1966; Clark *et al*. 1975; Wrigley and Cooney 1992; Shaw and Shah 1996). Domiciliary and social services, from both the statutory and voluntary sectors, should be encouraged for patients discharged into the community, patients receiving day care, and those living at home. Ideally, this should occur with supervision from the staff of geriatric medicine or geriatric psychiatry services. Home help and meals-on-wheels are of particular value. Relatives may find it difficult to continue providing support due to constant rebuff from the patient (MacMillan and Shaw 1966). About one-third of patients persistently refuse all offers of help (MacMillan and Shaw 1966; Shah 1992). Mental-health and other environmental-health legislation may be of value in managing these patients (Mulroy and Shah 1993; Shah 1995*b*).

The suicidal patient

The elderly account for up to 15% of all attempted suicides (Sendbuehler and Goldstein 1977; Pierce 1987; Hawton and Fagg 1990). Many will find their way into medical units as they often require resuscitation. Their recognition is important, as the prognosis is poor. Up to 18% of such people repeat their suicide attempt within a year (Pierce 1987; Hawton and Fagg 1990; Merrill and Owens 1990; Nowers 1993) and up to 8% of elderly attempters complete suicide within 1–3 years (Pierce 1987; Nowers 1993).

Attempted suicides are associated with being single, divorced, widowed, living alone, relationship difficulties, financial difficulties, unresolved grief, and belonging to a lower socioeconomic class (Pierce 1987; Hawton and Fagg 1990; De Leo *et al*. 1994; Draper 1994; Takahashi *et al*. 1995).

Up to 90% of people attempting suicide are clinically depressed (Pierce 1987; Draper 1994; Takahashi *et al.* 1995). Depressive symptoms (Draper 1994), psychotic symptoms, including mood congruent depressive delusions (Pierce 1987; Draper 1994), sleep disturbance (Draper 1994), and somatization (Takahashi *et al.* 1995) are important. Alcoholism and alcohol consumption before attempted suicide are common (Hawton and Fagg 1990; Draper 1994). Up to 26% have a secondary diagnosis of personality disorder (Draper 1994).

Several earlier studies showed that dementia was common (Batchelor and Napier 1953; O'Neal *et al.* 1956; Sendbuehler and Goldstein 1977). More recent studies, using standardized techniques, report lower prevalence in some studies (Pierce 1987; Lyness *et al.* 1992; Nowers 1993) and higher prevalence in others (Rifai *et al.* 1993; Draper 1994; Schmid *et al.* 1994; Takahashi *et al.* 1995). One study reported a higher prevalence of delirium in a group of patients who attempted suicide than in the comparison group (Takahashi 1995). Frontal lobe dysfunction for impulsive episodes (Draper 1994) and comorbid depression (Pierce 1987; Lyness *et al.* 1992; Draper 1994) are also important.

Serious physical illness and pain may lead to demoralization and attempted suicides (Pierce 1987; Draper 1994; Takahashi *et al.* 1995). Sendbeuhler and Goldstein (1977) suggested that many attempted suicides in late life are serious bids that have failed due to confusion resulting from physical illness, over-medication, and alcohol misuse. In contrast, Pierce (1987) reported that individuals with organic brain disease tended to make impulsive and hazardous attempts, often with more than one means, in the context of confusion, depression, and cerebral disinhibition.

Recent studies report drug overdoses as the most common self-harm method (up to 90%) (Pierce 1987; Hawton and Fagg 1990; Nowers 1993; Draper 1994; Takahashi *et al.* 1995). Drugs employed include minor tranquillizers, hypnotics, antidepressants, and analgesics (Pierce 1987; Hawton and Fagg 1990; Nowers 1993; Draper 1994). In recent years, barbiturate self-poisoning has declined with a concomitant increase in non-opiate analgesic poisoning, particularly paracetamol (Pierce 1987; Hawton and Fagg 1990). Self-injury methods (wrist-cutting, shooting, attempted drowning, jumping from heights, and attempted asphyxiation) are more common among men (Hawton and Fagg 1990). Self-poisoning is more common among women (Hawton and Fagg 1990).

Suicidal ideation is not static but changes with time; victims neither want to live nor die, but do both at the same time, usually one more than the other. Under-reporting of suicide is highest in old age because suicidal behaviours such as refusal to eat and drink, medication and treatment non-compliance, and social withdrawal are often unrecognized (Blazer *et al.* 1986; Hasegawa *et al.* 1992; Kishi *et al.* 1996*a*). They have been labelled as 'subintentional suicide', 'hidden suicide', and 'indirect self-destructive behaviour' (Nelson and Farberow 1980; Hasegawa *et al.* 1992). These covert suicidal behaviours often result in poor physical health (Nelson and Farberow 1980; Hill *et al.* 1988), which later may necessitate admission into a medical bed. Thus covert suicidal ideations may not infrequently be encountered in medically ill elderly inpatients (Nelson and Farberow 1980).

Overtly reported suicidal ideation has been examined in patients with strokes, both at onset and follow-up (Kishi *et al.* 1996*a,b*) in medically ill elderly inpatients (Shah *et al.* 1998, 2000) and in the primary-care setting (Callaghan *et al.* 1996). The prevalence of suicidal ideation was 1% in primary-care attenders (Callaghan *et al.* 1996); 7% in acute and 11% in chronic poststroke periods (Kishi *et al.* 1996*a,b*); 13% in acute geriatric inpatients; and 26% in continuing-care patients (Shah *et al.* 1998, 2000). Suicidal ideation is more common in those with younger age, social isolation, sensory impairment, functional impairment, and strokes with anterior and posterior cerebral lesions (Callaghan *et al.* 1996; Kishi *et al.* 1996*a,b*). Symptoms of early morning awakening, hopelessness, and depressive illness (Callaghan *et al.* 1996; Kishi *et al.* 1996a,b; Shah *et al.* 1998. 2000) increase the likelihood of suicidal ideation or activity. Substance misuse (Kishi *et al.* 1996*b*), and the prescription of psychotropic drugs, especially anxiolytics (Shah *et al.* 1998, 2000) are additional risk factors.

All doctors should be vigilant about the possibility of suicidal behaviour in elderly patients. Any patient with overt suicidal ideation, subintentional or hidden suicidal behaviour, or attempted suicide coming into contact with medical services should receive a formal assessment by the geriatric psychiatry service. Careful attention should be paid to the method and perceived fatality of the behaviour. Violent methods tend to be associated with an increased risk of successful suicide. The individual's current views on the acceptability of suicide as a personal option are also important. The person who has thought through their suicide plan in detail is at greater risk for successful completion as their self-harm efforts are generally more serious than impulsive attempts. Precautions taken to avoid being discovered and planning for a postdeceased future (funeral arrangements, wills and other related issues), are also important clues to the degree of intent. For more detail on the assessment of suicide risk, the reader is directed to Chapter 5.

Psychiatric disorder should be treated in its own right, as should any social or physical morbidity. Depending on the severity of the illness and the risk of suicide, the patient may need psychiatric admission after medical resuscitation. Sometimes, if safety is a major issue, detention under a Mental Health Act may be necessary.

Patients who do not eat

Nursing staff worry intensely when patients in their care will not eat, especially if they are losing weight. Patients refuse to eat for a number of reasons, including physical illness, psychiatric illness, side-effects of prescribed drugs, and occasionally for unclear reasons. Appetite loss is a common symptom of physical illnesses such as pneumonia, urinary tract infection, strokes, myocardial infarcts, and cancer.

Many drugs used to treat these illnesses can also directly or indirectly suppress appetite because they induce nausea, vomiting, constipation and other gastro-intestinal symptoms, lethargy, and confusion. Anorexia is a symptom of many psychiatric disorders including depressive illness, dementia, alcohol misuse, and late-onset schizophrenia. Characteristically, patients in liaison settings may have loss of appetite due to a combination of physical illness, its treatment, and concomitant psychiatric illness.

A careful history from the patient and other informants, mental state examination, physical examination, and special investigations will clarify the cause. If the aetiology is due to physical illness or its treatment then the medical referring team should be unequivocally informed. If psychiatric illness is identified then it should also be treated in the normal fashion, though it may be best to avoid the selective serotonin-reuptake inhibitors as they can suppress appetite.

Case study 11.5

Mr T.P was an 88-year-old widower who presented with weight loss and lethargy. After diagnosing a chest infection he was admitted to a medical ward. After the treatment with intravenous antibiotics he continued to loss weight because of a reluctance to eat. The patient saw little desire to continue with life and had a number of depressive symptoms. Treatment was initially commenced with fluoxetine by the geriatric team, but this caused his appetite to decrease further. An urgent psychiatric assessment was sought and major depression with melancholia was diagnosed. He was subsequently treated with electro-convulsive therapy. Mr P. made a rapid recovery and no longer wished to die.

If the aetiology is unclear, or the patient gives any indication of suicidal ideation or passive death wish, then passive suicidal behaviour should be considered. Refusal to eat may achieve high mortality from vulnerability to medical illness (Nelson and Farberow 1980). Objective data on this phenomenon is lacking, as this group of patients is reluctant to become involved in research (Shah 1998; Shah et al. 1998, 2000)

These patients cause distress among staff who require support to identify, under-stand, and manage them. An ongoing dialogue between the liaison geriatric psychiatry team and the medical teams on a consultation and liaison basis is essential

Psychiatric complications of prescribed and non-prescribed drugs

A careful enquiry should be made about the consumption of non-prescribed and prescribed drugs. The literature on elderly patients consuming non-prescribed drugs such as opiates, hallucinogens, cocaine, crack, and amphetamines is negligible. Anecdotally, the authors have rarely seen clinical referrals in liaison settings when these drugs are important in the presentation. However, this may change in the future as the post-World War II 'baby boom cohort', a generation who experimented with recreational drugs out of proportion to any preceding generation, grows old. Of more concern, at the present time, is the misuse of prescription drugs.

A large number of prescribed drugs, individually or as drug interactions, can produce neuropsychiatric disorders—including delirium, depression, mania, anxiety, and psychosis—as adverse effects (Ford and Folks 1985; Larson *et al.* 1987; Katzman *et al.* 1988; Katz *et al.* 1991; De and Shah 1998). Geriatric psychiatric liaison services are not infrequently asked to assess these patients (Ford and Folks 1985; De and Shah 1998). The common categories of medications involved in developing neuropsychiatric side-effects are listed in Table 11.2, with benzo-diazepines and drugs with anticholinergic properties being particularly implicated (Tune and Bylsma 1991).

A careful chronological history taken from the patient and other informants will be required to attribute the symptoms to drug prescription or drug interactions. Where possible, the offending drug should be stopped or its dose lowered. If this is not possible, or if the strategy fails, the subsequent neuropsychiatric disorder should be treated symptomatically.

Newly admitted patients who experience difficulty in sleeping in the hospital environment are too often prescribed benzodiazepine sedatives such as temazepam or nitrazepam, without adequate assessment of any other underlying cause. Sleep reduction may be associated with their physical illness, prescribed medication, change of environment, and understandable anxiety about the treatment procedures (e.g. surgery). Sometimes hypnotics may be necessary, but should not be a substitute for adequate reassurance, discussion of sleep problems, and simple sleep-hygiene strategies. Hypnotics should be used in the smallest doses for the shortest period possible.

Table 11.2 Prescribed drugs which have been reported to cause neuropsychiatric side-effects

Delirium:	Depression:
Antibiotics	Antibiotics
Anticonvulsants	Antihypertensives
Antihypertensives	Parkinson's drugs
Carcinogens	Steroids
Diabetic agents	Anticonvulsants
Parkinson's drugs	Antituberculous drugs
Steroids	Psychotropics
Anticholinergics	**Mania:**
Antihistamines	Anticonvulsants
Anti-inflammatories	Antidepressants
Cardiac drugs	Steroids
Opiate and non-opiate analgesics	
Psychotropics	

Alcohol-related problems

Surveys in the community indicate an approximately 1.5–2% prevalence of alcoholism in older males, and under 1% in females (Saunders *et al*. 1989). However, a greater proportion are seen in clinical settings. Up to 8% of medically ill elderly patients have a history of excessive alcohol consumption, and about 5% have an alcohol-dependence syndrome (Luttrell *et al*. 1997). Recognition of alcohol-related problems in medically ill elderly inpatients is low (Rosin and Glatt 1971; Curtis *et al*. 1989). Up to 7% of referrals to geriatric psychiatry liaison services are specifically for alcohol misuse (Scott *et al*. 1988; Wrigley and Loane 1991; Swanwick *et al*. 1994; Collinson and Benbow 1998). The precise prevalence of alcohol-related amnestic syndrome, alcohol-related dementia, alcoholic hallucinosis, and primary depression with secondary alcohol misuse in the liaison setting is unknown. The natural history and long-term outcome of alcohol-related problems and risk factors have been poorly studied in the elderly population.

Patients may present with medical, psychological, social, and forensic consequences of excessive alcohol intake (Ticehurst 1994). On medical wards, alcohol-related disorders may be coincidentally identified in patients with unrelated disorders, or they may be an important component of the medical presentation. Such medical presentations include falls, seizures, incontinence, burns, blackouts, liver dysfunction, haematemesis, malnutrition, ataxia, diabetes, acute confusion, and hypothermia (Schuckit and Pastor 1978; Wattis 1981). Psychological sequelae include pathological drunkenness, alcohol-dependence syndrome, alcohol withdrawal, alcoholic hallucinosis, amnestic syndrome, and alcoholic dementia or depression (for clinical features see Chapter 10).

Pathologically drunk patients can create major management difficulties by disrupting ward activities, interfering with the clinical care of other patients, and being aggressive and demanding. They may present major challenges if brought to a busy emergency room with other vulnerable patients in the vicinity. Staff and patients are often frightened of these situations, particularly if the patient is violent. Although, most units have protocols for dealing with disruptive drunken patients, the pathologically drunk, disruptive patient may be discharged from hospital prematurely to protect other patients and staff.

Patients with alcohol withdrawal syndrome or those at risk from withdrawal (as they may have discontinued drinking whilst in hospital) will need detoxification. Long-acting benzodiazepines such as diazepam are useful in alcohol withdrawal as their anticonvulsant action protects against withdrawal seizures. An alternative could be clomethiazole (chlormethiazole). Usually, patients also require supplementation with B-group vitamins, correction of any electrolyte imbalance, and treatment of any intercurrent medical problems (Chick 1989). Administration of parenteral thiamine may well avoid the development of irreversible neurological and psychiatric disability (Cutting 1978).

These patients may suffer from clinically significant, alcohol-related complications of one or more other organ systems. Patients with depression whilst drinking alcohol should be reassessed after detoxification to determine whether the depression was primary and independent of drinking or secondary to the alcohol problem.

These patients require counselling and guidance on how to remain abstinent if the urge to drink continues. Rehabilitation usually requires close liaison between the medical team, the liaison geriatric psychiatry team, and the alcohol-abuse service. The influence of cognitive impairment, either reducing or increasing the urge to drink alcohol, should always be considered.

Prolonged heavy use of alcohol can cause cognitive impairments and there is no doubt that neurotoxicity increases with age (Atkinson and Ganzini 1994). Alcohol overuse impairs memory, cognitive flexibility, and abstract reasoning. In mild alcohol abuse, these effects of alcohol can be quite subtle and are difficult to distinguish from those of normal ageing. Reversible cognitive impairment following acute excess alcohol use tends to be more severe and prolonged in the older person. It may persist in upwards of 10% of people, even after abstinence. Resolution of the cognitive problems can take months to years following abstinence, so it is worthwhile advising patients of this fact. Some alcohol-related cognitive deficits might be irreversible. Whether excessive and prolonged use of alcohol can cause a diffuse dementia, 'alcoholic dementia', is debatable. Other factors beside alcohol itself cause dementia. Cognitive impairment may be due to a reduced bioavailability of thiamine, hypertension, head injury from falls (Atkinson and Ganzini 1994, Fisman *et al.* 1996) or cigarette smoking. The advice to the patient is to stop drinking immediately, as abstinence may slow the progression of dementia.

The classical disorder of alcohol abuse is the acute alcohol amnestic disorder (Wernicke—Korsakoff syndrome). This syndrome is characterized by the impairment of consciousness, a memory deficit, disorientation, ataxia, and ophthalmoplegia. The disorder is a medical emergency and is discussed in more detail in Chapter 10.

Features of alcohol withdrawal in the elderly are no different from those seen in the young, although as they may be more physically frail, the withdrawal period may be more difficult to treat and there may be greater mortality.

References

Anderson, J. (1970). A study of disturbed behaviour in patients with dementia in two hospital populations. *Gerontologica Clinica*, **12**, 49–64.

Anonymous. (1969). The unwanted patient. *Medical Journal of Australia*, **2**, 469–70.

Anonymous. (1975). Diogenes' syndrome. *Lancet*, **i**, 515.

Atkinson, R. M. and Ganzini, L. (1994). Substance abuse. In *The American Psychiatric Press textbook of geriatric neuropsychiatry* (ed. E.C. Coffey and J.L. Cummings), pp. 297–321. American Psychiatric Press, Washington, DC.

Baheerathan. M. and Shah, A.K. (1999). The impact of two changes in service delivery on a geriatric psychiatry liaison service. *International Journal of Geriatric Psychiatry*, **14**, 767–75.

Batchelor, I.R.C. and Napier, M.B. (1953). Attempted suicide in old age *British Medical Journal*, **ii**, 1186–90.

Blazer, D.G., Bacher, J.R., and Manton, K.G. (1986). Suicide in late life: review and commentary. *Journal of the American Geriatrics Society*, **34**, 519–25.

Callaghan, C.M., Hendrie, H.C, Nienaber, N.A., and Tierney, W.M. (1996). Suicidal ideation among older primary care patients. *Journal of the American Geriatrics Society*, **44**, 1205–9.

Chick, J. (1989). Delirium tremens. *British Medical Journal*, **298**, 3–4.

Clark, A.N.G., Manikar, G.O., and Gray, I. (1975). Diogenes' syndrome: a clinical study of gross self-neglect in old age. *Lancet*, **i**, 366–8.

Collinson, Y. and Benbow, S.M. (1998). The role of an old age consultation liaison nurse. *International Journal of Geriatric Psychiatry*, **13**, 159–63.

Curtis, J.R., Geller, G., Stokes, E.J., Levine, D.M., and Moore, R.D. (1989). Characteristics, diagnosis and treatment of alcoholism in elderly patients. *Journal of the American Geriatrics Society*, **37**, 310–16.

Cutting, J. (1978). The relationship between Korsakoff's syndrome and alcoholic dementia. *British Journal of Psychiatry*, **132**, 240–51.

Cybulska, E. and Rucinski, J. (1986). Gross self neglect in old age. *British Journal of Hospital Medicine*, **36**, 21–4.

De, T. and Shah, A.K. (1998). Dementia: behavioural problems can be managed effectively. *Geriatric Medicine*, **28**, 60–4.

De Leo, D., Bille-Braha, U., Bjerke, T., and Lonnquvist, J. (1994). Parasuicide in the elderly: results from the WHO/Euro multicentre study 1989–1993. A short report. *IPA Bulletin*, **11**, 15–17.

Draper, B. (1994). Suicidal behaviour in the elderly. *International Journal of Geriatric Psychiatry*, **9**, 655–61.

Ewing, J.A. (1965). Handling the cantankerous patients. *Medical Times*, **93**, 1117–19.

Finkel, S. (1996). New focus on behavioral and psychological signs and symptoms of dementia. *International Psychogeriatrics*, **8**(Suppl. 3), 215–16.

Fisman, M., Ramsay, D., and Weiser, M. (1996). Dementia in the elderly male alcoholic: a retrospective clinicopathological study. *International Journal of Geriatric Psychiatry*, **11**, 209–18.

Foli, S. and Shah, A.K. (2000). Measurement of disturbed behaviour, non-cognitive features and quality of life. In *Dementia* (ed. J. O'Brien, D. Ames, and A. Burns), pp. 87–100. Chapman Hall, London.

Ford, C.V. and Folks, D.G. (1985). Psychiatric disorders in geriatric medical and surgical patients. *Southern Medical Journal*, **78**, 397–402.

Goldberg, R.J. and Goldberg, J. (1997). Risperidone for treating dementia related disturbed behaviour in nursing home residents: a clinical experience. *International Psychogeriatrics*, **9**, 65–8.

Hallberg, I.R., Edberg, A., and Nordmark, A. (1993). Daytime vocal activity in institutionalised severely demented patients identified as vocally disruptive by nurses. *International Journal of Geriatric Psychiatry*, **8**, 155–64.

Halliday, G., Banerjee, S. Philpot, M., and Macdonald, A. (2000). Community study of people who live in squalor *Lancet*, **355**, 882–6.

Hasegawa, K., Finkel, S.I., Bergener, M., and Cohen, G.D. (1992). Late life suicide. *International Psychogeriatrics*, **4**, 163.

Hawton, K. and Fagg, J. (1990). Deliberate self-poisoning and self injury in older people. *International Journal of Geriatric Psychiatry*, **5**, 367–3.

Hill, R.D., Gallagher, B., Thompson, L.W., and Ishida, T. (1988). Hopelessness as a measure of suicidal intent in the depressed elderly. *Psychology and Ageing*, **3**, 230–3.

Katz, I.R., Parmelee, P., and Brubaker, K. (1991). Toxic and metabolic encephalopathies in long-term care patients. *International Psychogeriatrics*, **3**, 337–47.

Katz, I.R., Jeste, D., Mintzer, J.E., Clyde, C., Napolitano, J., and Brecher, M. (1999). Comparison of risperidone and placebo for psychosis and behavioural disturbances associated with dementia: a randomised double blind trial. *Journal of Clinical Psychiatry*, **60**, 107–15.

Katzman, R., Lasker, R., and Bernstein, N. (1988). Advances in the diagnosis of dementia: accuracy of diagnosis and consequences of misdiagnosis of disorders causing dementia. *Aging and the Brain*, **32**, 17–62.

Kishi, Y., Robinson, R.G., and Kosier, J.T. (1996*a*). Suicidal plans in patients with acute stroke. *Journal of Nervous and Mental Diseases*, **284**, 274–80.

Kishi, Y., Robinson, R.G., and Kosier, J.T. (1996*b*). Suicidal plans in patients with strokes: comparison between acute-onset and delayed-onset suicidal plans. *International Psychogeriatrics*, **8**, 623–34.

Larson, E.B., Kukall, W.A., Buchner, D., and Reifler, B.V. (1987). Adverse drug reactions associated with global cognitive impairment in elderly patients. *Annals of Internal Medicine*, **107**, 169–73.

Luttrell, S., Watkin, V., Livingston, G., Walker, Z., D'Ath, P., Patel, P., *et al.* (1997), Screening for alcohol misuse in older people. *International Journal of Geriatric Psychiatry*, **12**, 1151–4.

Lyness, J.M., Conwell, Y., and Nelson, J.C. (1992). Suicide attempts in elderly psychiatric inpatients. *Journal of the American Geriatrics Society*, **40**, 320–4.

MacMillan, D. and Shaw, P. (1966). Senile breakdown in standards of personal and environmental cleanliness. *British Medical Journal*, **ii**, 1032–7.

Merrill, J. and Owens, J. (1990). Age and attempted suicide. *Acta Psychiatrica Scandinavica*, **82**, 385–8.

Moore, R. (1989). Diogenes' syndrome. *Nursing Times*, **83**, 46–8.

Mulroy, R. and Shah, A.K. (1993). Indescribable squalor. *Update*, **46**, 244–6.

Nelson, F.L. and Farberow, N.L. (1980). Indirect self-destructive behaviour in the elderly nursing home patient. *Journal of Gerontology*, **35**, 949–57.

Norman, A. (1985). *Triple jeopardy: growing old in a second homeland.* Centre for Policy on Ageing, London.

Nowers, M. (1993). Deliberate self-harm in the elderly: a survey of one London Borough. *International Journal of Geriatric Psychiatry*, **8**, 609–14.

O'Connor, M. (1987). Disturbed behaviour in dementia—psychiatric or medical problem. *Medical Journal of Australia*, **147**, 481–5.

O'Dowd, T.C. (1988). Five years of heart sink patients in general practice. *British Medical Journal*, **297**, 528–30.

O'Neal, P., Robins, E., and Schmidt, E.H. (1956). A psychiatric study of attempted suicide in persons sixty years of age. *Archives of Neurological Psychiatry*, **75**, 275–84.

Orrell, M.W., Sahakian, B.J., and Bergmann, K. (1989). Self-neglect and frontal lobe dysfunction. *British Journal of Psychiatry*, **155**, 101–5.

Papper, S. (1969). The undesirable patient. *Journal of Chronic Diseases*, **22**, 777–9.

Pierce, D. (1987). Deliberate self-harm in the elderly. *International Journal of Geriatric Psychiatry*, **2**, 105–10.

Rait, G., Burns, A., and Chew, C. (1996). Age, ethnicity and mental illness: a triple whammy. *British Medical Journal*, **313**, 1347.

Rifai, A.H., Mulsant, B.H., Sweet, R.A., Pasternak, R.E., Rosen, J., and Zubenko, G.S. (1993). A study of elderly suicide attempters admitted to an inpatient psychiatric unit. *American Journal of Geriatric Psychiatry*, **1**, 126–35.

Risse, S.C. and Barnes, R.I. (1986). Pharmacologic treatment of agitation associated with dementia. *Journal of the American Geriatrics Society*, **34**, 368–76.

Roe, P.F. (1977). Self neglect. *Age and Ageing*, **6**, 192–4.

Rosin, A.J. and Glatt, M.M. (1971). Alcohol excess in the elderly. *Quarterly Journal of Studies on Alcohol*, **32**, 53–9.

Saunders, P.A., Copeland, J.R.M., Dewey, M.E., Davidson, I.A., McWilliam, C., Sharma, V.K., *et al.* (1989). Alcohol use and abuse in the elderly: findings from the Liverpool longitudinal study of continuing health in the community. *International Journal of Geriatric Psychiatry*, **4**, 103–8.

Schmid, H., Manjee, K., and Shah, T. (1994). On the distinction of suicide ideation versus attempt in elderly psychiatric inpatients. *Gerontologist*, **34**, 332–9.

Schneider, L.S., Pollock, V.E., and Lyness, S.A. (1990). A meta-analysis of controlled trails of neuroleptic treatment in dementia. *Journal of the American Geriatrics Society*, **38**, 553–63.

Schuckit, M.A. and Pastor, P.A. (1978). The elderly as a unique population: alcoholism. *Alcoholism: Clinical and Experimental Research*, **2**, 31–8.

Scott, J., Fairbairn, A., and Woodhouse, K. (1988). Referrals to a psychogeriatric consultation-liaison service. *International Journal of Geriatric Psychiatry*, **3**, 131–5.

Sendbeuhler, J.M. and Goldstein, S. (1977). Attempted suicide among the aged. *Journal of the American Geriatrics Society*, **25**, 245–8.

Shah, A.K. (1990). Psychiatric Munchausen's syndrome. *British Journal of Social and Clinical Psychiatry*, **7**, 143–4.

Shah, A.K. (1992). Senile squalor syndrome: a small case-series. *Care of the Elderly*, **4**, 299–300.

Shah, A.K. (1995a). Squalor syndrome: a view point. *Australian Journal on Ageing*, **13**, 160–2.

Shah, A.K. (1995b). The use of legislation in squalor syndrome. *Medicine, Science and the Law*, **35**, 43–4.

Shah, A.K. (1998). Suicidal ideation: a preventative role for health professionals. *Geriatric Medicine*, **28**, 25–8.

Shah, A.K. (1999). Aggressive behaviour in the elderly. *International Journal of Psychiatry in Clinical Practice*, **3**, 85–103.

Shah, A.K. (2000). What are the necessary characteristics of behavioural and psychological signs of dementia rating scales. *International Psychogeriatrics*, **12**(Suppl. 1), 205–9.

Shah, A.K. and Allen, H. (1999). Is improvement possible in the measurement of behaviour disturbance? *International Journal of Geriatric Psychiatry*, **14**, 512–19.

Shah, A.K. and Ames, D. (1994). Behavioural problems in patients with dementia. *Modern Medicine*, **May**, 67–72.

Shah, A.K., Dighe-Deo, D., and Chapman, C. (1998). Suicidal ideation among acutely medically ill elderly inpatients. *Ageing and Mental Health*, **2**, 300–5.

Shah, A., Hoxey, K., and Mayadunne, V. (2000). Suicidal ideation in acutely medically ill elderly inpatients: prevalence correlates and longitudinal stability. *International Journal of Geriatric Psychiatry*. **15**, 162–9.

Shaw, T. and Shah, A.K. (1996). Study on squalor syndrome: squalor syndrome and psychogeriatric admissions. *International Psychogeriatrics*, **8**, 669–74.

Short, D. (1994). Difficult patients. *British Journal of Hospital Medicine*, **51**, 128–30.

Snowdon, J. (1987). Uncleanliness among persons seen by community mental health workers. *Hospital and Community Psychiatry*, **38**, 491–4.

Sunderland, T. and Silver, M.A. (1988). Neuroleptics in the treatment of dementia. *International Journal of Geriatric Psychiatry*, **3**, 784–90.

Swanwick, G.R.J., Lee, H., Clare, A.W., and Lawlor, B. (1994). Consultation-liaison psychiatry: a comparison of two service models for geriatric patients. *International Journal of Geriatric Psychiatry*, **9**, 495–9.

Takahashi, Y., Hirasawa, H., Koyama, K., Asakawa, O., Kido, M., Onose, H., *et al.* (1995). Suicide and ageing in Japan: an examination of treated elderly suicide attempters. *International Psychogeriatrics*, **7**, 239–51.

Tariot, P.N., Erb, R., Podgorski, C.A., Cox, C., Patel, S., Jakimovich, L., *et al.* (1998). Efficacy and tolerability of carbamazepine for agitation and aggression in dementia. *American Journal of Psychiatry*, **155**, 54–61.

Ticehurst, S. (1994). Substance use and abuse. In *Functional psychiatric disorders of the elderly* (ed. E. Chiu and D. Ames), pp. 269–84. Cambridge University Press, Cambridge.

Tune, L.E. and Bylsma, F.W. (1991). Benzodiazepine-induced and anticholinergic-induced delirium in the elderly. *International Psychogeriatrics*, **3**, 397–408.

Wattis, J.P. (1981). Alcohol problems in the elderly. *Journal of the American Geriatrics Society*, **24**, 131–4.

Wattis, J., MacDonald, A., and Newton, P. (1999). Old age psychiatry: a speciality in transition: results of the 1996 survey. *Psychiatric Bulletin*, **23**, 331–5.

Weiner, T. (1993). Lessons from an inconvenient patient. *North Carolina Medical Journal*, **54**, 573–4.

Wrigley, M. and Cooney, C. (1992). Diogenes syndrome—an Irish series. *Irish Journal of Psychological Medicine*, **9**, 37–41.

Wrigley, M. and Loane, R. (1991). Consultation-liaison referrals to the North Dublin old age psychiatry service. *Irish Medical Journal*, **84**, 89–91.

Section 4:
Treatment

12 Psychopharmacological management of the medically ill older person

Alastair J. Flint

Summary

This chapter reviews the pharmacological management of psychiatric disorders in older people with physical illness. It focuses on aspects of treatment that are most relevant to the psychiatrist who is consulting to medical, surgical, or rehabilitation services. The chapter starts by reviewing the effects of ageing, physical illness, and drug interactions on pharmacokinetics and pharmacodynamics. It also outlines the general principles of pharmacotherapy in the elderly. The bulk of the chapter is devoted to a review of the pharmacological management of the three 'Ds'—depression, dementia, and delirium. There is also discussion of the treatment of anxiety, mania, and schizophrenia and other psychoses.

Introduction

Psychiatric illness and physical illness frequently coexist in older people. Depression, dementia, and delirium are common disorders in elderly medical and surgical patients, and thus the treatment of these disorders is emphasized in this chapter. However, there is also discussion of the pharmacological management of anxiety, mania, schizophrenia, delusional disorder, and other psychoses. This chapter is not intended to be a comprehensive review of geriatric psychopharmacology; rather, it focuses on those aspects of treatment that are most relevant to the psychiatrist who is consulting to medical, surgical, or rehabilitation services. In keeping with this focus, the chapter is primarily concerned with acute aspects of treatment and little mention is made of strategies to prevent relapse or recurrence of symptoms. It is important to bear in mind, however, that most psychiatric disorders in later life are chronic or recurrent and require a long-term approach to treatment. Therefore, decisions regarding acute treatment need to be made in the context of a management plan that anticipates the future course of the illness. In this regard, appropriate follow-up should be arranged for patients who are to be continued on psychotropic medications following their discharge from hospital.

Pharmacokinetics and pharmacodynamics

Pharmacokinetics is that aspect of pharmacology pertaining to the absorption, distribution, metabolism, and elimination of drugs. Pharmacodynamics refers to the effects of drugs on the body. Pharmacokinetics and pharmacodynamics can change as a result of normal ageing, but concomitant physical disorders and drug–drug interactions can also alter them. As a result, there is tremendous variability between older persons in the way their bodies deal with and are affected by drugs and, in this respect, there is far more heterogeneity among the elderly than among the young.

Absorption

Ageing is associated with a reduction in stomach acid, diminished mesenteric blood flow, delayed gastric emptying, and decreased intestinal motility. However, these changes in gastrointestinal function have minimal effect on the absorption of psychotropic drugs (Catterson *et al.* 1997).

Distribution

Once in the systemic circulation, drugs distribute in tissue and organs where they exert their therapeutic and adverse effects. As people age, there is an increase in the proportion of body fat and a reduction in body water and muscle mass. As a consequence of increased adipose tissue, lipid-soluble drugs (which include all psychotropics except lithium) will have a larger volume of distribution in the elderly. This can result in a longer elimination half-life and, potentially, drug accumulation which increases the risk of adverse effects (Catterson *et al. 1997*).

Ageing is also associated with a reduction in the level of plasma albumin. In theory, drugs that are highly bound to albumin are more likely to show an increase in their free fraction which, in turn, can result in enhanced pharmacodynamic effects. However, an increase in the free drug is rapidly equilibrated by redistribution and elimination, thereby diminishing the effect of plasma-protein displacement (Rolan 1994). For this reason, drug–drug interactions involving the displacement of one highly protein-bound drug by another are rarely of clinical significance (Rolan 1994).

Metabolism

The metabolism of drugs generally takes place in the liver. A family of enzymes known as the cytochrome P450 (CYP) system is responsible for the biotransformation of a great many drugs, including psychotropic agents (Table 12.1). It is important to understand that there is not a uniform age-associated decline in liver metabolism and that a number of factors contribute to intraindividual and inter-individual variability. First, ageing has a variable effect on the activity of CYP isoenzymes. For example, the activity of CYP2D6 does not appear to change with age *per se*, whereas age-associated decrements in the function of CYP2C19 and CYP3A4 have been identified (Sweet and Pollock 1998). Second, approximately 7% of the White population is genetically deficient in CYP2D6 (Eichelbaum and Gross 1990), an isoenzyme that is involved in the metabolism of many psychotropic drugs. Plasma concentrations of drugs metabolized by this enzyme will be much higher in genetically deficient individuals than in non-deficient individuals who are given the same dose. Genetic deficiencies in CYPIA2 and CYP2C19 have also been identified (Sweet and Pollock 1998). Third, many drugs inhibit CYP isoenzymes and thus can potentially inhibit the metabolism of other drugs that undergo biotransformation by the same enzymes. Some drugs, such as fluoxetine and paroxetine, are such potent inhibitors of CYP2D6 that patients with normal 2D6 function who are given these medications can become the phenotypic equivalent of patients who are genetically deficient in this enzyme (Catterson *et al.* 1997). Since elderly people often take a number of drugs concurrently, it is important to be aware of the potential for these drug–drug interactions. Fourth, interindividual differences in drug metabolism are magnified by age-associated and illness-associated reductions in hepatic blood flow and hepatic mass. These changes can result in the reduced clearance of drugs, especially those that undergo extensive first-pass metabolism by the liver (Catterson *et al.* 1997).

Elimination

Ageing is associated with reduced renal clearance. This will result in the accumula-tion of active drugs (such as lithium) and active metabolites (such as hydroxylated metabolites of antidepressants or antipsychotics) that are subject to clearance by the kidneys (Catterson *et al.* 1997). Clearance of these compounds can be further impaired by renal disease.

Pharmacodynamics

Age-associated changes in cellular structure and function can render older people more vulnerable to the adverse effects of psychotropic medications. Ageing is associated with a progressive loss of dopamine D_2 receptors in the striatum of the brain, which probably explains the increased incidence of antipsychotic-induced parkinsonism and tardive dyskinesia in the elderly (Catterson *et al.* 1997). Older patients with antipsychotic-induced parkinsonism are at an increased risk of falls and urinary incontinence (Sweet and Pollock 1998). Patients with pathology of the striatum (e.g. Parkinson's disease, cerebrovascular disease, or certain types of

Table 12.1 A partial list of drugs metabolized by cytochrome P450 (CYP) isoenzymes 1A2, 2C, 2D6, and3A4

CYP1A2
Antidepressants—amitriptyline, clomipramine, fluvoxamine, imipramine, mirtazapine
Antipsychotics—clozapine, haloperidol, olanzapine
Beta-blockers—propranolol
Calcium-channel blockers—verapamil
Miscellaneous—acetaminophen, caffeine, phenacetin, tacrine, theophylline

CYP2C
Antidepressants—amitriptyline, citalopram, clomipramine, imipramine, moclobemide
Barbiturates—hexobarbital, mephobarbital
Benzodiazepines—diazepam
Beta-blockers—propranolol
Miscellaneous—omeprazole, phenytoin, proguanil, tolbutamide, warfarin

CYP2D6
Antiarrhythmics—encainide, flecainide, mexiletine, propafenone
Antidepressants—amitriptyline, clomipramine, desipramine, fluoxetine, imipramine, maprotiline, mCPP metabolite of nefazodone and trazodone, mirtazapine, nortriptyline, *N*-desmethyl-citalopram, paroxetine, trazodone, trimipramine, venlafaxine
Antipsychotics—clozapine, haloperidol, olanzapine, perphenazine, risperidone, thioridazine, zuclopenthixol
Beta-blockers—alprenolol, metoprolol, propranolol, timolol
Opiates—codeine, dextromethorphan, ethylmorphine
Miscellaneous—4-hydroxy-amphetamine, phenformin

CYP3A4
Antiarrhythmics—lidocaine (lignocaine), propafenone, quinidine
Antidepressants—amitriptyline, clomipramine, imipramine, mirtazapine, nefazodone, sertraline
Antihistamines—astemizole, terfenadine
Antipsychotics—clozapine, quetiapine
Benzodiazepines—alprazolam, midazolam, triazolam
Calcium-channel blockers—diltiazem, felodipine, nifedipine, verapamil
Opiates—dextromethorphan
Miscellaneous—carbamazepine, cortisol, cyclosporin, dexamethasone, erythromycin, ethinyloestradiol, tamoxifen, vinblastine

---

degenerative dementia) are even more sensitive to the extrapyramidal effects of neuroleptics. Ageing also involves the loss of cholinergic cells and the decreased activity of cholineacetyltransferase, the enzyme responsible for the synthesis of acetylcholine (Amenta *et al.* 1991). As a result, elderly people in general, but especially those with Alzheimer's disease, are at increased risk of experiencing cognitive impairment when taking drugs with anticholinergic activity (Catterson *et al.* 1997).

It is important to bear in mind that drug–drug interactions can occur at a pharmacodynamic level. These interactions may be direct (e.g. two or more drugs blocking muscarinic receptors and thereby worsening memory, or two or more drugs blocking α_1-adrenergic receptors and thereby causing hypotension), or indirect (e.g. the additive hypotensive effects of a tricyclic antidepressant (TCA) and a beta-blocker).

General principles of pharmacotherapy in the elderly

Before discussing the treatment of specific disorders, it is worth emphasizing a few principles regarding the use of psychotropic drugs in the elderly (Pollock and Mulsant 1998):

- One of the main goals of treatment is not only to alleviate symptoms, but also prevent them from recurring. Therefore, adhere to a schedule in administering medications and avoid an 'as needed' approach to pharmacotherapy.
- Whenever feasible, choose monotherapy over polytherapy.
- Before initiating therapy, define the short-term and long-term goals of treatment.
- Plan the duration of treatment.
- Start low, go slow, but do not undertreat.
- Monitor the patient on a regular basis for therapeutic and adverse effects. Carefully evaluate the effect of treatment on the overall quality of life and function of the patient, not just the target syndrome or symptoms.
- Document the outcomes of treatment.
- Be patient and persistent.

Delirium

Delirium is a common disorder in elderly medical and surgical inpatients (Jacobson 1997). The mainstay of management is the timely diagnosis and treatment of the physical condition(s) causing the delirium (Jacobson 1997). This includes tapering or discontinuing non-essential medications. Pharmacological treatment is under-taken, when required, to control associated agitation and psychosis (Jacobson 1997). Because of its minimal anticholinergic and hypotensive effects, haloperidol is usu-ally considered the antipsychotic of choice in the symptomatic treatment of delirium (Pollock and Mulsant 1995). Oral or intramuscular administration of low doses of haloperidol (for example, 0.5–1.0 mg two or three times a day) is recommended in elderly patients (Pollock and Mulsant 1995). Haloperidol can be given intravenously to patients who are unable to take medication by mouth and for whom multiple intra-muscular injections are inadvisable. In most cases, antipsychotic medication can be discontinued after 1–2 weeks. Withdrawal of the drug over 2–3 days rather than abrupt discontinuation is recommended.

The role of newer, atypical antipsychotic medications in the treatment of delirium has yet to be determined. Clozapine and olanzapine are antagonists of muscarinic receptors and so they have the potential to worsen delirium (Sweet and Pollock 1998). Risperidone lacks significant anticholinergic activity, but it has the capacity to produce postural hypotension (Sweet and Pollock 1998), so it is unclear whether it has advantages over low-dose haloperidol.

In general, benzodiazepines are reserved for the specific treatment of alcohol- or benzodiazepine-withdrawal delirium (Jacobson 1997). Benzodiazepines are not recommended in other types of delirium because they have the potential to worsen cognitive impairment, psychomotor impairment, and behavioural disinhibition (Breitbart et al. 1996).

Dementia

Behavioural disturbance

Behavioural disturbance is a common reason for psychiatric intervention in medical or surgical patients with dementia. Before embarking on symptomatic treatment, assess the patient for medications, physical problems (including constipation and pain), or depression that could be contributing to the behavioural disturbance and remedy as many of these factors as possible. Remember that patients with dementia are extremely vulnerable to developing delirium. Abrupt onset of insomnia, visual hallucinations, or agitation should alert the clinician to this possibility.

Medical treatment for dementia-related behavioural problems is indicated if they threaten the safety of the patient or others, compromise the patient's medical care or activities of daily living, cause significant patient distress, or interfere with his or her placement (Pollock and Mulsant 1998).

Antipsychotics (neuroleptics)

Antipsychotics have been the most extensively studied drugs for the treatment of behavioural disturbance in dementia. Several randomized, placebo-controlled studies have found that antipsychotic medications can result in statistically and clinically significant improvement in agitation, aggression, and psychosis (Petrie et al. 1982; Finkel et al. 1995; Devanand et al. 1998; Katz et al. 1999). There is no evidence that one antipsychotic drug is more efficacious than another in patients with dementia, therefore the choice of drug is based on its side-effect profile. Given the sensitivity of older persons to extrapyramidal and anticholinergic adverse effects, intermediate-potency drugs such as loxapine or perphenazine have traditionally been the antipsychotics of choice in the treatment of dementia (Pollock and Mulsant 1998). The usual dose range in these patients is 5–15 mg/day of loxapine (starting dose of 2.5–5 mg/day) or 4–16 mg/day of perphenazine (starting dose of 2–4 mg/day).

The role of atypical antipsychotics in the treatment of dementia requires much more study. Clozapine, olanzapine, quetiapine, and risperidone have side-effects that are potentially of concern in patients with dementia (Pollock and Mulsant 1998). All four drugs have the capacity for causing sedation and hypotension, and clozapine and olanzapine may worsen confusion as a result of the blockade of muscarinic receptors (Sweet and Pollock 1998). The use of clozapine is also limited by its capacity to cause agranulocytosis (a risk that may be increased in the elderly) (Alvir et al. 1993) and the consequent need for regular monitoring of a patient's white blood count. Risperidone can induce clinically significant extrapyramidal symptoms in patients with dementia at doses as low as 2 mg/day (Katz et al. 1999), and this author's experience is that extrapyramidal effects can develop with olanzapine at doses as low as 5 mg/day. Quetiapine appears to have a lower incidence of extrapyramidal effects (Sweet and et al. Pollock 1998), but there are few data pertaining to the use of this drug in the elderly. Jeste et al. (1999) recently reported that older patients treated with risperidone were less likely to develop tardive dyskinesia than those treated with haloperidol. This preliminary finding needs to be replicated in a double-blind, randomized, controlled trial, but it does raise the possibility that elderly patients with dementia may be at less risk of developing tardive dyskinesia with atypical antipsychotics than with typical agents.

Anticonvulsants

There is some evidence that carbamazepine is more effective than placebo in treating the behavioural symptoms of dementia (Cooney et al. 1996; Tariot et al. 1998a). In the studies showing positive results, the mean plasma level of carbamazepine was approximately 5 µg/ml (20 µmol/l), usually achieved with doses of 200–600 mg/day. At this plasma concentration, carbamazepine was generally well tolerated, but it has been suggested that adverse effects (including cognitive decline, sedation, dizziness, ataxia, and diplopia) are more likely to occur in the elderly when plasma concentrations are above 9 µg/ml (40 µmol/l) (Pollock and Mulsant 1998). The elderly are also susceptible to blood dyscrasias caused by carbamazepine, the incidence of which increase with advanced age (Cates and Powers 1998). Thus, patients treated with this drug should have complete blood counts checked on a regular basis. In rare instances, carbamazepine can cause liver toxicity. Carbamazepine is a potent *inducer* of CYP2D6 and, therefore, may diminish the activity of drugs that are metabolized by this enzyme.

Despite a lack of placebo-controlled data, valproate has become a popular alternative to carbamazepine in the treatment of agitation in dementia (Pollock and Mulsant 1998). In part, this popularity is based on the fact that valproate may have less potential for drug–drug interactions and may be better tolerated than carbamazepine (Pollock and Mulsant 1998). Nevertheless, valproate has the potential to cause sedation, tremor, ataxia, and dizziness, and it has also been associated with hepatic and haematological toxicity (Pollock and Mulsant 1998). Platelet counts should be monitored for possible thrombocytopenia. Valproate dose requirements have not been adequately characterized in patients with dementia, but there has been a tendency to use plasma levels established for the treatment of seizure disorders (50–100 μg/ml; 350–700 μmol/l). In the elderly, these levels are frequently attained with doses of 750–1500 mg/day.

Antidepressants

Placebo-controlled data on the use of antidepressant medications in the treatment of behavioural disturbance in dementia are limited and inconclusive. Citalopram was found to be more effective than placebo in reducing irritability, but not restlessness, in patients with Alzheimer's disease (Nyth and Gottfries 1990). However, two other selective serotonin-reuptake inhibitors (SSRIs) (alaproclate and fluvoxamine) were no more effective than placebo in controlling behavioural symptoms (Dehlin *et al.* 1985; Olafsson *et al.* 1992, respectively). Single studies found that trazodone given at a mean dose of 120 (± 35) mg/day and selegiline given at a dose of 10 mg/day resulted in statistically significant improvements in Brief Psychiatric Rating Scale (BPRS) total scores (Lawlor *et al.* 1994, 1997), but this does not necessarily imply improvement in agitation or aggression (Flint and Van Reekum 1998). Two other studies found no difference between selegiline and placebo on measures of behaviour. However, as subjects in these studies had few behavioural symptoms at baseline, this factor may have limited the investigators' ability to detect a drug effect (Burke *et al.* 1993; Tariot *et al.* 1998*b*).

Other medications

Benzodiazepines appear to be more effective than placebo but less effective than antipsychotics in the treatment of dementia-associated behavioural disturbance, although the data are of limited quality (American Psychiatric Association 1997). Benzodiazepines carry a number of risks for patients with dementia, including oversedation, ataxia, falls (and associated hip fractures), exacerbation of cognitive impairment and worsening of sleep-disordered breathing (American Psychiatric Association 1997). Because of the risks associated with benzodiazepines and the limited evidence regarding their benefit, benzodiazepines are generally not recommended as a first-line of treatment for patients with dementia.

Other drugs that have been proposed for the treatment of agitation or aggression include beta-blockers, buspirone, and lithium (Lantz and Marin 1996). Lithium is sometimes used when the behavioural disturbance has a manic-like quality. However, there are no placebo-controlled data regarding the efficacy or safety of these drugs in elderly patients with dementia, and none can be recommended with confidence. Case series suggest that medroxyprogesterone and related hormonal agents may sometimes be of benefit in male patients with disinhibited sexual behaviour (American Psychiatric Association 1997). Patients with dementia with Lewy bodies are susceptible to severe extrapyramidal side-effects with antipsychotic medication (McKeith and O'Brien 1999). Preliminary uncontrolled data suggest that pharmacotherapy with cholinesterase inhibitors, such as donepezil or rivastigmine, may be an effective and safer alternative to the use of antipsychotics in the treatment of psychosis or agitation in dementia with Lewy bodies (McKeith *et al.* 2000). This issue is currently being examined in a double-blind, placebo-controlled study (McKeith *et al.* 2000).

Choice of medication

To avoid the risk of drug-induced parkinsonism and tardive dyskinesia, some authors have advocated the use of a non-neuroleptic medication as the first line of treatment for behavioural symptoms associated with dementia (Pollock and Mulsant 1998). However, this approach may be less feasible for patients in acute hospital settings where prompt control of the behavioural disturbance is often the primary goal. Clinical experience suggests that antipsychotic medication may have a more rapid onset of effect than anticonvulsants or antidepressants.

Cognitive impairment

Cognitive impairment *per se* is seldom the primary reason for psychiatric referral of patients with dementia in medical or surgical settings. Nevertheless, a consultation liaison psychiatrist may recommend treatment for cognitive impairment as part of the overall management plan for these patients.

Currently, there are two approaches to the treatment of cognitive impairment in patients with Alzheimer's disease: symptomatic treatment, and treatment designed to slow the underlying disease process (Flint and Van Reekum 1998). Cholinesterase inhibitors (CEIs) are the class of drugs that have the best established efficacy in the symptomatic treatment of Alzheimer's disease (Flint and Van Reekum 1998). Uncontrolled data suggest that CEIs may also be useful in treating the cognitive impairment of dementia with Lewy bodies (Shea *et al.* 1998). These medications inhibit acetylcholinesterase and, thereby, increase the availability of brain intra-synaptic acetylcholine. There is no current evidence that they alter the course of the underlying disease process. For most patients, the cognitive-enhancing effects of CEIs are modest, although a minority of patients derive more substantial benefit. If a patient is treated with a CEI, he/she requires a minimum 12-week trial before a decision can be made about the drug's efficacy. Thus, if a trial of a CEI is initiated in hospital, it is important to arrange appropriate outpatient follow-up of the patient, so that the drug's effectiveness can be evaluated and a decision made about whether or not it should be continued.

For the most part, CEIs are well tolerated. The most common side-effects are nausea, loose stools, and disturbed sleep, which is sometimes associated with vivid dreams (Flint and Van Reekum 1998). Side-effects are dose-related and can be minimized by gradual titration of the dose (for example, give donepezil at 5 mg/day for the first 4 weeks of treatment and, if tolerated, increase the dose to 10 mg/day after that). Because of their cholinomimetic properties, CEIs may not be safe in patients with poorly controlled asthma or active peptic ulcer disease. In addition, CEIs can have vagotonic effects on the heart and should not be given to patients with sick sinus syndrome or other cardiac conduction abnormalities that could be exacerbated by slowing of the heart rate.

An important issue in the treatment of a progressive condition such as Alzheimer's disease is deciding when to stop CEI treatment. Lovestone *et al.* (1997) suggest that a cognitive-enhancing drug be stopped if: (1) the patient is poorly compliant; (2) there is continued cognitive deterioration at the pretreatment rate after 3–6 months of therapy; (3) there is accelerated deterioration after a period of stabilization; or (4) a drug-free period suggests that the drug is no longer working (i.e. there is no significant deterioration in cognitive function within a month of stopping the CEI).

With respect to medications given to slow the progression of Alzheimer's disease, research has examined the effect of antioxidants (selegiline and vitamin E), anti-inflammatories (non-steroidal anti-inflammatory drugs and prednisone), and exogenous oestrogen. At the current time, none of these therapies can be recommended for routine clinical practice. The authors of one randomized controlled study reported that either 2000 IU/day of vitamin E or 10 mg/day of selegiline were more effective than placebo in delaying the time to the occurrence of any of the following outcome variables: death, institutionalization, loss of ability to perform basic activities of daily living, or severe dementia (Sano *et al.* 1997). However, statistically significant results between active treatment and placebo were obtained only after the investigators adjusted for intergroup differences in baseline Mini-Mental State scores. In a small randomized controlled study, patients treated with 100–150 mg/day of indomethacin for 6 months had significantly less cognitive deterioration than those treated with placebo (Rogers *et al.* 1993). However, 20% of patients in the indomethacin group did not complete the study because of gastrointestinal side-effects. More recent trials with anti-inflammatory drugs (celecoxib 200 mg twice a day; prednisone 10 mg/day) (Sainati *et al.* 2000; Aisen *et al.* 2000, respectively) have not found that these drugs influence the course of Alzheimer's disease. Also, oestrogen replacement therapy has not been found to slow the progress of Alzheimers disease in women (Mulnard *et al.* 2000; Henderson *et al.* 2000).

Depression

It is well established that antidepressant medication is an effective treatment for major depression in elderly patients who do not have significant medical co-morbidity (Flint 1998*a*). Less is known about the efficacy and effectiveness of anti-depressant medication in depressed elderly people with medical illness, neurological disorders, or dementia, but the results of several placebo-controlled studies suggest that antidepressants can be of benefit in these populations

(Andersen, J. *et al.* 1980; Andersen, G. *et al.* 1994; Petracca *et al.* 1996; Roth *et al.* 1996; Evans *et al.* 1997).

There is no available evidence that one class of antidepressant medication is more efficacious than another in the treatment of late-life major depression. Therefore, selection of an antidepressant is based on other factors, including adverse effects and safety, the potential for drug–drug interactions, a patient's history of response or non-response to a particular drug, and cost-effectiveness. Space limitations preclude a discussion of each class of antidepressant medication (for a recent comprehensive review see Flint 1998*a*). This section of the chapter will focus on TCAs, SSRIs, and the more recently introduced antidepressants (mirtazapine, nefazodone, and venlafaxine).

Tricyclic antidepressants

Up until the 1990s, TCAs were the mainstay of antidepressant pharmacotherapy and, despite the availability of newer antidepressants, remain in widespread use among the elderly. TCAs have well-established efficacy and, indeed, there is an ongoing debate about whether TCAs are more effective than SSRIs in the treatment of severe or melancholic depression (Perry 1996; Hirschfeld 1999). However, a number of adverse effects can limit the use of TCAs in older persons, especially those with medical illness. The adverse effects of TCAs result from their blockade of central and peripheral cholinergic receptors (dry mouth, blurred vision, constipation, urinary hesitancy or retention, memory impairment, tachycardia), histaminergic receptors (sedation, body weight gain) and α-adrenergic receptors (orthostatic hypotension). Secondary amine TCAs, such as nortriptyline or desipramine, are less likely to induce these effects than tertiary amine drugs such as amitriptyline or imipramine (Preskorn and Burke 1992). Of the TCAs, nortriptyline has the least propensity for causing hypotension (Roose and Dalack 1992). Although nortriptyline is generally well tolerated by medically stable, cognitively intact, 'young-old' individuals (Georgotas *et al.* 1986; Rosen *et al.* 1993; Reynolds *et al.* 1995), it is less well tolerated by very old or frail patients (Katz *et al.* 1990), patients with stroke (Lipsey *et al.* 1984), and people with acute medical illness (Koenig and Breitner 1990). Because they slow intracardiac conduction, any of the TCAs may be hazardous in patients with bundle-branch block (Roose and Dalack 1992) and can be fatal when taken in overdose.

Nearly all the adverse effects associated with TCAs are concentration-dependent (Preskorn 1993). TCAs have a relatively narrow therapeutic index (margin between the therapeutic dose and a toxic dose) and, for a given dose, there is wide inter-individual variation in plasma concentrations (Preskorn 1993). Therefore, monitoring plasma TCA concentrations can be particularly helpful in order to maximize clinical response and minimize adverse effects. Nortriptyline has a reasonably well-established therapeutic window of 50–150 ng/ml (200–550 nmol/l) (Rockwell *et al.* 1988).

Selective serotonin-reuptake inhibitors

With the exception of paroxetine which may have a modest effect on cholinergic receptors (Thomas *et al*. 1987), the SSRIs have little affinity for adrenergic, histaminergic, or cholinergic receptors (Grimsley and Jann 1992). In selected physically healthy individuals, SSRIs lack significant cardiac effects and do not produce postural hypotension (Grimsley and Jann 1992). However, their safety in patients with cardiac disease has not been well studied (Sheline *et al*. 1997). A recent controlled trial found that paroxetine and nortriptyline had comparable efficacy in the treatment of major depression in patients with ischaemic heart disease, but paroxetine was associated with significantly fewer adverse cardiac events (Roose *et al*. 1998). Consistent with their apparent lack of cardiotoxicity, SSRIs have not proved fatal when taken alone in overdose. In contrast to TCAs, SSRIs have not been found to impair cognitive function (Hindmarch *et al*. 1990, 1994). Patients with dementia, therefore, may better tolerate SSRIs, although a direct comparison of an SSRI with an appropriately selected TCA (that is, a secondary amine drug) has not been undertaken in these patients. Thus, SSRIs lack many of the adverse effects associated with TCAs and, as a result, there are fewer barriers to their use in the elderly. However, SSRIs are not without adverse effects; although one may surmise that they are better tolerated than secondary amine TCAs by medically ill older patients, this hypothesis has not yet been tested in a randomized controlled trial.

The adverse effects of SSRIs primarily reflect central and peripheral serotonin-reuptake inhibition, including gastrointestinal upset (nausea, anorexia, flatus, frequent or loose stools), CNS dysfunction (insomnia, sedation, apathy, nervousness, restlessness, dizziness, tremor, headaches), and sexual dysfunction (decreased libido, anorgasmia, delayed ejaculation, and impotence) (Grimsley and Jann 1992).

A few side-effects appear to be more prevalent or disabling in older persons. SSRIs have been found to produce postural instability in older persons (Laghrissi-Thode *et al*. 1995) and, like many other psychotropic drugs, have been associated with an increased risk of falls and hip fractures in the elderly (Liu *et al*. 1998). Tremor may also be more problematic in older persons, especially if an SSRI is combined with lithium or a neuroleptic. However, open-label trials in patients with treated Parkinson's disease have not identified a worsening of motor symptoms with SSRI use (Meara *et al*. 1996; Hauser and Zesiewicz 1997). An infrequent, but potentially dangerous, adverse effect is the inappropriate secretion of antidiuretic hormone (SIADH) and hyponatraemia (Liu *et al*. 1996) which can present with confusion, fatigue, weakness, and falls. Most reported cases of SSRI-induced hyponatraemia have occurred within the first month of starting the drug (Liu *et al*. 1996). The hyponatraemia will resolve once the SSRI is discontinued (a short period of fluid restriction may also be necessary to correct the electrolyte imbalance), but may reoccur if the patient is rechallenged with the same or a different SSRI (Flint *et al*. 1996). Although SIADH has been associated with other classes of anti-depressants, it has been reported most frequently with SSRIs. However, it is not known whether this reflects a reporting bias or an increased incidence of this effect with SSRIs.

There are differences in the pharmacokinetics of SSRIs that have implications for their use in the elderly. Fluoxetine and its active metabolite norfluoxetine have a combined elimination half-life of approximately 2 weeks (Rickels and Schweizer 1990). As a result, it may take 2 months or more to achieve steady-state plasma concentrations of this drug, and there is the potential for ongoing side-effects and drug–drug interactions for many weeks after the drug is discontinued. Because of its long half-life, fluoxetine is potentially more problematic than citalopram, fluvoxamine, paroxetine, or sertraline, which have half-lives of 1–2 days and metabolites with little or no clinically significant activity (Grimsley and Jann 1992; Goodnick 1994). Fluoxetine and paroxetine have non-linear kinetics, and thus an increase in their dose can result in a disproportionate increase in plasma concentrations (Goodnick 1994). Therefore, the dosage of fluoxetine or paroxetine should not be increased by any more than 10 mg at a time in older patients. Age-related pharmacokinetic changes result in higher plasma concentrations and prolonged half-lives of citalopram and paroxetine, hence the starting dose and maximum dose of these drugs should be reduced in the elderly (Goodnick 1994) (Table 12.2). Age, *per se*, has not been shown to have a clinically significant effect on the pharmacokinetics of sertraline or fluvoxamine. Nevertheless, medically ill older persons may better tolerate these medications if they are started at a low dose and then titrated up to the minimum effective dose after a week or so (Table 12.2).

SSRIs also differ in their potency of inhibition of CYP isoenzymes (Nemeroff *et al.* 1996; Shader *et al.* 1996) (Table 12.3). It is important to note that the clinical significance of many potential SSRI–drug interactions is not known. Even when they are significant, there is tremendous interindividual variability in the severity of the clinical sequelae. Therefore, a potential drug–drug interaction does not necessarily preclude the use of an SSRI, but doses may need to be adjusted and the patient should be carefully monitored. Particular caution should be exercised when an SSRI is prescribed with a drug that has a narrow therapeutic index such as TCAs, antipsychotics, theophylline, phenytoin, carbamazepine, and tolbutamide

Table 12.2 Usual starting dose, minimum effective dose, and maximum dose of selective serotonin-reuptake inhibitors in elderly patients

SSRI	Usual starting dose (mg/d)	Minimum effective dose (mg/d)	Maximum dose (mg/d)
Citalopram	10	20	30
Fluoxetine	10	20	60
Fluvoxamine	25–50	100–150	300
Paroxetine	10	20	40
Sertraline	25–50	50–100	200

Table 12.3 Inhibitory effect of selective serotonin reuptake inhibitors on P450(CYP) isoenzymes*

Antidepressant	Isoenzyme 1A2	2C	2D6	3A4
Citalopram	0	0	+	0
Fluoxetine/norfluoxetine	0	++	+++	++
Fluvoxamine	+++	++	0	++
Paroxetine	0	0	+++	0
Sertraline	0	+	+/++	+

Potency of inhibition: 0 = none or minimal; + = mild; ++ = moderate; +++ = potent.
A rating of ++ or higher is usually necessary for inhibition to have clinical significance.
* Based on currently available in vitro and in vivo data (Crewe *et al.* 1992; Goodnick 1994; Harvey and Preskorn 1996; Nemeroff et al. 1996; Shader *et al.* 1996; Sproule *et al.* 1997).

(Nemeroff *et al.* 1996). SSRIs should be administered with caution, if at all, in patients taking type 1C antiarrhythmics (encainide, flecainide, propafenone) (Nemeroff *et al.* 1996).

SSRIs have a flat dose–response curve. For the majority of patients, increasing the dose beyond the minimum effective dose does not result in additional efficacy, but can produce more side-effects (Preskorn 1993). Thus, a patient should be monitored on the minimum effective dose for at least 4 weeks before an increase in dose is considered. If there are no signs of clinical improvement, the dose should then be gradually increased, guided by tolerability and efficacy.

Other antidepressants

Mirtazapine, nefazodone, and venlafaxine have minimal anticholinergic effects (Holm and Markham 1999; Robinson *et al.* 1996; Feighner 1994, respectively). In addition, they have not been found to have clinically significant effects on the heart, although there are few data pertaining to their use in patients with cardiovascular disease (Feighner 1994; Robinson *et al.* 1996; Holm and Markham 1999). Similar to SSRIs, they do not appear to be lethal when taken alone in overdose (Feighner 1994; Robinson *et al.* 1996; Holm and Markham 1999). Mirtazapine and venlafaxine do not cause orthostatic hypotension (Feighner 1994; Holm and Markham 1999).

Nefazodone is structurally related to trazodone. Like trazodone, it is a weak inhibitor of serotonin reuptake but a potent serotonin $5HT_2$ receptor antagonist (Goodnick 1994). Although nefazodone has affinity for α_1-adrenergic receptors, it is approximately five times less potent than trazodone in this regard (Taylor *et al.* 1995) and orthostatic hypotension is not a common complication (Goldberg 1997). Nefazodone can cause daytime sedation, but this effect is less marked than with trazodone (Robinson *et al.* 1996). Other side-effects include nausea, dry mouth, dizziness, constipation, and asthenia (Robinson *et al.* 1996). In contrast to SSRIs, nefazodone does not cause sexual dysfunction and unlike trazodone it does not cause priapism (Robinson *et al.* 1996). Nefazodone is a potent inhibitor of CYP3A4 (Nemeroff *et al.* 1996) and care should be taken when it is administered with other drugs metabolized by this isoenzyme. Ageing affects its pharmacokinetics, with the result that older patients require half the usual starting dose (50 mg twice a day), slower dose titration, and a lower therapeutic dose (200–400 mg/day) (Barbhaiya *et al.* 1996).

Venlafaxine inhibits serotonin and noradrenaline reuptake and, in this respect, is pharmacodynamically similar to TCAs (Feighner 1994). However, venlafaxine lacks TCAs unwanted affinity for cholinergic, histaminergic, and α_1-adrenergic receptors (Feighner 1994). The most common adverse effects of venlafaxine are nausea, somnolence, dry mouth, dizziness, nervousness, constipation, sexual dysfunction, sweating, and asthenia (Feighner 1994). A small number of patients experience modest elevations of blood pressure at higher doses of this medication and, as a result, blood pressure monitoring is recommended before and during venlafaxine therapy (Feighner 1994). However, as long as a patient's blood pressure is adequately controlled, a history of hypertension does not contraindicate the use of this drug. Venlafaxine is only a weak inhibitor of CYP2D6 and is much less likely than fluoxetine or paroxetine to interact with drugs metabolized by this isoenzyme (Nemeroff *et al.* 1996). Unlike SSRIs, venlafaxine does not have a flat dose–response curve, and higher doses of this drug are generally associated with a higher probability of response (Feighner 1994). However, the dose range is wide (75–375 mg/day) and the usual therapeutic dose for older patients has not been established. Furthermore, it has not been determined whether there is a therapeutic range of plasma concentrations for this drug. In older persons, a starting dose of 37.5 mg/day is recommended in order to avoid nausea.

Mirtazapine enhances noradrenergic and serotonergic transmission via blockade of α_2, $5HT_2$, and $5HT_3$ receptors (Holm and Markham 1999). Mirtazapine has a high affinity for histamine H_1 receptors and, as a result, can cause sedation, increased appetite, and body weight gain (Holm and Markham 1999). Interestingly, sedation may diminish at higher doses, possibly because of increased arousal associated with α_2 antagonism (Holm and Markham 1999). In contrast with other newer antidepressants, mirtazapine does not cause nausea, presumably because of $5HT_3$ blockade (Holm and Markham 1999). It has been suggested that, like nefazodone, mirtazapine's antagonism of $5HT_2$ receptors may facilitate anxiolytic and hypnotic effects (Holm and Markham 1999). Limited data suggest that mirtazapine has little impact on sexual function (Holm and Markham 1999). *In vitro* and *in vivo* studies indicate that mirtazapine is unlikely to affect the metabolism of drugs metabolized by CYPIA2, CYP2D6, and CYP3A4 (data are not available regarding CYP2C) (Holm and Markham 1999). Ageing does not appear to have a clinically significant effect on the pharmacokinetics of this drug, and the recommended starting dose (15 mg/day) and effective dose range (15–45 mg/day) are the same as those for younger adults (Holm and Markham 1999).

Stimulants

Uncontrolled data and the results of one small randomized, controlled, crossover study suggest that stimulants such as methylphenidate may be useful in the treatment of depression or apathy in medically ill patients (Satel and Nelson 1989; Wallace *et al*. 1995; Emptage and Semla 1996). At recommended doses (for example, 10–30 mg/day of methylphenidate) stimulants are generally well tolerated, with a rapid onset of action (often within days) reported (Satel and Nelson 1989; Emptage and Semla 1996). However, there are virtually no data on the medium-term or long-term efficacy of these drugs, in particular their ability to prevent relapse or recurrence of depression (Emptage and Semla 1996). Furthermore, there are no randomized controlled data on whether stimulants are as effective as conventional anti-depressants in the treatment of major depression in medically ill older patients (Emptage and Semla 1996). However, there are considerable data from controlled trials to show that stimulants are usually no more effective than placebo in the treatment of primary depression in people who are physically well (Satel and Nelson 1989). Therefore, in the opinion of this author, conventional antidepressants, rather than stimulants, are the drugs of choice for the treatment of major depression, regardless of whether physical illness is also present. Uncontrolled data suggest that methylphenidate may be useful in the treatment of apathy that is secondary to dementia (Galynker *et al*. 1997).

Treatment of non-responders

The goal of the acute phase of treatment is to achieve the remission of depressive symptoms. The first step is to ensure that the patient has received an adequate dose of antidepressant for a sufficient length of time (usually a minimum of 6 weeks). However, 30% of elderly patients do not respond to an initial adequate trial of antidepressant medication and require additional or alternative treatment (Schneider 1996). One approach is to augment the antidepressant with another drug, either a second antidepressant (for example, adding a TCA to an SSRI) or a medication that is not primarily an antidepressant (for example, adding lithium, tri-iodothyronine, methylphenidate, pindolol, buspirone, or valproate) (Flint 1995). The advantage of augmentation is that it does not require discontinuation of the original antidepressant and, therefore, patients who partially respond to treatment are not put at risk of returning to their baseline severity of depression. Also, response may at times be faster with augmentation than with a new trial of anti-depressant medication. The disadvantage of augmentation, especially in medically ill elderly patients, is that the combination of medications increases the risk of adverse effects and drug–drug interactions. Furthermore, there have been no controlled trials of augmentation in elderly people and, therefore, the effectiveness of this approach in treating geriatric depression has not been established (Flint 1995).

Refractory depression can also be managed by changing from one antidepressant medication to another. Generally, patients should be given a different class of antidepressant rather than another drug in the same class (Thase *et al.* 1994/1995). If a patient has failed to respond to an SSRI or nefazodone, then changing to an antidepressant with dual neurotransmitter action (for example, venlafaxine, mirtazapine, or nortriptyline) is a sensible strategy. Finally, electroconvulsive therapy (ECT) can be an efficacious and safe treatment for depression in medically ill older patients and should always be considered as an alternative to pharmacotherapy in this population (Greenberg 1997).

Anxiety

When anxiety develops in elderly patients with medical illness or neurological disorders it is frequently associated with depression (Flint 1994). Therefore, new-onset anxiety, especially if the symptoms are of generalized anxiety or panic, should always prompt a careful examination for an underlying depressive illness. If anxiety is found to be associated with depression, the most appropriate primary pharmacological treatment is antidepressant medication (Flint 1998*b*). Certain antidepressants can also be used as a first-line treatment for generalized anxiety disorder, panic disorder, obsessive–compulsive disorder, post-traumatic stress disorder and social phobia, even when depression is absent (Antony and Swinson 1996). SSRIs in particular have a broad spectrum of efficacy in the treatment of primary or secondary anxiety (Antony and Swinson 1996).

Benzodiazepines may at times be required as an adjunct to antidepressant medication in the treatment of anxiety. In addition, benzodiazepines may be used as a primary treatment for acute situational anxiety, generalized anxiety disorder or panic disorder that are not associated with depression, and social phobia (Antony and Swinson 1996). The benzodiazepines that are most appropriate for use in the elderly are lorazepam or oxazepam since they have relatively short half-lives (12–15 hours), no active metabolites, and do not undergo oxidative metabolism in the liver (and thus their clearance is unaffected by age or other drugs). As a result, these drugs do not have the potential for cumulative toxicity, which is a risk associated with longer acting agents such as diazepam or clonazepam (American Psychiatric Association 1990). The usual dose range in the elderly is 0.5–2 mg/day of lorazepam and 10–30 mg/day of oxazepam.

Although buspirone can be an effective treatment for generalized anxiety disorder (Steinberg 1994), it has a limited role in the management of anxiety in later life. Buspirone has a delayed onset of action of 2 weeks or more (Steinberg 1994) and so it is unsuitable for acute anxiety states. Furthermore, as already noted, generalized anxiety in the elderly is frequently associated with a depressive illness and, in this situation, antidepressant medication remains the drug of choice. Unlike benzodiazepines, buspirone does not cause sedation, psychomotor or cognitive impairment, or depressed respiratory drive (Steinberg 1994). Therefore, buspirone may be preferable to a benzodiazepine in the longer term management of generalized anxiety in non-depressed patients with chronic obstructive airways disease, sleep apnoea, or neurological disorders.

Bipolar disorder (mania)

Lithium has been the mainstay of the acute and maintenance treatment of bipolar disorder in late life (Eastham *et al.* 1998). However, there have been no controlled studies of its use in the elderly. Because of an age-related decline in renal clearance, older patients require lower doses of lithium to achieve therapeutic plasma levels (Eastham *et al.* 1998). The elderly are particularly sensitive to the neurological effects of lithium (tremor, ataxia, cognitive impairment) even at plasma concentrations considered to be therapeutic in younger adults (Flint 1993). This vulnerability is enhanced when lithium is combined with other medications that have neurological effects (for example, neuroleptics or anticonvulsants) or if the patient has neurological disease. As a result, plasma levels of 0.5–0.8 mmol/l have been recommended for use in the elderly (frequently achieved with doses in the range of 300 to 750 mg/day) (Eastham *et al.* 1998). Thiazide diuretics, angiotensin-converting enzyme (ACE) inhibitors, and non-steroidal anti-inflammatory drugs can interfere with the excretion of lithium, and caution should be exercised when these drugs are used in combination with lithium.

In recent years, valproate and carbamazepine have been widely used as alternatives or adjuncts to lithium in the treatment of mania and bipolar disorder (Baldessarini *et al.* 1996). These drugs have not been systematically studied in the elderly, but in younger individuals they have been shown to be effective therapies for mania, including mania that has failed to respond to lithium (Baldessarini *et al.* 1996). Controlled studies in mixed-age patients have found that carbamazepine is as effective as lithium in preventing recurrences of bipolar disorder, and uncontrolled trials have provided encouraging observations about the prophylactic effect of valproate (Baldessarini *et al.* 1996). Uncontrolled data suggest that valproate and carbamazepine may be more efficacious than lithium in the treatment of rapid cycling bipolar illness (Baldessarini *et al.* 1996). As previously noted, anecdotal evidence suggests that valproate may be better tolerated than carbamazepine in old age. The recommended plasma level for valproate in the treatment of bipolar disorder in the elderly is 50–100 µg/ml (350–700 µmol/l), and for carbamazepine the recommended plasma level is 4–12 µg/ml (17–50 µmol/l). Combination mood-stabilizer therapy (for example, lithium and valproate, or lithium and carbamazepine) is commonplace in the treatment of refractory bipolar disorder in younger individuals (Freeman and Stoll 1998). Although some elderly patients may tolerate combination therapy, adverse effects may limit this strategy in later life (Wils and Golüke-Willemse 1997).

Adjunctive treatment with antipsychotic medication is frequently required in acute mania, especially if psychosis or severe behavioural disturbance is present. There have been a number of reports of neurotoxicity resulting from the combination of lithium and antipsychotic medication (Freeman and Stoll 1998). Most of these cases of neurotoxicity were associated with the use of conventional antipsychotics (especially haloperidol), but the combination of lithium and risperidone can also carry some risk (Freeman and Stoll 1998). Therefore, care should be taken when combining lithium and a neuroleptic in the elderly, even if the antipsychotic is an atypical agent. Neurological side-effects may possibly be less of a risk with a valproate–antipsychotic combination (Freeman and Stoll 1998), but, nevertheless, patients should be closely monitored for adverse effects. Antipsychotic medication is seldom indicated in the maintenance treatment of geriatric bipolar disorder, and every effort should be made to withdraw an antipsychotic following resolution of the acute manic episode.

Although efficacy data are lacking, benzodiazepines are occasionally administered to elderly patients with acute mania. Low doses of lorazepam may be used to treat sleep disturbance or mild agitation when a mood stabilizer alone does not adequately control these symptoms. Clonazepam is frequently used as an adjunctive agent in the acute treatment of mania in younger patients. However, clonazepam is generally not recommended for older patients because it has a long elimination half-life and the potential for accumulation and toxicity. At dosages as low as 1 mg/day, clonazepam can cause clinically significant drowsiness and psychomotor impairment in the elderly, especially when it is combined with antipsychotics, lithium, or anticonvulsants.

Schizophrenia, delusional disorder, and other psychoses

Schizophrenia and delusional disorder

Irrespective of whether they are of early or late onset, schizophrenia and delusional disorder are typically chronic disorders requiring long-term treatment. Elderly patients are at high risk of developing tardive dyskinesia (Kane et al. 1988) and this is an important consideration in the selection of an antipsychotic in these disorders. Preliminary data suggest that older patients may be less likely to develop tardive dyskinesia with risperidone than with haloperidol (Jeste et al. 1999). Moreover, a study involving younger patients with schizophrenia found that the incidence of tardive dyskinesia was significantly lower with olanzapine than with haloperidol (Tollefson et al. 1997). Thus, in this respect, atypical antipsychotics may have a major advantage over conventional antipsychotics in the treatment of schizophrenia or delusional disorder in later life.

Psychotic depression

Studies involving young and middle-aged adults have found that depression with psychotic features (psychotic depression) is more likely to respond to a combination of tricyclic antidepressant and antipsychotic medications than to a tricyclic alone (Kroessler 1985). In some studies the rate of response to combination pharmaco-therapy was similar to that associated with ECT (Kroessler 1985; Spiker *et al.* 1985). In contrast, preliminary data suggest that a tricyclic–antipsychotic combination has limited efficacy in the treatment of psychotic depression in older patients (Meyers *et al.* 1985; Flint and Rifat 1998), and many psychiatrists consider ECT to be the treatment of choice for this condition in late life (Finlay-Jones and Parker 1993). Currently, there are no data on the efficacy or safety of newer antidepressants or antipsychotics in the treatment of psychotic depression in the elderly.

Psychosis associated with Parkinson's disease

Hallucinations and delusions can occur in patients with Parkinson's disease, usually in association with the drugs used to treat this disorder. If psychotic symptoms are troublesome, the first strategy is to attempt to reduce the dose of the antiparkinsonian drug or to use a different drug. However, this may not be feasible and antipsychotic medication may be required. Patients with Parkinson's disease are particularly sensitive to the extrapyramidal effects of antipsychotics. Atypical agents may be safer in this regard, but, once again, research data are limited. A recently published, randomized, double-blind trial found that low doses of clozapine (starting dose of 6.25 mg/day; dose range of 6.25–50 mg/day) was significantly more effective than placebo in the treatment of psychosis in patients with Parkinson's disease (The Parkinson Study Group 1999). At these doses, clozapine was generally well tolerated and had no deleterious effects on the severity of parkinsonism. In fact, interestingly, tremor improved with clozapine. Case reports suggest that low doses of quetiapine (a starting dose of 12.5–25 mg/day is recommended) may also be effective and well tolerated in these patients (Parsa and Bastani 1998).

References

Aisen, P.S., Davis, K.L., Berg, J.D., Schafer, K., Campbell, K., Thomas, R.G., *et al.* (2000). A randomized controlled trial of prednisone in Alzheimer's disease. Alzheimer's Disease Cooperative Study. *Neurology,* 54, 588–93.

Alvir, J.M., Lieberman, J.A., Safferman, A.Z., Schwimmer, J.L., and Schaaf, J.A. (1993). Clozapine-induced agranulocytosis. Incidence and risk factors in the United States. *New England Journal of Medicine,* **329**, 162–7.

Amenta, F., Zaccheo, D., and Collier, W.L. (1991). Neurotransmitters, neuroreceptors and aging. *Mechanics of Ageing and Development,* 61, 249–73.

American Psychiatric Association. (1990). *Benzodiazepine dependence, toxicity and abuse*. American Psychiatric Association, Washington, DC.

American Psychiatric Association. (1997). Practice guideline for the treatment of patients with Alzheimer's disease and other dementias of late life. *American Journal of Psychiatry,* **154** (Suppl.) 1–39.

Andersen, G., Vestergaard, L., and Lauritzen, L. (1994). Effective treatment of poststroke depression with the selective serotonin reuptake inhibitor citalopram. *Stroke,* **25**, 1099–104.

Andersen, J., Aabro, E., Gulmann, N., Hjelmsted, A., and Pedersen, H.E. (1980). Antidepressive treatment in Parkinson's disease. A controlled trial of the effect of nortriptyline in patients with Parkinson's disease treated with L-DOPA. *Acta Neurologica Scandinavica,* **62**, 210–19.

Antony, M.M. and Swinson, R.P. (1996). *Anxiety disorders and their treatment: a critical review of the evidence-based literature.* Health Canada, Ottawa.

Baldessarini, R.J., Tondo, L., Suppes, T., Faedda, G.L., and Tohen, M. (1996). Pharmacological treatment of bipolar disorder throughout the life cycle. In *Mood disorders across the life span* (ed. K.I. Shulman, M. Tohen, and S.P. Kutcher), pp. 299–338. Wiley, New York.

Barbhaiya, R.H., Buch, A.B., and Greene, D.S. (1996). A study of the effect of age and gender on the pharmacokinetics of nefazodone after single and multiple doses. *Journal of Clinical Psychopharmacology,* **16**, 19–25.

Breitbart, W., Marotta, R., Platt, M.M., Weisman, H., Derevenco, M., Grau, C., *et al.* (1996). A double-blind trial of haloperidol, chlorpromazine, and lorazepam in the treatment of delirium in hospitalized AIDS patients. *American Journal of Psychiatry,* **153**, 231–7.

Burke, W.J., Roccaforte, W.H., Wengel, S.P., Bayer, B.L., Ranno, A.E., and Willcockson, N.K. (1993). L-deprenyl in the treatment of mild dementia of the Alzheimer type: results of a 15-month trial. *Journal of the American Geriatrics Society,* **41**,1219–25.

Cates, M. and Powers, R. (1998). Concomitant rash and blood dyscrasias in geriatric psychiatry patients treated with carbamazepine. *Annals of Pharmacotherapy,* **32**, 884–7.

Catterson, M.L., Preskorn, S.H., and Martin, R.L. (1997). Pharmacodynamic and pharmacokinetic considerations in geriatric psychopharmacology. *Psychiatric Clinics of North America,* **20**, 205–18.

Cooney, C., Mortimer, A., Smith, A., Newton, K., and Wrigley, M. (1996). Carbamazepine use in aggressive behaviour associated with senile dementia. *International Journal of Geriatric Psychiatry,* **11**, 901–5.

Crewe, H.K., Lennard, M.S., Tucker, G.T., Wood, F.R., and Haddock, R.E. (1992). The effect of selective serotonin re-uptake inhibitors on cytochrome P450 2D6 (CYP2D6) activity in human liver microsomes. *British Journal of Clinical Pharmacology,* **34**, 262–5.

Dehlin, O., Hedenrud, B., Jansson, P., and Norgard J. (1985). A double-blind comparison of alaproclate and placebo in the treatment of patients with senile dementia. *Acta Psychiatrica Scandinavica,* **71**, 190–6.

Devanand, D.P., Marder, K., Michaels, K.S., Sackeim, H.A., Bell, K., Sullivan, M.A., *et al.* (1998). A randomized, placebo-controlled dose-comparison trial of haloperidol for psychosis and disruptive behaviors in Alzheimer's disease. *American Journal of Psychiatry,* **155**, 1512–20.

Eastham, J.H., Jeste, D.V. and Young R.C. (1998). Assessment and treatment of bipolar disorder in the elderly. *Drugs and Aging,* **12**, 205–24.

Eichelbaum, M. and Gross, A.S. (1990). The genetic polymorphism of debrisoquine/sparteine metabolism—clinical aspects. *Pharmacology and Therapeutics,* **46**, 377–94.

Emptage, R.E. and Semla, T.P. (1996). Depression in the medically ill elderly: a focus on methylphenidate. *Annals of Pharmacotherapy,* **30**, 151–7.

Evans, M., Hammond, M., Wilson, K., Lye, M., and Copeland, J. (1997). Placebo-controlled treatment trial of depression in elderly physically ill patients. *International Journal of Geriatric Psychiatry,* **12**, 817–24.

Feighner, J.P. (1994). The role of venlafaxine in rational antidepressant therapy. *Journal of Clinical Psychiatry,* **55** (9 Suppl. A), 62–8.

Finkel, S.I. Lyons, J.S., Anderson, R.L., Sherrell, K., Davis, J., Cohen-Mansfield, J., *et al.* (1995). A randomized, placebo-controlled trial of thiothixene in agitated, demented nursing home patients. *International Journal of Geriatric Psychiatry,* **10**, 129–36.

Finlay-Jones, R. and Parker, G. (1993). A consensus conference on psychotic depression. *Australian and New Zealand Journal of Psychiatry,* **27**, 581–9.

Flint, A.J. (1993). Ageing as a risk factor for lithium neurotoxicity at therapeutic serum levels. *British Journal of Psychiatry,* **163**, 555–6.

Flint, A.J. (1994). Epidemiology and comorbidity of anxiety disorders in the elderly. *American Journal of Psychiatry,* **151**, 640–9.

Flint, A.J. (1995). Augmentation strategies in geriatric depression. *International Journal of Geriatric Psychiatry,* **10**, 137–46.

Flint, A.J. (1998a). Choosing appropriate antidepressant therapy in the elderly. A risk–benefit assessment of available agents. *Drugs and Aging,* **13**, 269–80.

Flint, A.J. (1998b). Management of anxiety in late life. *Journal of Geriatric Psychiatry and Neurology,* **11**, 194–200.

Flint, A.J. and Rifat, S. L. (1998). The treatment of psychotic depression in later life: a comparison of pharmacotherapy and ECT. *International Journal of Geriatric Psychiatry,* **13**, 23–8.

Flint, A.J. and Van Reekum, R. (1998). The pharmacologic treatment of Alzheimer's disease: a guide for the general psychiatrist. *Canadian Journal of Psychiatry,* **43**, 689–97.

Flint, A.J., Crosby, J., and Genik, J.L. (1996). Recurrent hyponatremia associated with fluoxetine and paroxetine. *American Journal of Psychiatry,* **153**, 134.

Freeman, M.P. and Stoll, A.L. (1998). Mood stabilizer combinations: a review of safety and efficacy. *American Journal of Psychiatry,* **155**, 12–21.

Galynker, I., Ieronimo, C., Miner, C., Rosenblum, J., Vilkas, N., and Rosenthal, R. (1997). Methylphenidate treatment of negative symptoms in patients with dementia. *Journal of Neuropsychiatry and Clinical Neurosciences,* **9**, 231–9.

Georgotas, A., McCue, R.E., Hapworth, W., Friedman, E., Kim, O.M., Welkowitz, J., *et al.* (1986). Comparative efficacy and safety of MAOIs versus TCAs in treating depression in the elderly. *Biological Psychiatry,* **21**, 1155–66.

Goldberg, R.J. (1997). Antidepressant use in the elderly. Current status of nefazodone, venlafaxine and moclobemide. *Drugs and Aging,* **11**, 119–31.

Goodnick, P.J. (1994). Pharmacokinetic optimisation of therapy with newer antidepressants. *Clinical Pharmacokinetics,* **27**, 307–30.

Greenberg, R.M. (1997). ECT in the elderly. *New Directions for Mental Health Services,* **76**, 85–96.

Grimsley, S.R. and Jann, M.W. (1992). Paroxetine, sertraline and fluvoxamine: new selective serotonin reuptake inhibitors. *Clinical Pharmacy,* **11**, 930–57.

Harvey, A.T. and Preskorn, S.H. (1996). Cytochrome P450 enzymes: interpretation of their interactions with selective serotonin reuptake inhibitors. Part II. *Journal of Psychopharmacology,* **16**, 345–55.

Hauser, R.A. and Zesiewicz, T.A. (1997). Sertraline for the treatment of depression in Parkinson's disease. *Movement Disorders,* **12**, 756–9.

Henderson, V.W., Paganini-Hill, A., Miller, B.L., Elble, R.J., Reyes, P.F., Shoupe, D., *et al.* (2000). Estrogen for Alzheimer's disease in women: randomized, double-blind, placebo-controlled trial. *Neurology,* **54**, 295–301.

Hindmarch, I. and Kerr, J.S. (1994). Effects of paroxetine on cognitive function in depressed patients, volunteers and elderly volunteers. *Medical Science Research,* **22**, 669–70.

Hindmarch, I., Shillingford, J., and Shillingford, C. (1990). The effects of sertraline on psychomotor performance in elderly volunteers. *Journal of Clinical Psychiatry,* **51**(12 Suppl. B), 34–6.

Hirschfeld, R.M. (1999). Efficacy of SSRIs and newer antidepressants in severe depression: comparison with TCAs. *Journal of Clinical Psychiatry,* **60**, 326–35.

Holm, K.J. and Markham, A. (1999). Mirtazapine. A review of its use in major depression. *Drugs,* **57**, 607–31.

Jacobson, S.A. (1997). Delirium in the elderly. *Psychiatric Clinics of North America,* 20, 91–110.

Jeste, D.V., Lacro, J.P., Bailey, A., Rockwell, E., Harris, M.J., and Caligiuri M.P. (1999). Lower incidence of tardive dyskinesia with risperidone compared with haloperidol in older patients. *Journal of the American Geriatrics Society,* **47**, 716–19.

Kane, J.M., Woerner, M., and Lieberman, J. (1988). Tardive dyskinesia: prevalence, incidence and risk factors. *Journal of Clinical Psychopharmacology*, **8**(4 Suppl.), 52S–56S.

Katz, I.R., Simpson, G.M., Curlik, S.M., Parmelee, P.A., and Muhly, C. (1990). Pharmacologic treatment of major depression for elderly patients in residential care settings. *Journal of Clinical Psychiatry*, **51**(Suppl. 7), 41–7

Katz, I.R., Jeste, D.V., Mintzer, J.E., Clyde, C., Napolitano, J., *et al.* for the Risperidone Study Group. (1999). Comparison of risperidone and placebo for psychosis and behavioral disturbances associated with dementia: a randomized, double-blind trial. *Journal of Clinical Psychiatry*, **60**, 107–15.

Koenig, H.G. and Breitner, J.C.S. (1990). Use of antidepressants in medically ill older patients. *Psychosomatics*, **31**, 22–32.

Kroessler, D. (1985). Relative efficacy rates for therapies of delusional depression. *Convulsive Therapy*, **1**, 173–82.

Laghrissi-Thode, F., Pollock, B.G., Miller, M., Altieri, L., and Kupfer, D.J. (1995). Comparative effects of sertraline and nortriptyline on body sway in older depressed patients. *American Journal of Geriatric Psychiatry*, **3**, 217–28.

Lantz, M.S. and Marin, D. (1996). Pharmacologic treatment of agitation in dementia: a comprehensive review. *Journal of Geriatric Psychiatry and Neurology*, **9**, 107–19.

Lawlor, B.A., Radcliffe, J., Molchan, S.E., Martinez, R.A., Hill, J.L., and Sunderland, T. (1994). A pilot placebo-controlled study of trazodone and buspirone in Alzheimer's disease. *International Journal of Geriatric Psychiatry*, **9**, 55–9.

Lawlor, B.A., Aisen, P.S., Green, C., Fine, E., and Schmeidler J. (1997). Selegiline in the treatment of behavioural disturbance in Alzheimer's disease. *International Journal of Geriatric Psychiatry*, **12**, 319–22.

Lipsey, J.R., Robinson, R.G., Pearlson, G.D., Rao, K., and Price, T.R. (1984). Nortriptyline treatment of post-stroke depression: a double-blind study. *Lancet*, **1**, 297–300.

Liu, B.A., Mittmann, N., Knowles, S.R., and Shear, N.H. (1996). Hyponatremia and the syndrome of inappropriate secretion of antidiuretic hormone associated with the use of selective serotonin reuptake inhibitors: a review of spontaneous reports. *Canadian Medical Association Journal*, **155**, 519–27.

Liu, B., Anderson, G., Mittmann, N., To, T., Axcell, T., and Shear, N. (1998). Use of selective serotonin reuptake inhibitors and tricyclic antidepressants and risk of hip fractures in elderly people. *Lancet*, **351**, 1303–7.

Lovestone, S., Graham, N., and Howard, R. (1997). Guidelines on drug treatments for Alzheimer's disease. *Lancet*, **350**, 232–3.

McKeith, I. and O'Brien, J. (1999). Dementia with Lewy bodies. *Australian and Zealand Journal of Psychiatry*, **33**, 800–8.

McKeith, I.G., Grace, J.B., Walker, Z., Byrne, E.J., Wilkinson, D., Stevens, T. *et al.* (2000). Rivastigmine in the treatment of dementia with Lewy bodies:

preliminary findings from an open trial. *International Journal of Geriatric Psychiatry,* **15**, 387–92.

Meara, R.J., Bhowmick, B.K., and Hobson, J.P. (1996). An open uncontrolled study of the use of sertraline in the treatment of depression in Parkinson's disease. *Journal of Serotonin Research,* **4**, 243–9.

Meyers, B.S., Greenberg, R., and Mei-Tal, V. (1985). Delusional depression in the elderly In *Treatment of affective disorders in the elderly* (ed. C.A. Shamoian), pp. 19–28, American Psychiatric Press, Washington, DC.

Mulnard, R.A., Cotman, C.W., Kawas, C., van Dyck, C.H., Sano, M., Doody, R., *et al.* (2000). Estrogen replacement therapy for treatment of mild to moderate Alzheimer disease: a randomized controlled trial. Alzheimer's Disease Cooperative Study. *Journal of the American Medical Association,* **283**, 1007–15.

Nemeroff, C.B., DeVane, C.L., and Pollock, B.G. (1996). Newer antidepressants and the cytochrome P450 system. *American Journal of Psychiatry,* **153**, 311–20.

Nyth, A.L. and Gottfries, C.G. (1990). The clinical efficacy of citalopram in treatment of emotional disturbances in dementia disorders. A Nordic multicentre study. *British Journal of Psychiatry,* **157**, 894–901.

Olafsson, K., Jorgensen, S., Jensen, H.V., Bille, A., Arup, P., and Andersen J. (1992). Fluvoxamine in the treatment of demented elderly patients: a double-blind, placebo-controlled study. *Acta Psychiatrica Scandinavica,* **85**, 453–6.

Parsa, M.A. and Bastani, B. (1998). Quetiapine (Seroquel) in the treatment of psychosis in patients with Parkinson's disease. *Journal of Neuropsychiatry and Clinical Neurosciences,* **10**, 216–19.

Perry, P.J. (1996). Pharmacotherapy for major depression with melancholic features: relative efficacy of tricyclic versus selective serotonin reuptake inhibitor antidepressants. *Journal of Affective Disorders,* **39**, 1–6.

Petracca, G., Tesón, A., Chemerinski, E., Leiguarda, R., and Starkstein, SE. (1996). A double-blind placebo-controlled study of clomipramine in depressed patients with Alzheimer's disease. *Journal of Neuropsychiatry and Clinical Neurosciences,* **8**, 270–5.

Petrie, W.M., Ban, T.A., Berney, S., Fujimori, M., Guy, W., Ragheb, M., *et al.* (1982). Loxapine in psychogeriatrics: a placebo- and standard-controlled clinical investigation. *Journal of Clinical Psychopharmacology,* **2**, 122–6.

Pollock, B.G. and Mulsant B.H. (1995). Antipsychotics in older patients. A safety perspective. *Drugs and Aging,* **6**, 312–23.

Pollock, B.G. and Mulsant, B.H. (1998). Behavioral disturbances of dementia. *Journal of Geriatric Psychiatry and Neurology,* **11**, 206–12.

Preskorn, S.H. (1993). Recent pharmacologic advances in antidepressant therapy for the elderly. *American Journal of Medicine,* **94**(Suppl. 5A), 2S–12S.

Preskorn, S. and Burke, M. (1992). Somatic therapy for major depressive disorder: selection of an antidepressant. *Journal of Clinical Psychiatry,* **53**(Suppl. 9), 5–18.

Reynolds, C.F. 3rd, Frank, E., Perel, J.M., Miller, M.D., Paradis, C.F., Stack, J.A., *et al.* (1995). Nortriptyline side effects during double-blind, randomized, placebo-controlled maintenance therapy in older depressed patients. *American Journal of Geriatric Psychiatry,* **3**, 170–5.

Rickels, K. and Schweizer, E. (1990). Clinical overview of serotonin reuptake inhibitors. *Journal of Clinical Psychiatry,* **51**(12, Suppl. B), 9–12.

Robinson, D.S., Roberts, D.L., Smith, J.M., Stringfellow, J.C., Kaplita, S.B., Seminara, J.A., *et al.* (1996). The safety profile of nefazodone. *Journal of Clinical Psychiatry,* **57**(Suppl. 2), 31–8.

Rockwell, E., Lam, R.W., and Zisook, S. (1988). Antidepressant drug studies in the elderly. *Psychiatric Clinics of North America,* **11**, 215–33.

Rogers, J., Kirby, L.C., Hempelman, S.R., Berry, D.L., McGeer, P.L., Kaszniak, A.W., *et al.* (1993). Clinical trial of indomethacin in Alzheimer's disease. *Neurology,* **43**,1609–11.

Rolan, P.E. (1994). Plasma protein binding displacement interactions—Why are they still regarded as clinically important? *British Journal of Clinical Pharmacology,* **37**, 125–8.

Roose, S.P. and Dalack, G.W. (1992). Treating the depressed patient with cardiovascular problems. *Journal of Clinical Psychiatry,* **53**(Suppl. 9), 25–31.

Roose, S.P., Laghrissi-Thode, F., Kennedy, J.S., Nelson, J.C., Bigger, J.T. Jr, Pollock, B.G., *et al.* (1998). Comparison of paroxetine and nortriptyline in depressed patients with ischemic heart disease. *Journal of the American Medical Association,* **279**, 287–91.

Rosen, J., Sweet, R., Pollock, B.G., and Mulsant, B.H. (1993). Nortriptyline in the hospitalized elderly: tolerance and side effect reduction. *Psychopharmacology Bulletin,* **29**, 327–31.

Roth, M., Mountjoy, C.Q., Amrein, R., and the International Collaborative Study Group (1996). Moclobemide in elderly patients with cognitive decline and depression. An international double-blind, placebo-controlled trial. *British Journal of Psychiatry,* **168**, 149–57.

Sainati, S.M., Ingram, D.M., Talwalker, S., and Geis, G.S. (2000). Results of a double-blind, randomized, placebo-controlled study of celecoxib in the treatment of progression of Alzheimer's disease. *Sixth International Stockholm/Springfield Symposium on Advances in Alzheimer Therapy Abstract Book,* 180. Stockholm, 2000.

Sano, M., Ernesto, C., Thomas, R.G., Klauber, M.R., Schafer, K., Grundman, M., *et al.* (1997). A controlled trial of selegiline, alpha-tocopherol, or both as treatment for Alzheimer's disease. *New England Journal of Medicine,* **336**, 1216–22.

Satel, S.L. and Nelson, J.C. (1989). Stimulants in the treatment of depression: a critical overview. *Journal of Clinical Psychiatry,* **50**, 241–9.

Schneider, L.S. (1996). Pharmacologic considerations in the treatment of late-life depression. *American Journal of Geriatric Psychiatry,* **4**(Suppl. 1), S5I–S65.

Shader, R.I., von Moltke, L.L., Schmider, J., Harmatz, J.S., and Greenblatt D.J. (1996). The clinician and drug interactions—an update. *Journal of Clinical Psychopharmacology,* **16**, 197–201.

Shea, C., MacKnight, C., and Rockwood, K. (1998). Donepezil for treatment of dementia with Lewy bodies: a case series of nine patients. *International Psychogeriatrics,* **10**, 229–38.

Sheline, Y.I., Freedland, K.E., and Carney, R.M. (1997). How safe are serotonin reuptake inhibitors for depression in patients with coronary heart disease? *American Journal of Medicine,* **102**, 54–9.

Spiker, D.G., Weiss, J.C., Dealy, R.S., Griffin, S.J., Hanin, L., Neil, J.F., *et al.* (1985). The pharmacological treatment of delusional depression. *American Journal of Psychiatry,* **142**, 430–6.

Sproule, B.A., Naranjo, C.A., Bremner, K.E., and Hassan, P.C. (1997). Selective serotonin reuptake inhibitors and CNS drug interactions. A critical review of the evidence. *Clinical Pharmacokinetics,* **33**, 454–71.

Steinberg, J.R. (1994). Anxiety in elderly patients. A comparison of azapirones and benzodiazepines. *Drugs and Aging,* **5**, 335–45.

Sweet, R.A. and Pollock, B.G. (1998). New atypical antipsychotics. Experience and utility in the elderly. *Drugs and Aging,* **12**, 115–27.

Tariot, P.N., Erb, R., Podgorski, C.A., Cox, C., Patel, S., Jakimovich, L., *et al.* (1998*a*). Efficacy and tolerability of carbamazepine for agitation and aggression in dementia. *American Journal of Psychiatry,* **155**, 54–61.

Tariot, P.N., Goldstein, B., Podgorski, C.A., Cox, C., and Frambes, N. (1998*b*). Short-term administration of selegiline for the mild-to-moderate dementia of the Alzheimer's type. *American Journal of Geriatric Psychiatry,* **6**,145–54.

Taylor, D.P., Carter, R.B., Eison, A.S., Mullins, U.L., Smith, H.L., Torrente, J.R., *et al.* (1995). Pharmacology and neurochemistry of nefazodone, a novel antidepressant drug. *Journal of Clinical Psychiatry,* **56**(Suppl. 6), 3–11.

Thase, M.E., Rush, A.J., Kasper, S., and Nemeroff, C.B. (1994/1995). Tricyclics and newer antidepressant medications: treatment options for treatment-resistant depressions. *Depression,* **2**,152–68.

The Parkinson Study Group. (1999). Low-dose clozapine for the treatment of drug-induced psychosis in Parkinson's disease. *New England Journal of Medicine,* **340**, 757–63.

Thomas, D.R., Nelson, D.R., and Johnson, A.M. (1987). Biochemical effects of the antidepressant paroxetine, a specific 5-hydroxytryptamine uptake inhibitor. *Psychopharmacology (Berlin),* **93**, 193–200.

Tollefson, G.D., Beasley, C.M., Tamura, R.N., Tran, P.V., and Potvin, J.H. (1997). Blind, controlled, long-term study of the comparative incidence of treatment-emergent tardive dyskinesia with olanzapine or haloperidol. *American Journal of Psychiatry,* **154**, 1248–54.

Wallace, A.E., Kofoed, L.L., and West, A.N. (1995). Double-blind, placebo-controlled trial of methylphenidate in older, depressed medically ill patients. *American Journal of Psychiatry*, **152**, 929–31.

Wils, V. and Golüke-Willemse, G. (1997). Extrapyramidal syndrome due to valproate administration as an adjunct to lithium in an elderly manic patient. *International Journal of Geriatric Psychiatry*, **12**, 272.

13 ECT in older patients with physical illness

James D. Tew Jr, Benoit H. Mulsant, and Adele Towers

Summary

This chapter discusses the administration of electroconvulsive therapy (ECT) and the immediate physiological response. ECT in the context of specific cardiac conditions such as hypertension, coronary artery disease, cardiac arrhythmia/atrial fibrillation, congestive heart failure (CHF), aneurysms, and pacemakers is also covered.

ECT in relation to specific neurological conditions, e.g. seizure disorder, cerebrovascular malformation, cerebral aneurysm, stroke, and intracranial mass, is examined. In addition, this chapter considers the place of ECT in dementia and other physical conditions such as chronic obstructive pulmonary disease, anticoagulation, glaucoma, gastro-oesophageal reflux disease, electrolyte disturbances, and endocrine disorders. Recommendations for evaluation prior to initiating ECT in an older patient with physical illness are also given.

Introduction

Electroconvulsive therapy (ECT) is one of the treatments of choice in older patients who present with severe depression and comorbid medical conditions, or a history of poor tolerance to psychotropic medications. It is considered the preferred treatment for psychotic depression or depression associated with marked disability. In the 1940s and 1950s, ECT was widely used, without general anaesthesia, in the treatment of most psychiatric disorders. By the 1950s, ECT was recognized to be particularly effective for the treatment of mood disorders. However, at that time the advent of effective pharmacotherapy, combined with a growing public perception that ECT was crudely administered and unacceptably dangerous, led to a steady decline in its use. The advent of modified ECT (i.e. ECT performed under general anaesthesia with oxygenation) led to a reduction in its adverse effects. The improved

295

safety of ECT, combined with some technical advances and the realization that a subgroup of patients respond poorly to medications, has led to a renewed interest in the it's use. Recent data indicate that, in the United States, nearly 10% of all adult patients admitted to hospitals with recurrent major depression were treated with ECT (Olfson *et al.* 1998), with over 100 000 patients treated annually (Hermann *et al.* 1995).

ECT is now indicated in the treatment of all subtypes of major depression. It is also used to treat other conditions in patients who have failed to respond to pharmacotherapy, including all forms of catatonia, schizophrenia, and other psychoses, and prominent depressive symptoms associated with dementia (American Psychiatric Association, 2001). Benefits of ECT include a faster rate of symptom remission (vitally important in emergency cases), a high treatment-response rate, and proven efficacy in many patients with a history of treatment-refractory depression (Flint and Rifat 1998).

The elderly now represent more than half of those treated with ECT (Olfson *et al.* 1998). The indications for ECT are the same in older as in younger adults. Numerous studies have shown that elderly depressed patients demonstrate an equal or better acute response to ECT than younger patients with a similar diagnosis (Alexopoulos *et al.* 1984; Burke *et al.* 1987; Wilkinson *et al.* 1993; Zielinski *et al.* 1993; Rice *et al.* 1994; Tew *et al.* 1999). In most cases, patients are referred for ECT only after failing to respond to or tolerating psychotropic agents (American Psychiatric Association, 2001). The typical response time for antidepressant pharmacotherapy is from 4–6 weeks, but many older patients have a longer response time (Thase *et al.* 1997). Conversely, patients begin to benefit from ECT within the first two treatments, and a complete treatment course typically involves eight to twelve treatments. Thus, with ECT administered three times a week, clinical remission of depressed symptoms can often be achieved in half the time of pharmacotherapy (Flint and Rifat 1998). For this reason alone, ECT is often the preferred 'first line' treatment in frail older patients with psychotic depression, catatonia, poor food and fluid intake, or marked psychomotor retardation, even before medication is prescribed.

As with any medical intervention, appropriate screening procedures should be performed to minimize the potential hazards and maximize the benefits of treatment. Almost all patients can be treated safely. US data from 1990 indicate that the mortality rate associated with ECT is only 0.28/10 000 individual treatments, no higher than the expected mortality associated with general anaesthesia (Kramer 1985). Up to a few years ago, many older patients who were too physically ill to tolerate pharmacotherapy with tricyclic antidepressants were referred for ECT. As a result, older patients treated with ECT in the 1980s and early 1990s typically presented with a higher burden of physical illness than patients who were treated with psychotropic medications (Kroessler and Fogel 1993). In spite of this, numerous studies have documented that ECT can be administered safely to older patients even in the presence of significant comorbid physical illness or dementia

(Mulsant *et al.* 1991; Knos and Sung 1993; Zielinski *et al.* 1993; Rice *et al.* 1994). To whit, the American Psychiatric Association (APA) Task Force on ECT (2001) concluded 'there are no absolute contraindications for ECT'. However, understanding the physiological changes associated with ECT and the specific risks in patients presenting with specific physical problems is essential to the safe management of older patients who receive ECT.

This chapter first briefly reviews the administration of ECT, focusing on the risks associated with general anaesthesia and the haemodynamic changes that occur during ECT. The next two sections discuss the management of patients with cardiovascular or other specific physical disease and the potential effects of concurrent medication use during ECT. Finally, we propose a systematic approach to the screening of ECT candidates, with an emphasis on assessing physical illness that may require treatment modifications to minimize the risks of ECT.

Administration of ECT

ECT procedure

Prior to ECT, the patient takes nothing by mouth for at least 6 hours, except for medications that can be given with a sip of water. Intravenous access is secured and patients are asked to breathe 100% oxygen through a face mask. Throughout the procedure, cardiac rhythm and heart rate, blood pressure, and oxygen saturation are monitored. Prior to the administration of general anaesthesia, selected patients are premedicated with glycopyrrolate, atropine, or curare (see below). Typically, a short-acting barbiturate (e.g. methohexital) 0.5–1.0 mg/kg is administered intravenously. Alternatively, in patients who have a very high seizure threshold or for whom the arrhythmogenic effects of barbiturate may be problematic, etomidate (0.02 mg/kg) can be used. Succinylcholine (0.5–1 mg/kg), an agent that depolarizes the neuromuscular junction, is the paralysing agent of choice to prevent the tonic and clonic movements of an unmodified generalized seizure (Gaines and Rees 1986). Prior to paralysis, the administration of succinylcholine initially produces muscular fasciculations that can result in muscle pain lasting several hours. Pretreatment with low-dose (3–4.5 mg) curare can be used to prevent these fasciculations. Also, in those rare patients who suffer from familial pseudocholinesterase deficiency, succinylcholine can result in prolonged paralysis requiring intubation and mechanical ventilation. Thus, in patients with a past history or family history of this complication, atracurium should be used (Davis *et al.* 1991). Isolation of a single limb (typically, the right lower extremity) with an arterial tourniquet prior to the administration of succinylcholine allows the psychiatrist to observe tonic–clonic movements in that limb, and thus to measure the duration of the motor seizure. Once paralysed, the patient is ventilated with 100% oxygen delivered by a bag-valve and a mask. A mouthpiece is inserted between the patient's jaw to prevent mouth injuries that could result from clenching of the jaw induced by the direct electrical stimulation of the masseter muscles (i.e. bypassing the neuromuscular junction).

The ECT stimulus is delivered using an ECT device that transforms AC/DC current to a brief pulse, square-wave current of fixed intensity. Older ECT devices that use sine-wave stimuli should no longer be used since they are more likely to induce severe cognitive impairment (Abrams 1997; American Psychiatric Association, 2001). Various protocols have been designed to optimize the charge (or energy) of the ECT stimulus. The systematic determination of each patient's seizure threshold during the first treatment is preferred, since it has been shown to improve efficacy and to decrease cognitive impairment (Sackheim *et al.* 1993). To minimize the risks of interictal confusion, treatment in older patients can be initiated with unilateral ECT (i.e. with electrodes placed over the non-dominant hemisphere). Exceptions are patients who have previously responded to bilateral but not to unilateral ECT, or those who are so sick that the most definitive treatment is needed (e.g. a catatonic patient refusing fluids and food). If a patient shows no or minimal improvement after five or six unilateral treatments, the electrodes should be switched to bilateral (i.e. bitemporal) placement.

Typically, ECT treatments are administered two or three times a week. Mood and cognition should be carefully assessed on the days post-ECT. If significant interictal confusion persists on the days post-ECT, any psychotropic medications the patient is still receiving should be discontinued, further ECT treatment should be withheld until the confusion resolves, and, upon resuming ECT, treatments should be given no more than twice a week (Lerer *et al.* 1995). ECT is typically discontinued once a patient's mood is back to baseline or when it reaches a plateau after two consecutive treatments. Generally, an ECT course consists of 8–12 treatments, though some patients (in particular schizophrenic patients) may require more.

Immediate physiological response to the ECT stimulus

The delivery of the ECT stimulus induces a brief parasympathetic response, followed by a more sustained sympathetic reaction and an increase in cerebral blood flow and intracranial pressure (see Table 13.1). Delivery of the ECT charge activates the parasympathetic centre in the brainstem producing a brief (i.e. 10–15 seconds) increase in vagal tone with a sharp increase in acetylcholine outflow. This can result in sinus bradycardia and hypotension. Not infrequently, transient asystole is observed (Burd and Kettl 1998). The effects of vagal outflow can be prevented or dampened by the administration of an anticholinergic drug such as atropine or glycopyrrolate (see Table 13.2). However, in most cases, this is unnecessary since this brief parasympathetic response is usually followed by a sustained sympathetic reaction (see below). Thus, the APA Task Force on ECT recommends an individualized approach to the use of anticholinergic drugs (e.g. use only when sympathetic blocking agents are also being administered, or when prior treatment has resulted in profound bradyarrhythmia). Though complications resulting from vagal response

Table 13.1 Physiological changes associated with ECT

TIME	5 s	10 s	20 s	30 s	40 s	60s	2 min	4 min	10 min	30 min
Electric seizure characteristic	RECRUITMENT		POLYSPIKE AND SLOW WAVE				POST-ICTAL SUPPRESSION			
Motor seizure characteristic	TONIC		CLONIC				RECOVERY			
Vagal/sympathetic tone	VAGAL		SYMPATHETIC					VAGAL/SYMPATHETIC		
ACTH	nl	nl	↑	↑	↑	↑	↑↑↑↑	↑↑↑↑	↑↑	↑
Serum cortisol	nl	nl	Nl	nl	nl	nl	nl	↑	↑↑	↑↑↑↑
Epi./NE	?	?	↑	↑	↑↑	↑↑	↑↑↑↑	↑↑↑	↑	nl
Blood pressure	↓↓↓↓	↓↓	↑	↑	↑↑↑	↑↑↑↑	↑↑↑↑	↑↑↑↑	nl	nl
Pulse	↓↓↓↓	↓↓	↑	↑↑	↑↑↑	↑↑↑↑	↑↑↑↑	↑↑	↑↓	↑
Cerebral blood flow	↓	↑	↑↑	↑↑	↑↑	↑↑	↑↑	↑↑	↑	↑↑
Cerebral metabolism and ICP	?	↑	↑↑	↑	↑	↑	↑↑	↑↑	↑	nl
Pv_{O_2}	?	?	↑	↑	↑	↑	↓	↓	→	↑
Pa_{CO_2}	nl	nl	nl	nl	nl	nl	nl	nl	nl	nl

Epi, epinephrine (adrenaline); NE, norepinephrine (noradrenaline); Pv_{O_2}, partial pressure O_2 (venous); Pa_{CO_2}, partial pressure CO_2 (arterial); nl, normal. Permission granted by *Anaesthesiology* (Lippincott Wilkins and Williams).

Table 13. 2 APA Task Force dose recommendations for use of anticholinergic medications during ECT

Anticholinergic	Dose	Administered
Atropine	0.4–1.0 mg IV	2–3 min prior to treatment
Atropine	0.3–0.6 mg SC or IM	30–60 min prior to treatment
Glycopyrrolate	0.2–0.4 mg IV, IM, or SC	30–60 min prior to treatment

IV, intravenous; IM, intramuscular; SC, subcutaneous.

are rare, they may be more frequent with subconvulsive electrical stimuli (i.e. electrical stimulations that do not result in a seizure and its associated sympathetic reaction). Consequently, some authors have recommended systematic premedication with atropine when electrical stimulus titration is used to a determine a patient's seizure threshold (Sackheim *et al.* 1993).

As the patient starts to seize, a discharge of catecholamines from the adrenal medulla is observed. Increases of plasma epinephrine (adrenaline) and nor-epinephrine (noradrenaline) concentrations up to 15-fold and 3-fold, respectively, have been observed. In turn, this results in a rise in heart rate (e.g. up to 200 beats/min or more) and arterial blood pressure (e.g. systolic blood pressure up to 240 mmHg or more) associated with an increase in left ventricular afterload and an increase in myocardial oxygen demand (Gaines and Rees 1986). Maximal cardio-vascular stress occurs from the time immediately following the seizure, but typically resolves within 20 minutes (Howie *et al.* 1990, 1992). Myocardial ischaemia can result from this increase in myocardial oxygen demand if it is not associated with a proportionate increase in oxygen supply (e.g. in a patient with coronary artery disease or significant anaemia). In turn, ischaemia is the major cause of arrhythmia. The primary preventive measure for these complications is adequate ventilation and oxygenation. In addition, several classes of drugs can be used to manage the effects of the sympathetic response to ECT (see Table 13.3). Two effective medications are the beta-blocker esmolol and the alpha/beta-blocker labetalol. Administration of either drug with anaesthesia prior to treatment has been shown to reduce ECT-induced tachycardia and blood pressure elevation (Stoudemire *et al.* 1990; Zvara *et al.* 1997). Of note, while these may blunt the severity of oxygen debt, definitive evidence that they reduce the overall incidence of myocardial ischaemia is still lacking (Zvara *et al.* 1997). In combination with, or as an alternative to, beta-blockers, calcium-channel blockers or nitrates can be used to improve coronary blood flow and control the haemodynamic changes associated with ECT (Abrams 1997).

Table 13.3 Medications used to blunt the sympathetic response associated with ECT

Drug class	Agents used	Dose	Route administered
β₂-receptor blocker	Esmolol	100–200 mg	IV push, with anaesthesia
β₁/α-blocker	Labetalol	10–20 mg	IV push, with anaesthesia
Nitrates	Nitroglycerin ointment	5 cm (2 inches) of 2% ointment	Applied to chest 45 min prior to ECT
Calcium-channel blocker	Nifedipine	Contents of 10 mg capsule	Sublingual, 20 min prior to ECT induction

One difficulty in determining the exact frequency of ECT-related complications associated with cardiovascular disease is due to the variable definitions of ischaemic events used by different practitioners. A recent review of the literature reveals that there is wide variation in the frequency of reports of ECT-induced myocardial ischaemia and related complications (see Table 13.4). Nevertheless, it is apparent that patients with coronary artery disease or other cardiac risk factors are at increased risk for myocardial ischaemia and arrhythmia.

Table 13.4 Occurrence of electrocardiographic and regional wall motion abnormality during ECT

Authors	Cardiovascular change	N	% Occurrence
Green and Woods 1955	ISCH	105	11
Gerring and Shields 1982	ISCH or arrhythmia	42	28
		17*	70
Dec et al. 1985	ISCH	85	0
Hay 1989	Arrhythmia	90	0
		45*	10
Guttmacher and Greenland 1990	Arrhythmia	8*	0
Messina et al. 1992	RWMA	11	45
	ISCH	—	27
Zielinski et al. 1993	ISCH or arrhythmia	40*	55
Rice et al. 1994	ISCH	26*	19.2
		27	7.4
Ruwitch et al. 1994	RWMA	10*	67
Castelli et al. 1995	ISCH	90*	0
O'Connor et al. 1996	RWMA	26	4
	ISCH	—	0

Arrhythmia: significant new atrial or ventricular arrhythmia other than sinus tachycardia.
ISCH, ECG changes indicative of myocardial ischaemia; RWMA, regional wall motion abnormality; N, number of subjects.
*Treatment of patients identified by author as 'high cardiac risk population'.
Permission granted by *Convulsive Therapy* (Lippincott Wilkins and Williams).

ECT is also associated with transient increases in intracranial, intraocular, and intragastric pressure. The electrical stimulus administered to the patients' temples causes a brief cerebrovascular contraction. This contraction, combined with a 1.5- to 7-fold increase in cerebral blood flow (due to the catecholamine-induced increase in cardiac output), results in a moderate rise in intracranial pressure. An increase in intragastric pressure results from forced expiration against a closed glottis, as occurs during the initial parasympathetic surge following the administration of the electrical stimulus. Ordinarily, these temporary changes are tolerated without incident. However, in the presence of certain physical conditions, a patient may be at increased risk for treatment-related complications and specific precautions may need to be taken (see below).

ECT and specific cardiac conditions

The autonomic cardiovascular response to ECT described above is short-lived, but can be significant. It has been the source of most major complications, including myocardial infarction. While these haemodynamic changes may place the elderly patient with cardiac disease at increased risk for complications, such risks can be minimized with appropriate medical management. In general, most adverse events can be prevented or limited by ensuring adequate oxygenation and strict control of the heart rate and blood pressure. Specific cardiovascular conditions associated with increased risk during ECT, along with interventions designed to minimize complications, are discussed below.

Hypertension

Hypertension is the most prevalent cardiac risk factor among patients referred for ECT. Patients with pre-existing hypertension are at increased risk for marked blood pressure elevations during treatment, which can lead to myocardial ischaemia or cerebrovascular complications. Good control of hypertension prior to the initiation of ECT is the most effective way to prevent these complications. Acutely, patients who present to the ECT suite with an elevated blood pressure can be managed with short-acting intravenous blocking agents (see Table 13.3). Patients who fail to respond to these agents may benefit from augmentation with calcium-channel blockers or nitrates. The APA Task Force on ECT suggests that patients receiving sympathetic blocking agents should be additionally treated with an anticholinergic agent to prevent prolonged, unopposed parasympathetic effects such as bradycardia and asystole (American Psychiatric Association, 2001). After each treatment, the patient's blood pressure should be monitored until haemodynamic stability is observed.

Coronary artery disease

Patients with coronary artery disease should receive a careful cardiac evaluation to assess their specific risks. Patients with a history of recent myocardial infarction (MI) are at a very high risk of death in case of reinfarction (Rao *et al.* 1983). Usually, ECT is not given within 6 months of a myocardial infarction. However, a proper evaluation of cardiac function in all patients with coronary artery disease is essential, since a severe infarction 12 months ago may present substantially greater risks than a mild, more recent infarction. Critical elements of cardiac function that should be evaluated include ejection fraction, valvular function, conduction pattern, vascular supply, contractility, and stress tolerance. Electrocardiography and echocardiography provide effective non-invasive means of evaluating conduction pattern, ejection fraction, and valve function. Additionally, exercise or pharmacological stress tests and cardiac catheterization are useful in the assessment of ischaemic risk and functional capacity.

The management of patients with coronary artery disease focuses on minimizing the increase in myocardial oxygen demand during and after ECT. Beta-blockers should be considered for all patients with underlying coronary artery disease, as long as there are no contraindications to their use. Contraindications may include congestive heart failure (CHF), chronic obstructive pulmonary disease (COPD), diabetes mellitus, or conduction abnormalities. Other agents such as calcium-channel blockers and nitrates have also been shown to be effective, though recently there is some concern about the use of short-acting, calcium-channel blockers and the risk of MI (due to rapid lowering of the blood pressure and decreased coronary blood flow).

Cardiac arrhythmia/atrial fibrillation

In some susceptible patients, ECT may trigger an arrhythmia. These arrhythmias are usually precipitated by cardiac ischaemia. Thus, the best preventive treatment in these patients is proper ventilation and oxygenation, and control of hypertension. When they occur, arrhythmias usually respond to vigorous oxygenation and anti-hypertensive agents. Typical antiarrhythmic agents (e.g. beta-blockers, lidocaine (lignocaine), digoxin, and verapamil) can also be used as the situation warrants. However, lidocaine should not be given routinely prior to ECT since it increases the seizure threshold and may decrease the effectiveness of ECT. Pre-existing cardiac arrhythmias, when identified, are usually treatable and should not prevent the safe administration of ECT. It is particularly important to identify atrial fibrillation prior to initiation of treatment, as published case series have demonstrated that ECT can convert atrial fibrillation to normal sinus rhythm (Petrides and Fink 1996). While some of these cases were treated without incident in the absence of anticoagulation treatment, heparin or warfarin administration is recommended due to the potential for thrombotic embolism. ECT may also unmask a previously occult arrhythmia. For instance, patients with sick-sinus syndrome may require the insertion of a pace-maker to continue to receive ECT safely.

Congestive heart failure (CHF)

Patients with CHF and low cardiac output (ejection fraction < 25%) are at increased risk for pulmonary oedema during ECT. Such risks can be reduced with the use of vasodilators, calcium-channel blockers, and, in selected cases, the use of beta-blockers. Stern et al. (1997) described a protocol using nitroglycerin, sublingual nifedipine, labetalol, and the avoidance of anticholinergic agents to successfully treat a small series of patients with low cardiac output (left ventricular ejection fractions between 20% and 26%, as determined by echocardiography). Pulmonary oedema, when it does occur, is usually transient, and typically responds to oxygen, nitrates, and furosemide (frusemide) within 15–30 minutes (Welch 1993).

Aortic aneurysms

All aortic aneurysms should be assessed for operability prior to ECT, due to the serious risk of arterial wall rupture associated with an increase in blood pressure. Complications tend to be associated with abdominal or thoracic aortic aneurysms larger than 4 cm. However, there are several case reports on the successful use of ECT among patients with inoperable cardiovascular lesions, including aneurysms (Alexopoulos and Francis 1980; Rosenfeld et al. 1988; Devanand et al. 1990). Care of patients with unstable aortic aneurysms requires aggressive control of blood pressure (e.g. nitroprusside by intravenous (IV) drip). ECT should be conducted with a large-bore IV line in place and several units of blood available for immediate transfusion in the event of a wall rupture. Consultation and ongoing monitoring by an experienced vascular surgeon is essential. Additionally, it is important to recognize that patients with aortic aneurysms have a significantly increased risk of coronary artery and carotid artery disease (Jeffrey et al. 1983). Thus, these patients should be evaluated similarly to patients with a known history or risk of coronary artery and carotid artery disease.

Cerebrovascular malformation, cerebral aneurysm, and stroke

Patients with cerebrovascular malformation, cerebral aneurysms, or recent stroke are at increased risk for intracranial bleeding due to the significant increase in blood pressure associated with ECT (see above). Typically, ECT is not performed in patients with a recent stroke (i.e. within 4–8 weeks). In patients with minor vascular malformations, the management of risks focuses on tempering the cardiac response to ECT via beta-blocking agents (see Table 13.3) (Farah et al. 1996).

There are anecdotal reports of successful ECT performed on patients with cerebral aneurysms (Farah et al. 1996; Hunt and Kaplan 1998; Najjar and Guttmacher 1998).

These reports emphasize the strict control of blood pressure and oxygenation. Currently, there are no recommendations regarding the size of an aneurysm and the safety of ECT. In general, patients with a known cerebral aneurysm should be evaluated by an experienced neurosurgeon and anaesthetist prior to ECT.

Pacemakers

Numerous case reports support the safety of ECT in patients with pacemakers (Abrams 1997). Due to the high resistance of body tissue, the ECT electrical stimulus rarely reaches myocardial tissue. However, given the increasing complexity of programmable pacemakers, a cardiologist or electrophysiologist should be involved in the management of these patients. As a minimum, a chest radiograph and electrophysiological testing should be ordered to evaluate appropriate pacemaker placement and functioning. Pacemaker wires should be checked to ensure intact insulation, as a breach could provide a low-resistance energy pathway capable of disrupting the pacemaker.

ECT and specific neurological conditions

Seizure disorder

Epilepsy does not represent a significant risk factor for ECT as long as it is diagnosed and treated, and underlying structural or vascular lesions are excluded. It has been well documented that over a course of ECT, the seizure threshold increases (Sackheim *et al.* 1983). Thus, while epilepsy is not of itself an indication for ECT, there have been case reports of patients with seizure disorders experiencing temporary alleviation of symptoms after ECT (Sackheim 1983). Anticonvulsants increase the seizure threshold and shorten the ECT-induced seizure duration. Adjustment of anticonvulsant dosage may be necessary to obtain therapeutic seizures. However, it is unnecessary to discontinue all antiseizure medication to obtain a therapeutic response to ECT; even a slow tapering of all anticonvulsant medications increases the risk of status epilepticus (Hauser 1983) and spontaneous seizures occurring between treatment ('tardive seizures'). Thus, in a patient with a seizure disorder, anticonvulsants should initially be maintained at a therapeutic dosage/level and carefully decreased if an adequate seizure cannot be elicited.

Intracranial mass

The early literature on ECT clearly documented that space-occupying lesions constitute a major risk for neurological deterioration and death (Maltbie *et al.* 1980). Indeed, patients with increased intracranial pressure from any cause are at a major risk of cerebral herniation and death when exposed to the increase in intracranial pressure observed during ECT. However, a series of cases documenting the successful and safe use of ECT in patients with small intracranial masses (e.g. meningiomas) with no or minimal peripheral oedema have been published over the past two decades (Abrams 1997). Thus, all space-occupying lesions are no longer considered an absolute contraindication to ECT. Nevertheless, great caution should be used with these patients. Neuroimaging and consultation with a neurosurgeon are necessary to assess the risks of ECT and whether any treatment can decrease these risks (e.g. use of steroids or mannitol to decrease cerebral oedema prior to the initiation of ECT).

Dementia

A substantial proportion of patients with dementia develop significant depressive symptoms (Mulsant *et al.* 1997). ECT has been shown to be an effective treatment of depression in patients with dementia (Price and McAllister 1989; Nelson and Rosenberg 1991). In these patients, ECT can be associated with a significant (even if temporary) improvement of cognition and function (Mulsant *et al.* 1991). However, such patients are at a higher risk for confusion; this acute confusion associated with ECT is typically transient and gradually resolves after the conclusion of treatment. In patients with dementia, ECT should begin with unilateral stimulations, as right unilateral (RUL) (or non-dominant hemisphere) ECT has been shown to induce less significant cognitive side-effects than bilateral ECT (Sackheim *et al.* 1993).

Of note, it is increasingly recognized that late-onset depression can be a prodrome for an irreversible dementia (Chen *et al.* 1999). Thus, the successful treatment with ECT of depressive symptoms in an older person may reveal an underlying incipient dementia. Patients and their family may misinterpret this complex clinical situation and believe that ECT actually 'caused' the underlying dementia. When clinicians suspect that a patient may be in the early stages of a dementia, they should document it and warn the patient and the family of this possibility **prior** to the initiation of ECT.

ECT and other physical conditions

Anticoagulation

As mentioned above in the discussion about patients with atrial fibrillation, many older patients are treated chronically with warfarin or heparin to reduce the risk of thromboembolization. Theoretically, these patients are at an increased risk of un-controlled cerebral bleeding due to the increased blood pressure associated with ECT. Conversely, inadequate anticoagulation may be associated with pulmonary or systemic embolization during ECT. Thus, a target INR (international normalized ratio) of at least 2 and at most 3.5 may be optimal during ECT. Unless a patient has been treated with a stable anticoagulant regimen for a long period, appropriate laboratory tests should be checked prior to each treatment. Numerous case reports have shown that well-monitored anticoagulated patients can receive safe, effective courses of ECT without complication (Petrides and Fink 1996; Abrams 1997).

Chronic obstructive pulmonary disease

Patients with chronic pulmonary diseases, such as emphysema or asthma, are at an increased risk for developing significant hypoxaemia during general anaesthesia. These patients should have their pulmonary function optimized prior to initiating an ECT course.

To minimize airway reactivity, patients with reversible airway obstruction should be treated with two or three puffs of a b_2-selective bronchodilator, such as aerosolized albuterol or terbutaline, prior to each treatment (Knos and Sung 1993). Theophylline is a xanthine compound, used to control bronchospasm. It decreases seizure threshold and has been associated with prolonged ECT-induced seizures (Rasmussen and Zorumski 1993). Therefore, theophylline use during ECT increases the risk of status epilepticus and, if possible, theophylline should be discontinued and other bronchodilators substituted.

Glaucoma

Brief intraocular pressure increases are observed with the administration of succinylcholine and with the motor seizure phase of ECT (Edwards *et al.* 1990). An insignificant event in normal patients, this increase presents a theoretical risk in patients with poorly controlled open-angle glaucoma, though such a complication has yet to be reported (Van den Berg and Honjol 1998). While the use of regular antiglaucoma medications during the ECT course is recommended, anti-cholinesterase ophthalmic solutions may prolong the effects of succinylcholine, resulting in long apnoea. In the rare cases when these older agents are still used, alternative antiglaucoma treatments should be substituted for these agents throughout the ECT course.

Gastro-oesophageal reflux disease

Reflux and the subsequent aspiration of stomach contents during ECT have been associated with aspiration pneumonitis, a very serious complication with a 28% mortality rate. The advent of muscle relaxants has drastically reduced the incidence of aspiration pneumonitis in ECT (Bynum and Pierce 1976). However, all patients should be 'nil by mouth' for a minimum of 6 hours prior to treatment. In addition, patients with gastro-oesophageal reflux disease, hiatus hernia, obesity, or pregnancy who are at increased risk of reflux should receive additional treatment with an H_2-receptor blocker or a proton-pump inhibitor. Alternatively, these patients can be given 30 ml of a bicitrate solution orally shortly before the induction of anaesthesia. Proper ventilation also decreases the likelihood of reflux. In the most severe cases, endotracheal intubation and cuff inflation prior to the electrical stimulus effectively seals the trachea.

Electrolyte disturbances

Hyponatraemia and hyperkalaemia can be associated with specific complications with ECT. These electrolyte imbalances can be fairly common in older patients who are treated with diuretics or who are on renal dialysis. Hyponatraemia is also fairly common in patients with psychiatric disorders (Critchlow 1998). Moreover, many psychotropic medications (including most antidepressants and anticonvulsants) have been associated with hyponatraemia, particularly in older patients (Ball and Herzberg 1994). Hyponatraemic patients have a lower seizure threshold and are at risk for prolonged seizures and status epilepticus (Finlayson *et al*. 1989; Greer and Stewart 1993). Hyperkalaemia alone is arrhythmogenic and, in combination with the depolarizing muscle relaxant succinylcholine, may be cardiotoxic. Whenever possible, electrolyte disturbances should be corrected prior to the initiation of treatment. If possible, patients on renal dialysis should be treated with ECT the day after dialysis. When the hyperkalaemia cannot be fully corrected prior to ECT, a non-depolarizing muscle relaxant should be used.

Endocrine disorders

Depression in diabetic patients has been associated with poor compliance with behavioural interventions, an increase of complications, and an increased incidence of hyperglycaemia (Leedom *et al*. 1991; Williams *et al*. 1992; Goodnick *et al*. 1995). Therefore, vigilant glucose monitoring and control is essential when considering ECT for a diabetic patient. Attempts should be made to ensure that a patient is euglycaemic (as determined by 'finger-stick' glucose testing) prior to each treatment. Typically, diabetic patients are held 'nil by mouth' for at least 6 hours and their morning insulin or oral agents withheld prior to each ECT treatment. These patients should be scheduled as the first to be treated, early in the morning. After recovering from anaesthesia and eating a liquid breakfast, they receive their antidiabetic medication. ECT may be associated with a transient increase in plasma glucose and insulin levels, which can affect diabetes management (Williams *et al*. 1992). In addition, in some patients, normalization of the hypothalamo–pituitary–adrencortical (HPA) axis associated with the successful treatment of severe depression may result in a decreased requirement for insulin or oral agents. An internist or endocrinologist should be included in the management of diabetic patients receiving ECT to optimize appropriate glucose management and insulin requirements.

Little information has been published on the use of ECT in patients with hyper-thyroid disorders. Though a case has yet to be described in the literature, the possibility of a thyroid storm during treatment places these patients are at an increased risk of complications with ECT (Farah *et al.* 1995). In addition, hyper-thyroid patients are at increased risk for arrhythmia. Thus, hyperthyroid patients should be stabilized to the extent possible prior to initiating ECT. The APA Task Force on ECT recommends the use of beta-blockers when thyroid control is sub-optimal. Hypothyroidism, hypoparathyroidism, and pseudohypoparathyroidism have not been associated with increased risks during ECT (American Psychiatric Association, 2001). However, it is prudent to optimize any metabolic abnormality prior to the initiation of ECT. Due to the physiological stress associated with ECT, patients with Addison's disease or other adrenocortical deficiency should receive an increased dose of steroid prior to receiving ECT. Cushing's disease has not been found to require treatment modifications or to increase the risk of ECT-related complications.

Recommended evaluation prior to initiating ECT in an older patient with physical illness

In addition to a thorough psychiatric evaluation (including a detailed history of previous treatment) that establishes and documents the indications for ECT, an assessment of cognitive function prior to treatment helps to monitor potential cognitive changes induced by ECT. Minimally, it should include a general cognitive screening test such as Folstein's Mini-Mental Status Examination (Folstein *et al.* 1975), a test of attention such as the Trail Making Test (Reitan 1958), and measures of remote and recent memory.

To assess adequately the risk:benefit ratio of ECT and to optimize the patient's condition to decrease the medical risks associated with ECT, a minimal physical work-up is recommended prior to initiating ECT in an older person. In all patients, this work-up should include a careful history and physical examination by a clinician familiar with ECT and its physiological effects. Investigations should include a battery of blood tests (serum electrolytes, blood urea nitrogen (BUN), creatinine, full blood count (FBC) with a differential smear, liver function tests, metabolic profile, and thyroid-stimulating hormone (TSH)); an electrocardiogram (ECG); a chest radiograph; and brain imaging (computed tomography (CT) scan or magnetic resonance imaging (MRI)) if it has not been obtained since the onset of the psychiatric disorder being treated. Further assessment may be needed in some patients. For instance, spinal radiographs can be used to detect and document the severity of pre-existing vertebral compression fractures or osteoporosis, which put a patient at higher risk for a new compression fracture. A cardiologist familiar with ECT and its specific cardiac risks can be consulted to assist in the assessment and management of patients with significant cardiac disease.

References

Abrams, R. (1997). *Electroconvulsive therapy* (3rd edn). Oxford University Press, New York.

Alexopoulos, G.S. and Frances, R.J. (1980). ECT and cardiac patients with pacemakers. *American Journal of Psychiatry*, **137**, 1111–12.

Alexopoulos, G.S., Shanoian, C.J., Lucas, J., Weiser, N., and Berger, H. (1984). Medical problems of geriatric psychiatric patients and younger controls during electroconvulsive therapy. *Journal of the American Geriatrics Society*, **32**, 651–4.

American Psychiatric Association Committee on Electroconvulsive Therapy (2001), *The practice of Electroconvulsive Therapy: Recommendations for treatment, training and privileging (2nd Edition)*. American Psychiatric Association, Washington, D.C.

Ball, C.J. and Herzberg, J. (1994). Hyponatraemia and selective serotonin reuptake inhibitors. *International Journal of Geriatric Psychiatry*, **9**, 819–22.

Burd, J. and Kettl, P. (1998). Incidence of asystole in electroconvulsive therapy in elderly patients. *American Journal of Geriatric Psychiatry*, **6**, 203–11.

Burke, W.J., Rubin, E.H., Zorumski, C.F., and Wetzel, R.D. (1987). The safety of ECT in geriatric psychiatry. *Journal of the American Geriatric Society*, **35**, 516–21.

Bynum, L.J. and Pierce, A.K. (1976). Pulmonary aspiration of gastric contents. *American Review of Respiratory Disease*, **114**, 1129–36.

Castelli, I., Steiner, L.A., Kauffman, M.A., Alfille, P.H., Schouten, R., Welch, C.A., *et al.* (1995). Comparative effects of esmolol and labetalol to attenuate hyperdynamic states after electroconvulsive therapy. *Anesthesia and Analgesia*, **80**, 557–61.

Chen, P., Ganguli, M., Mulsant, B.H., and DeKosky, S.T. (1999). The temporal relationship between depressive symptoms and dementia: a community-based prospective study. *Archives of General Psychiatry*, **56**, 261–6.

Critchlow, S. (1998). Hyponatremia in elderly psychiatric inpatients. *International Journal of Geriatric Psychiatry*, **13**, 816–18.

Davis, J.M., Janicak, P.G., Sakkas, P., Gilmore, C., and Wang, Z. (1991). Electroconvulsive therapy in the treatment of neuroleptic malignant syndrome. *Convulsive Therapy*, **7**, 111–20.

Dec, G.W. Jr, Stern, T.A., and Welch, C. (1985). The effects of electroconvulsive therapy on serial electrocardiograms and serum cardiac enzyme values. A prospective study of depressed hospitalized inpatients. *Journal of the American Medical Association*, **253**(17), 2525–9.

Devanand, D.P., Malitz, S., and Sackheim, H.A. (1990). ECT in a patient with aortic aneurysm. *Journal of Clinical Psychiatry*, **51**, 255–6.

Dolinski, S.Y. and Zvara, D.A. (1997). Anesthetic considerations of cardiovascular risk during electroconvulsive therapy. *Convulsive Therapy*, **13**, 157–64.

Edwards, R.M., Stoudemire, A., Vela, M.A., and Morris, R. (1990). Intraocular pressure changes in nonglaucomatous patients undergoing electroconvulsive therapy. *Convulsive Therapy*, **6**, 209–13.

Farah, A., McCall, W. (1995). ECT administration to a hyperthyroid patient. *Convulsive Therapy*, **11**, 126–8.

Farah, A., McCall, W.V., and Amundson, R.H. (1996). ECT after cerebral aneurysm repair. *Convulsive Therapy*, **12**, 165–70.

Finlayson, A.J.R., Vieweg, W.V.R., Wilkey, W.D., and Cooper, A.J. (1989). Hyponatremic seizure following ECT. *Canadian Journal of Psychiatry*, **34**, 463–4.

Flint, A.J. and Rifat, S.L. (1998). The treatment of psychotic depression in later life: a comparison of pharmacotherapy and ECT. *International Journal of Geriatric Psychiatry*, **13**, 23–8.

Folstein, M.F., Folstein, S.E., and McHugh, P.R. (1975). Mini mental state: a practical method for grading the cognitive state of patients for the clinician. *Journal of Psychiatric Research*, **12**, 189–98.

Gaines, G.Y. and Rees, D.I. (1986). Electroconvulsive therapy and anesthetic considerations. *Anesthesia and Analgesia*, **5**, 1345–56.

Gerring, J.P. and Shields, H.M. (1982). The identification and management of patients with a high risk of cardiac arrhythmias during modified ECT. *Journal of Clinical Psychiatry*, **43**, 140–3.

Goodnick, P.J., Henry, J.H., and Buki, V.M.V. (1995). Treatment of depression in patients with diabetes mellitus. *Journal of Clinical Psychiatry*, **56**, 128–36.

Green, R. and Woods, A. (1955). Effects of modified ECT on the electrocardiogram. *British Journal of Psychiatry*, **1**, 1503–5.

Greer, R.A. and Stewart, R.B. (1993). Hyponatremia and ECT. *American Journal of Psychiatry*, **150**, 1272.

Guttmacher, L.B. and Greenland, P. (1990). Effects of electroconvulsive therapy on the electrocardiogram in geriatric patients with stable cardiac disease. *Convulsive Therapy*, **6**, 5–12.

Hauser, W.A. (1983). Status epilepticus: frequency, etiology, and neurological sequelae. *Advances in Neurology*, **34**, 3–14.

Hay, D.P. (1989). Electroconvulsive therapy in the medically ill elderly. *Convulsive Therapy*, **5**, 8–16.

Hermann, R.C., Dorwat, R.A., Hoover, C.W., and Brody, J. (1995). Variation in ECT use in the United States. *American Journal of Psychiatry*, **152**, 869–75.

Howie, M.B., Black, H.A., Zvara, D., McSweeney, T.D., Martin, D.J., and Coffman, J.A. (1990). Esmolol reduces autonomic hypersensitivity and length of seizure induced by electroconvulsive therapy. *Anesthesia and Analgesia*, **71**, 384–8.

Howie, M.B., Heistand, D.C., Zvara, D., Kim, P.Y., McSweeney, T.D., and Coffman, J.A. (1992). Defining the dose range for esmolol used in electroconvulsive therapy hemodynamic attenuation. *Anesthesia and Analgesia*, **75**, 805–10.

Hunt, S.A. and Kaplan, E. (1998). ECT in the presence of a cerebral aneurysm. *Journal of ECT*, **14**, 123–4.

Jeffrey, C.C., Kunsman, J., Cullen, D.J., and Brewster, D.C. (1983) A prospective evaluation of cardiac risk index. *Anesthesiology*, **58**, 462–4.

Knos, G.B. and Sung, Y.F. (1993). ECT anesthesia strategies in the high risk medical patient. In *Psychiatric care of the medical patient* (ed. A. Stoudemire and B.S. Fogel), pp. 225–40. Oxford University Press, New York.

Kramer, B.A. (1985). Use of ECT in California, revisited. *Convulsive Therapy*, **12**, 76.

Kroessler, D. and Fogel, B.S. (1993). Electroconvulsive therapy for major depression in the oldest old. *American Journal of Geriatric Psychiatry*, **1**, 30–7.

Leedom, L., Meehan, W. P., Procci, W., and Zeidler, A. (1991). A. Symptoms of depression in patients with Type II diabetes mellitus. *Psychosomatics*, **32**, 280–6.

Lerer, B., Shapira, B., Calev, A., Tubi, N., Drexler, H., Kindler, S., *et al.* (1995). Antidepressant and cognitive effects of twice-versus three-times-weekly ECT. *American Journal of Psychiatry*, **152**, 564–70.

Maltbie, A.A., Wingfield, M.S., Volow, M.R., Weiner, R.D., Sullivan, J.L., and Cavenar, J.O., Jr. (1980). Electroconvulsive therapy in the presence of brain tumor. Case reports and an evaluation of risk. *Journal of Nervous and Mental Disease*, **168**, 400–5.

Messina, A.G., Paranicas, M., Katz, B, Markowitz, J., Yao, F.S., and Deveraux, R.B. (1992). Effects of electroconvulsive therapy on the electrocardiogram and echocardiogram. *Anesthesia and Analgesia*, **75**, 511–14.

Mulsant, B.H., Rosen, J., Thornton, J.E., and Zubenko, G.S. (1991). A prospective naturalistic study of electroconvulsive therapy in late-life depression. *Journal of Geriatric Psychiatry and Neurology*, **4**, 3–13.

Mulsant, B.H., Pollock, B.G., Nebes, R.D., Hoch, C.C., and Reynolds, C.F. (1997). Depression in Alzheimer's dementia. In *Progress in Alzheimer's disease and similar conditions* (ed. L.L. Heston), pp. 161–75. American Psychiatric Press, Washington DC.

Najjar, F. and Guttmacher, L.B. (1998). ECT in the presence of intracranial aneurysm. *Journal of ECT*, **14**, 266–71.

Nelson, J.P. and Rosenberg, D.R. (1991). ECT treatment of demented elderly patients with major depression: a restrospective study of efficacy and safety. *Convulsive Therapy*, **7**, 157–65.

O'Connor, C.J., Rothen, D.M., Soble, J.S., Macioch, J.E., McCarthy, R., Neumann, A., *et al.* (1996). The effect of esmolol pretreatment on the incidence of regional wall motion abnormalities during electroconvulsive therapy. *Anesthesia and Analgesia*, **82**, 143–7.

Olfson, M., Marcus, M., Sackheim, H.A., Thompson, J., and Pincus, H.A. (1998). Use of ECT for the inpatient treatment of recurrent major depression. *American Journal of Psychiatry*, **155**, 22–9.

Petrides, G. and Fink, M. (1996). Atrial fibrillation, anticoagulation, and electroconvulsive therapy. *Convulsive Therapy*, **12**, 91–8.

Price, T.R. and McAllister, T.W. (1989). Safety and efficacy of ECT in depressed patients with dementia: a review of clinical experience. *Convulsive Therapy*, **5**, 61–74.

Rao, T.L.K., Jacobs, K.H., and El-Etr, A.A. (1983). Reinfarction following anesthesia in patients with myocardial infarction. *Anesthesiology*, **59**, 499–505.

Rasmussen, K.G. and Zorumski, C.F. (1993). Electroconvulsive therapy in patients taking theophylline. *Journal of Clinical Psychiatry*, **54**, 427–31.

Reitan, R.M. (1958). Validity of the trailmaking test as an indicator of organic brain damage. *Perceptual and Motor Skills*, **8**, 271–6.

Rice, E.H., Sombrotto, L.B., Markowitz, J.C., and Leon, A.C. (1994). Cardiovascular morbidity in high-risk patients during ECT. *American Journal of Psychiatry*, **151**, 1637–41.

Rosenfeld, J.E., Glassberg, S., and Sherrid, M. (1988). Administration of ECT 4 years after aortic aneurysm dissection. *American Journal of Psychiatry*, **145**, 128–9.

Ruwitch, J.F., Perez, J.E., Miller, T.R., Gropler, R.J., and Rasmussen, K.G. (1994). Myocardial ischemia induced by electroconvulsive therapy. *Circulation*, **90**, 2034.

Sackheim, H.A., Decina, P., Prohovnik, I., Malitz, S., and Resor, S.R. (1983). Anticonvulsant and antidepressant properties of electroconvulsive therapy: a proposed mechanism of action. *Biological Psychiatry*, **18**, 1301–10.

Sackheim, H.A., Prudic, J., Devanand, D.P., Kiersky, J.E., Fitzsimons, L., Moody, B.J., *et al.* (1993). Effects of stimulus intensity and electrode placement on the efficacy and cognitive effects of electroconvulsive therapy. *New England Journal of Medicine*, **328**, 839–46.

Selvin, B.L. (1987). Electroconvulsive therapy—1987. *Anesthesiology*, **67**, 367–85.

Stern, L., Hirschmann, S., and Grunhaus, L. (1997). ECT in patients with major depressive disorder and low cardiac output. *Convulsive Therapy*, **13**, 68–73.

Stoudemire, A., Knos, G., Gladson, M., Markwalter, H., Sung, Y.F., Morris, R. and Cooper, R. (1990). Labetalol in the control of cardiovascular responses to electroconvulsive therapy in high-risk depressed medical patients, *Journal of Clinical Psychiatry*, **51**, 508–12.

Tew, J.D., Mulsant, B.H., Haskett, R.F., Prudic, J., Thase, M.E., Crowe, R., *et al.* (1999). Acute efficacy of ECT in the treatment of major depression in the old-old. *American Journal of Psychiatry*, **156**, 1865–70.

Thase, M.E., Greenhouse, J.B., Frank, E., Reynolds, C.F. 3rd, Pilkonis, P.A., Hurley, K., *et al.* (1997). Treatment of major depression with psychotherapy or psychotherapy–pharmacotherapy combinations. *Archives of General Psychiatry*, **54**, 1009–15.

Van Den Berg, A.A. and Honjol, N.M. (1998). Electroconvulsive therapy and intraocular pressure. *Middle East Journal of Anesthesiology*, **14**, 249–58.

Welch, C.A. (1993). ECT in medically ill patients. In *The clinical science of electroconvulsive therapy* (ed. C.E. Coffey), pp. 167–82. American Psychiatric Press, Washington, DC.

Wilkinson, A.M., Anderson, D.N., and Peters, S. (1993). Age and the effects of ECT. *International Journal of Geriatric Psychiatry*, **8**, 401–6.

Williams, K., Smith, J., Glue, P., and Nutt, D. (1992). The effects of electroconvulsive therapy on plasma insulin and glucose in depression. *British Journal of Psychiatry*, **161**, 94–8.

Zielinski, R.J., Roose, S.P., Devanand, D.P., Woodring, S., and Sackheim, H.A. (1993). Cardiovascular complications of ECT in depressed patients with cardiac disease. *American Journal of Psychiatry*, **150**, 904–9.

Zvara, D., Brooker, R.F., McCall, W.V., Foreman, A.S., Hewitt, B.S., Murphy, B.A., *et al.* (1997). The effect of esmolol on ST-segment depression and arrhythmias after electroconvulsive therapy. *Convulsive Therapy*, **13**, 165–74.

14 Non-biological therapies

Julia Payne and Ken Wilson

Summary

In this chapter, we will describe the evidence for non-biological treatments in older patients with mental health problems, with reference to their possible use in non-psychiatric settings. The first part of the chapter reviews the literature concerning formal psychotherapeutic interventions. In the second part, we examine the literature concerning less structured psychosocial, supportive, and other interventions. In this part, we also explore the role of non-drug interventions in the context of specific clinical situations. Lastly, we review aspects of the literature concerning family and domestic issues.

Introduction

The old age psychiatrist has a role to play in the recommendation and implementation of psychosocial treatments in non-psychiatric settings. These can range from management of a specific behavioural problem to a comprehensive and formal psychotherapeutic involvement. Psychosocial treatments can be with an individual, a family, a group, or with a caregiving system. Liaison services also provide valuable input by helping staff to understand the psychological, behavioural, and emotional problems encountered by older, physically ill patients.

In this chapter, we will describe the evidence for non-biological treatments in older patients with mental health problems, with reference to their possible use in non-psychiatric settings. The first part of the chapter reviews the literature concerning formal psychotherapeutic interventions. In the second part, we examine the literature concerning less structured psychosocial, supportive, and other interventions. In this part, we also explore the role of non-drug interventions in the context of specific clinical situations. Lastly, we review aspects of the literature concerning family and domestic issues.

Psychotherapy and the older person

The growing interest in the psychotherapeutic treatment of older people is reflected in the increasing numbers of manuals, case studies, and clinical and randomized controlled trials. Studies include examples of cognitive–behavioural interventions, interpersonal psychotherapy, problem-solving techniques, and self-help therapies. Despite the relatively few, high-quality, randomized controlled trials, the cumulative evidence strongly supports the role of psychotherapeutic and social interventions in the management of older, mentally ill people across a broad range of conditions.

Psychotherapeutic therapies in a liaison setting

The clinical diversity encountered in older people predicates a flexible and often eclectic approach to psychotherapies. However, it is evident that physical illness presents particular obstacles for both patient and therapist in an acute hospital setting. The institutional or hospital environment frequently exacerbates difficulties encountered by the therapist. Medical and surgical ward routine is subject to the specific physical needs of the patient, with little acknowledgment of any psycho-social issues. The requirement to discharge people as quickly as possible limits the potential for planned psychosocial rehabilitation. Lack of privacy on general wards inhibits the opportunity to form psychotherapeutic relationships. Frequent changes of staff, the use of temporary nursing staff, and locum doctors who are unfamiliar with the specific needs of the patient, impose further problems. Lack of expertise and 'psychotherapeutic awareness' of both nursing and medical staff, serving acute medical and surgical wards, compounds the difficulties. At first encounter, these problems can seem overwhelming. However, through adopting a systematic approach, couched in education, developing personal relationships with ward staff, and demonstrating the effectiveness of specific interventions, some of the barriers can be broken down.

Frequent, recurrent admissions of vulnerable older people to medical and surgical wards present liaison services with considerable challenges. Untreated depression is one of the major risk factors for readmission. Consequently, physically frail, chronically depressed, older people are particularly vulnerable to 'the revolving door' problem. Despite their obvious frailty, these patients will often respond to multidisciplinary team support in a community setting (Banerjee *et al.* 1996). Care packages are often complex, reflecting the longevity, severity, and composite nature of problems experienced by this group of patients. If inadequately recognized or treated, chronicity of both physical and psychiatric symptoms may lead to heavily entrenched maladaptive lifestyles, with an elaborate network of re-enforcers main-taining the status quo and contributing to frequent readmissions. For example, a depressed individual's isolative behaviour may influence the response of significant others. The immediate carers experience rejection and become alienated from the patient, thus exaggerating the individual's emotional and physical isolation (Bandura 1977). This predicament may be compounded by unrewarding input from helping agencies, leading to the passive resistance of further intervention (Steuer *et al.* 1984), and promoting the likelihood of hospitalization or long-term care. To avoid such scenarios, it is important to involve significant others who are possibly contributing towards maintenance of the depression, and who may provide an important therapeutic resource in the management and rehabilitation of the patient. The need for longer term community involvement for the appropriate rehabilitation of this vulnerable group of patients is self-evident. It is incumbent upon the liaison team to facilitate follow-up after the patient has been discharged from the institution.

There is no doubt that formal psychotherapies have the potential to play a significant role in the treatment and management of a wide range of conditions encountered by older people. These interventions require skill, and are most appropriately delivered by a therapist who has experience with older people. The therapist should have access to the expertise of a skilled multidisciplinary clinical team catering for the physical and psychopharmacological needs of the patient. In practice, these therapies require planning, the involvement of significant family, carers, and staff, and careful monitoring.

Behavioural therapies

Behavioural programmes are easily adapted for older people and utilized in both the management of depression (Thompson *et al.* 1987; Lichtenberg *et al.* 1996) and dementia (Burgio *et al.* 1996). The principles of behavioural therapies are well founded. First, there is an assessment of the targeted behaviour through examining the antecedents, behaviour, and consequences (**ABC**). Second, having analysed the targeted behaviour, possible solutions are generated through brainstorming techniques. Third, the solution is planned, rehearsed, and implemented. Finally, the entire process is evaluated, difficulties identified, and further solutions developed.

Loneliness is a common experience of older depressed people. Behavioural therapy offers an easily adaptable model of intervention. A return to social isolation at home is likely to promote patterns of depressive behaviour and associated cognition. These issues are readily identified through enabling the patient to examine their current lifestyle. A wide-ranging approach is encouraged with a view to emphasizing the most important and readily solvable issues concerning the patient. Solutions can be generated through working with the patient, carers, social services, and local community. The programme of resocialization is planned in a stepwise fashion. This might include the introduction of domiciliary services, home helps, and carer involvement. Attendance at day centres, local clubs, and involvement in religious organizations may be developed. Continued reassessment and evaluation is essential and can be readily conducted through follow-up clinics, community agencies, and carers working in collaboration with patient.

Behavioural therapy can be useful in the treatment of challenging behaviours encountered in some dementia sufferers. Manchip (1998) describes a systematic and practical approach to the management of these problems:

1. Define the specific problem as above.
2. Exclude delirium and physical causes.
3. Exclude and treat any underlying psychiatric problems.
4. Assess the role of carers and the environment in causing or perpetuating the symptoms, and manage these accordingly.

Proctor *et al.* (1999) demonstrated how nursing and residential-home staff could use behavioural interventions to manage patients. In their study, a psychiatric nurse implemented an educational programme to support the staff whilst undertaking a randomized controlled trial of behavioural interventions. The authors demonstrated improved depression scores, less cognitive deterioration, and fewer visits from the general practitioner, in the index group. Various behavioural and environmental interventions have their advocates for the treatment of behavioural excesses (disruptive vocalizations, wandering, and physical and verbal aggression) and behavioural deficits (excess dependency, lack of engagement in therapeutic activity, social interaction, and communication). Allen-Burge *et al.* (1999) provide a selective review of the research evidence for some of these interventions. They also discuss a programme for training nursing staff in the use of behavioural management skills and a motivational system for long-term use. Although behaviour therapies make intuitive sense to clinicians, there are few controlled trials examining the efficacy of behavioural therapy in patients with dementia. The therapy is also labour-intensive and, accordingly, has resource implications for institutions.

Behavioural therapies have been employed for the treatment of disorders other than dementia. Examples include the rehabilitation of older depressed people (Wilson *et al.* 1995). Graded task assignment, activity scheduling, and desensitization are some of the techniques employed, and these can be useful adjuvants to pharmacotherapy in the treatment of depression. What evidence there is suggests that both these and other psychotherapeutic approaches (Schneider *et al.* 1994) significantly contribute to the prevention of relapse and recurrence of depression.

Cognitive–behavioural therapy

The majority of studies have adapted cognitive and behavioural psychotherapeutic interventions to suit the specific needs of the particular populations under investigation (Lincoln *et al.* 1997). Yost *et al.* (1986) recommend specific adaptations for working with older depressed people. Sessions should be subdivided into sections, each with a beginning and an end, accompanied by verbal and visual cues. Frequent cueing of attention and memory is recommended. Advance notification of tasks (allowing preparation) is important. Homework is helpful to reinforce concept retention between sessions. Most manuals and descriptions of cognitive–behavioural therapy (CBT) and related interventions acknowledge other important features. These include the need to work in the context of a clinical team catering for physical and psychopharmacological needs of the patient. Involvement of family and carers in the psychotherapeutic process is desirable.

Cognitive–behavioural techniques can be tailored to the needs of older people with pronounced physical illness. Examples include the cognitive approaches developed by Rybarczyk *et al.* (1992). Specific recommendations include targeting and resolving the barriers to participation, accepting depression as a separate and reversible problem (from the physical illness), limiting excess disability, and counteracting loss in social roles and autonomy. Rybarczyk (1992) suggested that the therapist can help the elderly person to manage physical problems. A psycho-educational approach is strongly advocated, enabling the subject to make explicit the responsibilities and choices that are available for the management of their physical illness (Rybarczyk *et al.* 1992). The therapy helps the patient to recognize and modify dysfunctional thoughts, limit inappropriate and poorly informed anxiety-generating discussion, and reduce negative reinforcing activities. Patients are encouraged to adopt distraction techniques and to progress their coping skills. The therapist explains the importance of compliance with prescribed management plans. The behavioural management of pain, anxiety, and the restructuring of activities of the physically ill older person contribute substantially towards overall clinical treatment (Ewedemi and Linn 1987).

Self-help therapies may utilize some CBT techniques. Scrogin *et al.* (1989, 1990) found that 'bibliotherapy' was an accessible alternative to formal CBT in the treatment of older patients with mild or moderate depression. 'Bibliotherapy' involves encouraging the older person to read self-help and explanatory literature, provided by the therapist. However, Landreville and Bissonnette (1997) found that biblio-therapy (with minimal therapist contact) was ineffective in physically disabled older adults. They suggest that therapist involvement is crucial. The authors recommended close therapist support through telephone or personal contact when undertaking bibliotherapy or other related self-help techniques, in accordance with the suggestions of Glasgow and Rosen (1980).

Other psychotherapies

Preliminary evidence supporting the role of other psychotherapeutic techniques is less robust but promising. Problem-solving therapies have been adapted for use in rehabilitation settings (Godbole and Verinis 1974). All patients had major physical illnesses and either 'reactive depression' or a 'life-situation reaction'. Patients, randomized into a problem-solving group, showed a significant improvement over a non-treatment control group. Mossey *et al.* (1996) examined the efficacy of inter-personal counselling (IPC) in older medically ill patients. The IPC group showed some improvement in terms of the Geriatric Depression Score and self-rated health, but not on physical or social functioning. More recently, Reynolds *et al.* (1997) demonstrated the efficacy of interpersonal psychotherapy in preventing relapse and recurrence. These therapies are based on psychodynamic concepts. The therapist focuses on interpersonal issues, including the changing of roles, disputes, deficits, and grief. The model is readily adaptable to older people frequently experiencing loss, changes in life, and disability.

Recent research has established formal psychotherapeutic treatment (particularly IPT and CBT) as an important contribution to the management of mental illness in older people. Therapies have been adapted to cater for the clinical diversity encountered in older populations, including the needs of people with severe and chronic physical illness. The relatively few studies conducted in this population give reason for optimism. However, the difficulties in employing these interventions in the context of acute medical and surgical inpatient settings must not be under-estimated. Even if the liaison staff have a limited knowledge of some of the more basic principles of underpinning these interventions, fostering relationships and educating staff can do valuable preparatory work.

Other non-biological therapies

In this section, we describe other non-biological therapies sometimes employed in non-psychiatric settings. Much of the evidence of efficacy is based on descriptive studies and uncontrolled clinical trials. There are relatively few randomized controlled trials of significant scientific rigour. We have not attempted to provide an exhaustive review of the evidence. In each case, we have referred to one or two of the better quality studies with a view to illustrating the particular therapeutic approach.

Spiritual and pastoral therapy and the physically ill older person

It is important not to confuse spirituality and religion. An individual may have spiritual beliefs that they find comforting without being part of a recognized religious group or taking part in religious activity. Religion and, or spirituality may be important coping mechanisms. An American study interviewed elderly, hospital-ized, or institutionalized men and found an association between intrinsic religious activity (prayer) and life satisfaction (Ayele *et al.* 1999). They concluded that physicians need to recognize their own as well as their patients' spirituality if they are to reap the potential benefits for health. More specifically, Braam *et al.* (1997) found that religiosity (personal importance of religion) was significantly associated with recovery from depression in older patients living in the community. This association was particularly strong in those suffering from poor physical health.

The evidence suggests that the spiritual and religious needs of patients are rarely assessed. In a survey of patients given palliative care (Catterall *et al.* 1998), 40 out of 45 said that they found their own spiritual belief helpful or comforting, and this included some atheists and agnostics. The authors concluded that it is preferable to support individual beliefs rather than attempting to change or resolve spiritual idio-syncrasies. Methods of supporting patients' beliefs include the provision of quiet areas, places to worship, and making spiritual-care persons such as chaplains available. The role of the nurse can be particularly important. Espeland (1999) advocates the use of reflective questions to support patients' exploration and development of their own spiritual wellness. Particular issues that can be addressed through this approach include the meaning of life, relationship with a higher power, hope, encouragement; caring, meditation, striving for growth, and forgiveness. Reflective questions might include: 'What drives you?' 'What brings you joy?' and 'What do you want to be remembered for?' Grey (1994) has written a comprehensive paper on spirituality in palliative care with suggestions for how staff can assist their patients in approaching death.

Pet therapy

Fritz *et al.* (1995) sent a questionnaire to the primary caregivers of 146 patients with Alzheimer's disease who were still living at home. Regular contact with a companion animal was reported in 53% of the respondents. Significantly less anxiety and verbal aggression was described in the pet-exposed group. Greater attachment to the pet was associated with fewer mood disorders but not psychiatric or psychomotor symptoms. No significant differences were found between the dog- and cat-exposed patients for non-cognitive symptoms. Churchill *et al.* (1999) used a within-subject, repeat-measurement design to look at the use of a therapy dog to alleviate the agitation and desocialization of people with Alzheimer's disease. They found that the presence of the Labrador–Golden Retriever crossbreed improved socialization and decreased agitation amongst inpatients in a specialist unit during sundown hours. This was unrelated to the severity of the dementia. They concluded this therapy might be a useful adjunct. The mechanism by which improvements are achieved is still unclear. It may be due to relaxation, distraction, companionship, and affection or a combination of these. There are few controlled studies involving pets and more are required before generalizable recommendations can be adopted.

Psychomotor activation programme

Hopman-Rock *et al.* (1999) report the results of a randomized control trial looking at a psychomotor activation programme (PAP) in groups of cognitively impaired elderly living in nursing homes. PAP focuses on communication, reactivation, resocialization, and effective functioning. Activities and games are used to stimulate cognitive and psychosocial functions. PAP was administered in groups, two or more times per week for six months, by trained staff. The control group took part in usual activities. Despite difficulties in implementing the programme, because of heavy staff workload, they were able to demonstrate a statistically significant improvement in cognitive functioning and a trend towards reduced non-social activity in the PAP group. Unfortunately, the study suffered from a high drop out rate and inability to blind the observers to the treatment condition. Consequently, although PAP has clinical face validity the approach requires further evaluation.

Light therapy

Bright-light therapy has been suggested as an intervention for agitation in dementia related to disturbances in circadian rhythm or limited sunlight exposure. Lyketsos *et al.* (1999) used a randomized control trial to look at the possible benefits of exposing patients to 1 hour of bright light each morning. After 4 weeks, there was a statistically significant increase in sleep from baseline in the intervention group, but the increase in sleep as compared to the control group was not significant. There were no significant differences in the scores for behaviour and depression. The authors acknowledge the small size and duration of their study as one possible explanation for lack of benefit.

Music therapy

Music in the healthcare setting can aid reduction in stress, anxiety, and pain. Covington and Crosby (1997) described the use of a music-therapy group for men aged 18 to 90 years resident in a veterans psychiatric inpatient unit. In this study, a nurse facilitated the therapy. If the facilitator is unable to play an instrument then tapes, records, or compact discs are used. The type of music chosen depends on the goals of the group such as mood modulation, relaxation, or thought provocation. Koger and Brotons (1999) undertook a Cochrane Review of music therapy in dementia. Of the 79 studies identified, none were randomized controlled trials and they all had significant methodological problems. However, there were no apparent adverse effects and the evidence suggested a possible beneficial effect on non-cognitive symptoms of dementia.

Exercise therapy

Physical exercise has been suggested to have benefits on mood, cognitive functioning, and morale in the elderly, as well as the presumed benefits to physical health. Singh *et al.* (1997) conducted a randomized controlled trial of progressive resistance training (PRT) in elderly depressed patients. After 10 weeks the exercise group had significantly reduced depression, improved quality of life, and increased strength when compared with the control group. No significant adverse events were reported.

In summary

All these therapies have strong advocates. In the absence of substantial evidence of effectiveness, the psychiatric services should be circumspect in supporting their development in liaison settings.

Interventions used for specific problems

A number of clinical studies and case descriptions provide some evidence supporting the role of informal, psychosocial, and nursing techniques in the management of
specific conditions. However, the scientific evidence for their efficacy is mostly
small, contradictory, or difficult to generalize. Despite the lack of evidence, some
interventions for specific circumstances are worthy of mention.

Death, dying, and loss

Loss is a common issue in hospital settings particularly amongst the elderly. The
medically frail, older people can encounter loss of independence, support, and
function during their hospitalization. In addition, they may have to cope with other
losses such as the loss of significant others or the prospect of their own imminent
death. Parkes (1985) describes both normal and pathological grief and emphasizes
the relationship between grief and physical health. The immunological response is
transiently lowered following bereavement and there appears to be a positive
association between bereavement and death from heart disease. Clayton (1979)
reviewed studies into conjugal bereavement and found that certain conditions are
associated with increased rates of psychiatric consultation after bereavement,
including alcohol problems and dementia. Evidence also suggests that older men
have an increased mortality in the first 6 months after the loss of their spouse
(Clayton 1979).

Pathological grief usually takes the form of either delayed or avoided grief. Risk
factors include the type of death, characteristics of the relationship, characteristics
of the survivor, and social circumstances. There are various techniques to prevent
pathological grief in patients at risk. These include anticipatory guidance, techniques of breaking bad news, counselling, or befriending after death. Worden
(1991) provides a handbook for grief counselling and therapy that is a useful guide
for any member of the caring professions. The process of grief counselling is
essentially the same for all bereaved, but Worden highlights the need for special
consideration with the elderly, because of the potential for multiple losses, personal
death awareness, and loneliness. The latter problem may make group support and
counselling particularly relevant. It is important to remember that the grief
experience also extends to relatives, friends, and staff and they may need appropriate support (Parkes 1999).

For those who are unable to attend the funeral of a loved one (due to physical ill
health), a parallel funeral service may be appropriate. These can be held at the
bedside at the same time as the main service with one or two significant others
and a chaplain. They usually last 10–15 minutes. The involvement of nursing staff
and family members tangibly demonstrates acknowledgment of the event and
provides the ill patient with appropriate emotional and spiritual support (Wrapson
1999).

Delirium

Delirium, particularly of the agitated type, is a common reason for referral to the psychogeriatric team, usually because the patient is severely confused, agitated, disruptive to other patients in the ward, or confusion is compromising care. Between one-quarter and one-third of older people admitted to hospital can suffer from the syndrome (Mulligan and Fairweather 1997). Delirium has significant adverse outcomes, including prolonged hospital stay, increased risk of admission to long-stay care, and increased mortality. The management of delirium requires a confirmed diagnosis, treatment of underlying causes, provision of a predictable environment, orientation, and sedation with pharmacological agents (see Chapter 10).

The causes of delirium are multifactorial, with a single factor identified in less than 50% of cases (O'Keeffee 1999). Sedation with some psychotropic medications causes anticholinergic or sedative side-effects that can exacerbate the problem, and consequently these drugs should be avoided whenever possible. The importance of environmental and nursing strategies is self-evident. Meagher *et al.* (1996) conducted a prospective analysis of 46 consecutive referrals with delirium to a consultation service in a large Dublin hospital. They looked at the use of medication and eight basic nursing strategies:

- frequent observations (at least 4-hourly or more frequently);
- efforts by staff to orientate the patient to their surroundings;
- avoidance of excessive staff changes;
- single room;
- uncluttered environment around the bed;
- individual night-light;
- efforts to minimize noise levels (for example, from radio or television); and
- requesting relatives and friends to visit regularly, to enhance reorientation.

They found that simple environmental manipulation was frequently underused (half the measures were not used in more than half the patients). In addition, the frequency of interventions (pharmacological and environmental) was higher in Meagher's hyperactive group compared to his hypoactive group, irrespective of the severity of confusion.

Other suggested strategies include minimizing sensory deprivation by providing spectacles and hearing aids where appropriate. The use of clear, slow, and simple instructions, and adopting a calm and friendly approach with frequent reassurance and reorientation are recommended, especially when painful or unpleasant procedures are undertaken (Meagher and Quinn 1996). A combination of regular reassurance, reorientation, sleep hygiene, early mobilization, provision of sensory aids, and the avoidance of dehydration may prevent delirium in high-risk patients (Inouye *et al.* 1999).

Psychological therapies for dementia

Various psychological therapies have been tried with patients suffering from dementia. These include reminiscence, validation, and reality orientation therapy (Twining 1998). More eclectic approaches, for example memory aids (lists, notices, or instructions in appropriate places), have also been tried (Twining 1998).

Reminiscence therapy involves groups of elderly patients meeting regularly to talk about past events, assisted by aids such as videos, pictures, and music. Its use in dementia was suggested because remote memory is usually preserved until later in the disease process. It is hypothesized that it may encourage socialization as well as stimulating memory and thus have a beneficial effect on behaviour and cognition (Spector et al. 1999).

Validation therapy is based on a collection of principles that include the premise that everyone is unique and valuable, and that there are reasons that can explain the behaviour of the disorientated elderly. The techniques used include focusing on the individual, reminiscing, and non-verbal support through tone of voice, eye contact, and touch. The therapy's hypothesized benefits for the patient include increased self-worth and communication, and reduced withdrawal and anxiety (Neal and Briggs 1999).

There are two main types of reality orientation therapy (RO). Informal RO is continuous and involves reminding the patient about whom, when, and where he is, as well as information about his environment. Formal RO takes place in regular groups with a therapist. Information related to orientation is provided, for example the date, time, location, and name of participants, and this is then expanded upon during the session. Powell-Proctor and Miller (1982) performed a review of studies into RO and concluded that it has 'an effect which is more than just the non-specific consequences of instituting some form of intervention'. However, the benefits are modest and do not generalize well. The secondary benefits may include increased staff morale and reduced employment turnover. A Cochrane review of classroom (i.e. formal), reality orientation therapy (Spector et al. 1998) examined outcomes including cognition and behaviour. They found eight randomized control trials that met their inclusion criteria (total of 67 subjects and 58 controls). They concluded that RO has significant positive effects on both cognition and behaviour without any reported side-effects. However, although the short-term benefits seem clear there is insufficient evidence to draw any conclusions about long-term benefits. Baines et al. (1987) compared RO and reminiscence therapy in a crossover study in residents of local authority homes. Both forms of therapy helped the staff to get to know their confused residents better. Staff and residents enjoyed the sessions and the groups continued after completion of the study. The group that had RO before reminiscence therapy showed the greatest improvement. Although the improvements in orientation were lost after 1 month, the improvements in behaviour were maintained.

Vocally disruptive behaviour

Vocally disruptive behaviour (shouting and screaming) can cause distress to carers, other patients, and staff. The behaviour is most commonly associated with dementia, but it can also be related to depression and psychosis. It is positively correlated with severe impairment of activities of daily living, pain, and poor communication. Important environmental factors include social isolation, non-involvement in activities, quality of staff interactions, and inadvertent reinforcement by staff. It is important to recognize that the aetiology is likely to be multifactorial and, often, a combination of biological and non-biological strategies is indicated. Various techniques have been described. These include the use of 'white noise,' music therapy, validation therapy, and behavioural interventions (Meares and Draper 1999). The involvement of nursing staff is crucial to the management of these disruptive behaviours. This includes monitoring the target behaviour, identifying antecedents and consequences associated with the behaviour, and manipulating the environment accordingly. Vocally disruptive behaviour is distressing and the caring staff or families require explanations and reassurance. The problem is difficult to treat and a residual level of vocally disruptive behaviour may need to be part of the realistic goal (Meares and Draper 1999).

Sexual disorders

Sexual disorders may become known because of complaints by either the patient or their partner. Sexually disinhibited behaviour towards staff and other patients may also precipitate a referral. It is important to remember that about half of men and a third of women aged 70 report continued sexual intercourse (Kellett 1994). Patients may find it difficult to volunteer the presence of sexual difficulties and clinicians will need to employ tactful questioning to elicit them. They may be related to physical illness, psychiatric illness, the side-effects of treatment, or any combination of the above. Angina and recent cardiac disease is a common cause of concern regarding sexual activity. Careful counselling, advice concerning medication, and reassurance may play an important role in promoting quality of life and relationships in the context of potentially very frightening circumstances. Treatments are varied and dependent on the cause. Simple reassurance maybe effective, however counselling by experienced therapists may be indicated.

In the case of dementia, patients may not lose their sexual appetite until late in the disorder. This can either enhance the nature of the relationship or cause significant problems for the carer. When sexual relationships between the dementia sufferer and their spouse are no longer appropriate, the spouse may need non-judgemental counselling and possibly 'permission' to involve extramarital partners for their own psychological well-being (Higson 1999). New relationships may develop in institutions, causing jealousy amongst other residents and consternation amongst relatives and sometimes staff. The relationship choices of consenting adults need to be accepted and appropriate privacy provided, where possible. Unwanted sexual advances towards staff can usually be managed with environmental and behavioural interventions, for example the provision of same gender helpers for bathing. Carers should indicate that the person's need is understood, but can not be responded to as they wish, thus maintaining mutual respect (Oppenheimer 1997).

Driving

The psychiatrist may be asked for advice regarding an elderly patient who is still driving, especially if the family have raised concerns. In the UK, as in many other countries, a person has an obligation to inform the Driver and Vehicle Licensing Agency (DVLA), or equivalent agency, of any medical condition that may affect their fitness to drive. In addition, drivers over the age of 70 may have to produce a medical certificate attesting their fitness to drive or (in some countries) pass a practical driving test before their licence to drive a motor vehicle can be renewed. Licensing is ultimately the DVLA's responsibility, but the attending physician has a duty to inform the patient if their condition, including any prescribed medication, could adversely affect their driving (Johnson and Bouman 1997). The doctor should record any such advice in the case notes in case of later legal problems. However, the difficulty arises when the patient refuses to take advice or is incapable of understanding the information. Unfortunately, revoking the driving licence may not be sufficient to prevent the patient from driving and the family or police may need to be involved. Although families have no legal obligations, they may play an essential role in preventing the patient from driving, particularly when insight is an issue (Johnson and Bouman 1997).

The decision about when a patient with dementia is no longer fit to drive is a difficult one. Unfitness to drive is largely a clinical decision, based on the history and interdisciplinary assessment. No clear direct correlation has been found between neuropsychological tests and crash risk (O'Neill 1996). Drivers with dementia who drive accompanied have fewer crashes than those who drive alone, although the mechanism behind this is unclear (O'Neill 1996). The doctor should routinely ask about driving, speak to the carer, ask about recent problems (for example, accidents or getting lost), and consider the influence of other illnesses and medication. Then, if appropriate, advise the patient to stop driving and, if necessary, speak to the appropriate authorities. This can be a difficult issue between the patient and doctor and may threaten their therapeutic relationship if not handled carefully. O'Neill (1996) recommends taking a collaborative approach, exploring with the patient their feelings and fears about the consequences.

Families and carers

The liaison team has a role in identifying both patients and carers not already receiving the support of specialist services. They may be the first psychiatric contact that both the family and patient have encountered. Family members and carers play an influential role in determining both the short- and long-term management of older, mentally ill people admitted to medical and surgical wards. Their involvement in a successful management plan is essential. If family members consider themselves to have been marginalized in the medical process, the liaison team may encounter considerable stress and sometimes hostility. Carers of dementia sufferers are particularly vulnerable (Gilleard 1998) with reported rates of depression ranging from 14 to 40% (Morris *et al.* 1988). Donaldson *et al.* (1997) concluded that non-cognitive features of dementia (psychotic symptoms, mood disturbance, and behavioural problems) are positively related to caregiver burden and psychological disturbance. The caregiving relationship, carer's attribution and coping styles, and availability of support (both formal and informal) all contribute towards stress experienced by the carer. Caregivers are most likely to be depressed if they feel a loss of control over the sufferer's behaviour, inability to cope with the impact of caring, or if the situation is perceived as unchanging and universal (Morris *et al.* 1988). An acute medical or surgical admission may exacerbate these issues. Particular care should be taken to identify vulnerable carers so as to maintain supporting relationships, avoid potential elder abuse, and establish robust management plans (Gilleard 1998). Warning signs of depression in carers include repeated requests for reassessment when there has been no change, unreasonable complaints about the patient's care, and lack of co-operation from the carer.

The liaison services may provide the first opportunity for carers and families to discuss these and related issues. Individual therapy, education, practical advice, stress management, local support groups, and national organizations (Twining 1998) can provide effective support. The value of recruiting informal support for carers should not be underestimated. Carers with larger social networks of support feel less need for formal support and make fewer demands on services. Informal support may reduce feelings of isolation and the restriction on activities that frequently accompany caring (Morris *et al.* 1988). Carers can learn behavioural techniques and use these to reduce problematic behaviours. They also enjoy participation in supportive and psychoeducational groups. These can have beneficial effects on the carers' well-being, and may reduce depression, agitation, and delay institutionalization in the dementia sufferers (Teri 1999). Dementia training programmes for carers aim to reduce their burden and thus help the sufferer. The evidence suggests that while educational programmes increase the carer's knowledge about dementia, they have little impact on the burden. Programmes that are more comprehensive do appear to have outcomes that are more positive by reducing stress and delaying institutionalization. However, considerable resources are required (Gormley 2000). Relatives support groups can reduce the subjective burden, isolation, and depression in carers and increase their feelings of control. The information as well as the support they provide is useful (Morris *et al.* 1988). The paucity of research concerning the efficacy of these and other interventions in relieving carer stress (Thompson and Thompson 1999) is a cause for concern. Donaldson *et al.* (1997) draws attention to the need for further studies examining the effectiveness of such interventions in the prevention of institutionalization.

Chronic illness, psychiatric as well as physical, has repercussions throughout the family. Support from families becomes increasingly important as people age. Benbow and Marriott (1997) have written a summary of the theory and application of family therapy with elderly people. Unfortunately, little research has been published into the effectiveness of formal or informal family therapy. Although formal family therapy is unlikely to be available within the current resources of a consultation-liaison service, knowledge of the principles may be useful in managing issues that arise in relation to older people's family systems. It is important to recognize that the reasons for referral may be related to changes within the family, or their perceptions of changes, rather than differences in the patient's health. Hence, the importance of having an assessment that includes the family. On hospital wards, the inclusion of the family at meetings before discharge allows the airing of concerns and increases openness with all interested parties.

Conclusions

The problems facing a liaison team are considerable. Most services are young and relatively under-resourced. Medical and surgical teams are usually unfamiliar with even the most fundamental of psychological principles. Psychosocial interventions are labour-intensive and difficult to deliver in a potentially inhospitable environment. Not only is it impossible, but it would be inappropriate for the liaison team to provide these labour-intensive services. However, it is the role of a liaison service to provide information, education, and facilitate appropriate follow-up for this vulnerable group of older people.

In broadening the definition of liaison to include services catering for residents in nursing and residential care, non-biological approaches play an important, if not critical role in the management of mentally ill, older people. Education of staff and carers in the context of advice and care planning will contribute to both primary and secondary prevention of functional and behavioural disorders in mentally ill, older people. The role of well-established multiprofessional teams in supporting physically, frail older people living in the community has been clearly illustrated through Bannerjee's work (1996). In this study a specialist community team was shown to have proven efficacy in the treatment of depression in older, frail people living in the community, compared to non-specialized care. A minority was treated with antidepressant medication, emphasizing the importance of non-biological therapies in the treatment of depression in physically ill, older people. Specialized community teams are frequently involved in providing crisis intervention in community settings, and they play an important role in supporting both patients and staff of institutional settings, thus preventing increased dependency and medical-ization.

In writing this chapter we have attempted to provide the liaison services with a brief résumé of the literature concerning the more common psychosocial interventions. The résumé is far from exhaustive and is highly selective in the interventions and evidence examined. Despite this, we hope that we have emphasized the possible role of the non-biological therapies in the management of a wide range of conditions, and highlighted that they do have the potential for use in non-psychiatric settings and work with physically ill, older people.

References

Allen-Burge, R., Stevens, A.B., and Burgio, L.D. (1999). Effective behavioural interventions for decreasing dementia-related challenging behaviour in nursing homes. *International Journal of Geriatric Psychiatry*, **14**, 213–32.

Ayele, H., Mulligan, T., Gheorghiu, S., and Reyes-Ortiz, C. (1999). Religious activity improves life satisfaction for some physicians and older patients. *Journal of the American Geriatrics Society*, **47**, 453–5.

Baines, S., Saxby, P., and Ehler, K. (1987). Reality orientation and reminiscence therapy: a controlled crossover study of elderly confused people. *British Journal of Psychiatry*, **151**, 222–31.

Bandura, A. (1977). *Social learning theory*. Englewood Cliffs, Prentice Hall, NJ.

Banerjee, S., Shamash, K., MacDonald, A., and Mann, A. (1996). Randomised controlled trial of effect of intervention by psychogeriatric team on depression on frail elderly people at home. *British Medical Journal*, **313**, 1058–1061.

Benbow, S.M. and Marriott, A. (1997). Family therapy with elderly people. *Advances in Psychiatric Treatment*, **3**, 138–45.

Braam, A.W., Beekman, A.T.F., Deeg, D.J.H., Smit, J.H., and Tilburg, W. Van. (1997). Religiosity as a protective or prognostic factor of depression in later life: results from a community survey in The Netherlands. *Acta Psychiatrica Scandinavica*, **96**, 199–205.

Burgio, L.D., Cotter, E.M., and Stevens, A.B. (1996). Treatment in residential settings. In *Psychological treatment of older adults* (ed. M. Hersen and V.B. Van Hasselt), pp. 127–45. Plenum Press, New York.

Catterall, R.A., Cox, M., Greet, B., Sankey, J., and Griffiths, G. (1998). The assessment and audit of spiritual care. *International Journal of Palliative Nursing*, **4**, 162–8.

Churchill, M., Safaoui, J., McCabe, B.W., and Baun, M.M. (1999). Using a therapy dog to alleviate the agitation and desocialisation of patients with Alzheimer's disease. *Journal of Psychosocial Nursing*, **37**, 16–22.

Clayton, P.J. (1979). The sequelae and non-sequelae of conjugal bereavement. *American Journal of Psychiatry*, **136**, 1530–4.

Covington, H. and Crosby, C. (1997). Music therapy as a nursing intervention. *Journal of Psychosocial Nursing*, **35**, 34–7.

Donaldson, C., Tarrier, N., and Burns, A. (1997). The impact of symptoms of dementia on caregivers. *British Journal of Psychiatry*, **170**, 62–8.

Espeland, K. (1999). Achieving spiritual wellness: using reflective questions. *Journal of Psychosocial Nursing*, **37**, 36–40.

Ewedemi, F. and Linn, M.L. (1987). Health hassles in older and younger men. *Journal of Clinical Psychology*, **43**, 347–53.

Fritz, C.L., Farver, T.B., Kass, P.H., and Hart, L.A. (1995). Association with companion animals and the expression of non-cognitive symptoms in Alzheimer's patients. *Journal of Nervous and Mental Disorders*, **183**, 459–63.

Gilleard, C. (1998). Carers. In *Seminars in old age psychiatry* (ed. R. Butler and B. Pitt), pp. 279–90. Gaskell, London.

Glasgow, R.E. and Rosen, G.M. (1980). Behavioural bibliotherapy: a review of self help behavioural manuals. *Psychological Bulletin*, **85**, 1–23.

Godbole, A. and Verinis, J.S. (1974). Brief psychotherapy in the treatment of emotional disorders in physically ill geriatric patients. *The Gerontologist*, **14**, 143–8.

Gormley, N. (2000). The role of dementia training programmes in reducing caregiver burden. *Psychiatric Bulletin,* **24**, 41–2.

Grey, A. (1994). The spiritual component of palliative care. *Palliative Medicine*, **8**, 215–21.

Higson, N. (1999). Sex and psychiatric illness in the elderly. *Geriatric Medicine*, **29**, 39–40.

Hopman-Rock, M., Staats, P.G.M., Tak, E.C.P.M., and Dröes, R.M. (1999). The effects of a psychomotor activation programme for use in groups of cognitively impaired people in homes for the elderly. *International Journal of Geriatric Psychiatry*, **14**, 633–42.

Inouye, S.K., Bogardus, S.T., Charpentier, P.A., Leo-Summers, L., Acampora, D., Holford, T.R., *et al.* (1999). A multicomponent intervention to prevent delirium in hospitalised older patients. *New England Journal of Medicine*, **340**, 669–76.

Johnson, H. and Bouman, W. (1997). Driving a cause for concern in dementia. *Geriatric Medicine*, **27**(6), 59–60.

Kellett, J.M. (1994). Sexual disorders. In *Principles and practice of geriatric psychiatry* (ed. J.R.M. Copeland, M.T. Abou-Saleh, and D.G. Blazer), pp. 825–9. Wiley, Chichester.

Koger, S.M. and Brotons, M. (1999). Music therapy for dementia (Cochrane Review). In *The Cochrane Library*, Issue 1, Update Software, Oxford.

Landreville, P. and Bissonnette, L. (1997). Effects of cognitive bibliotherapy for depressed older adults with a disability. *Clinical Gerontologist*, **17**, 35–55.

Lichtenberg, P.A., Kimbarrow, M.L., Morris, P., and Vangel, S.J. (1996). Behavioural treatment of depression in predominantly African–American medical patients. *Clinical Gerontologist*, **17**, 15–33.

Lincoln, N.B., Flannaghan, T., Sutcliffe, L., and Rother, L. (1997). The evaluation of cognitive–behavioural treatment for depression after stroke: a pilot study. *Clinical Rehabilitation*, **11**, 114–22.

Lyketsos, C.G., Veiel, L.L., Baker, A., and Steele C. (1999). A randomised control trial of bright light therapy for agitated behaviours in dementia patients residing in long-term care. *International Journal of Geriatric Psychiatry*, **14**, 520–5.

Manchip, S. (1998). The assessment of behavioural problems in dementia. *Geriatric Medicine*, **28**, 39–42.

Meagher, D. and Quinn, J. (1996). Practical issues in the management of delirium. *Geriatric Medicine*, **26**, 52–4.

Meagher, D., O'Hanlon, D., O'Mahony, E., and Casey, P. (1996). The use of environmental strategies and psychotropic medication in the management of delirium. *British Journal of Psychiatry*, **168**, 512–15.

Meares, S. and Draper, B. (1999). Treatment of vocally disruptive behaviour of multifactorial aetiology. *International Journal of Geriatric Psychiatry*, **14**, 285–90.

Morris, G.M., Morris, L.W., and Britton, P.G. (1988). Factors affecting the emotional wellbeing of the caregivers of dementia sufferers. *British Journal of Psychiatry*, **153**, 147–56.

Mossey, J., Knott, K., Higgins, M., and Talerico, K. (1996). Effectiveness of a psychosocial intervention, interpersonal counselling for sub-dysthymic depression in medically ill elderly. *Journal of Gerontology*, **51a**, m172–m178.

Mulligan, I. and Fairweather, S. (1997). Delirium—the geriatrician's perspective. In *Psychiatry in the elderly* (2nd edn) (ed. R. Jacoby and C. Oppenheimer), pp. 507–26. Oxford University Press, Oxford.

Neal, M. and Briggs, M. (1999). Validation therapy for dementia (Cochrane Review). In *The Cochrane Library*, Issue 4. Update Software, Oxford.

O'Keeffee, S.T. (1999). Delirium in the elderly. *Age and Ageing*, **28** (Suppl. 2), 5–8.

O'Neill, D. (1996). Dementia and driving: screening, assessment and advice. *Lancet*, **348**, 1114.

Oppenheimer, C. (1997). Sexuality in old age. In *Psychiatry in the elderly* (2nd edn) (ed. R. Jacoby and C. Oppenheimer), pp. 689–708. Oxford University Press, Oxford.

Parkes, C.M. (1985). Bereavement. *British Journal of Psychiatry*, **146**, 11–17.

Parkes, C.M. (1999). Coping with loss: the consequences and implications for care. *International Journal of Palliative Nursing*, **5**, 250–4.

Powell-Proctor, L. and Miller, E. (1982). Reality orientation: a critical appraisal. *British Journal of Psychiatry*, **140**, 457–63.

Proctor, R., Burns, A., Stratton-Powell, H., Tarrier, N., Faragher, B., Richardson, G., *et al.* (1999). Behavioural management in nursing and residential homes: a randomised control trial. *Lancet*, **354**, 26–9.

Reynolds, C.F., Frank, E., Houck, P.R., Mazumdar, S., Dew, M.A., Comes, C., *et al.* (1997). Which elderly patients with remitted depression remain well with continued interpersonal psychotherapy after discontinuation of antidepressant medication? *American Journal of Psychiatry*, **154**, 958–62.

Rybarczyk, B., Gallagher, T., Dolores, R., Rodman, J., Zeiss, A., Gantz, S.E., *et al.* (1992). Applying cognitive–behavioural psychotherapy to the chronically ill elderly: treatment issues and case illustration. *International Psychogeriatrics*, **4**, 127–39.

Schneider, L., Reynolds, C., Lebowitz, B., and Friedhoff, A. (1994). *Diagnoses and treatment of depression in late life: results of the NIH Consensus Development Conference.* American Psychiatric Press, Washington DC.

Scrogin, F., Jamison, C., and Gochneaur, K. (1989). Comparative efficacy of cognitive and behavioural bibliotherapy for mildly and moderately depressed older adults. *Journal of Consulting and Clinical Psychology*, **57**, 403–7.

Scrogin, F., Jamison, C., and Davies, N. (1990). Two year follow up of bibliotherapy for depression in older adults. *Journal of Consulting and Clinical Psychology*, **58**, 665–7.

Singh, N.A., Clements, K.M., and Fiatarone, M.A. (1997). A randomised controlled trial of progressive resistance training in depressed elders. *Journal of Gerontology*, **52**, M27–M35.

Spector, A., Orrell, M., Davies, S., and Woods, B. (1998). Reality orientation for dementia (Cochrane Review). In *The Cochrane Library*, Issue 1. Update Software, Oxford.

Spector, A., Orrell, M., Davies, S., and Woods, R.T. (1999). Reminiscence therapy for dementia (Cochrane Review). In *The Cochrane Library*, Issue 4. Update Software, Oxford.

Steuer, J.L., Mintz, J., and Hammen, C. (1984). Cognitive–behavioural and psychodynamic group psychotherapy in the treatment of geriatric depression. *Journal of Consulting and Clinical Psychology*, **55**, 385–90.

Teri, L. (1999). Training families to provide care: effects on people with dementia. *International Journal of Geriatric Psychiatry*, **14**, 110–19.

Thompson, C. and Thompson, G. (1999). Support for carers of people with Alzheimer's type dementia (Cochrane Review). In *The Cochrane Library*, Issue 1. Update Software, Oxford.

Thompson, L.W., Gallagher, D., and Breckenbridge, J. (1987). Comparative effectiveness of psychotherapies for depressed elders. *Journal of Consulting and Clinical Psychology*, **55**, 385–90.

Twining, C. (1998). Psychological treatments. In *Seminars in old age psychiatry* (ed. R. Butler and B. Pitt), pp. 265–78. Gaskell, London.

Wilson, K.C.M., Scott, M., Abou-Saleh, M., Burns, R., and Copeland, J.R.M. (1995). Long-term effects of cognitive–behavioural therapy and lithium therapy on depression in the elderly. *British Journal of Psychiatry*, **167**, 653–8.

Worden, J.W. (1991). *Grief counselling and grief therapy: a handbook for the mental health practitioner* (2nd edn). Routledge, London.

Wrapson, D. (1999). Parallel funeral services. *Age and Ageing*, **28**, 501–2.

Yost, E., Beutler, L., Corbishley, M., and Allender, J. (1986). Group cognitive therapy. A treatment approach for depressed older adults. *Psychology Practitioner Guidebooks*, Pergamon Press, New York, USA.

Section 5:
Ethical and legal issues

Sr Nessage.

Imanage Laser-Stars.

fedd of line an accident

No Trash

905-729-6019

15 Ethical issues in geriatric psychiatry liaison

Christine J. Perkins

Summary

This chapter begins with a general discussion of the principles of medical ethics and their particular relevance to older people with psychiatric illness. The focus there-after is on practical problems encountered in the liaison situation. These include: assessment of capacity including the ability to give informed consent: end-of-life issues such as truth-telling, denial, disagreements over treatment, depression, and treatment refusal and euthanasia. The section on confidentiality discusses how to deal with the family, non-psychiatric staff, third parties, and writing the ward notes. The chapter covers the old age liaison psychiatrist's role as an advocate for the indi-vidual patient and family, and the wider issue of advocacy for the mentally ill elderly patient. Advocacy involves ensuring optimal treatment for the hospitalized older person, balancing patient and family needs, deciding on long-term care, elder abuse and the use of restraint, and the rationing of healthcare resources on the basis of age.

General principles

The traditional principles of medical ethics are those of autonomy, beneficence, non-maleficence, and justice. Ethical problems arise when these principles are in conflict. In the clinical setting, they need to be constantly balanced against one another. Ethical problems in liaison psychiatry are no different from those applying generally to the older person with a mental disorder. However, there are different emphases when the person is away from his or her usual community situation. This chapter deals with ethical issues as they arise in the hospital setting.

Autonomy

Autonomy refers to the individual's right to be self-governing, that is, to exercise self-direction, freedom, and moral independence. While some sections of society have achieved a good deal of autonomy, elderly mentally ill people, particularly those with dementia, may still be subjected to unjustified paternalism, for example, when doctors discuss the management of an older person with their family rather than fully consulting the patient, or when nurses in the inpatient setting impose a rigid regime that does not allow for individual variation.

Autonomy is currently highly prized, but it is not always a principle that older people themselves hold so dearly. Older women in particular may have had little experience in making decisions for themselves. For some cultural groups the concept of personal autonomy may be alien and ultimately disempowering. Some older people (and younger ones) may be respectful of physicians as authority figures or experts and prefer decisions to be made by them.

Patient autonomy is often an impossible goal. There is increasing acknowledgment that humans exist in interdependent relationships and social groups; there is no such thing as *total* autonomy. The involved parties such as family or care staff have competing values and interests that also must be considered (Hesse 1993). In some settings, such as long-term care institutions, residents may simply not have the options available to act on their desire for certain types of care. Furthermore, many older people, especially when ill, lack the capacity to make autonomous decisions. An important part of the liaison psychiatrist's work is the determination of the individual's ability to make decisions, especially the giving of informed consent to medical management.

Beneficence

Beneficence is doing good or conferring benefits that enhance personal or social well-being. The converse is *non-maleficence*: doing no harm. At times these two principles conflict, perhaps most obviously in the use of therapeutic drugs which have significant side-effects. Not doing harm also includes not rejecting a patient who takes actions that the doctor thinks are ill-advised. Doctors dealing with the elderly are usually not old themselves, and their views may differ from those of their elders as to what constitutes harm or good. An example is the differing values placed on the ongoing investigation of unexplained symptoms in a very old person.

Justice

Justice is about fairness and impartiality and attempts to find a balance between conflicting interests. The needs of carers of older people must be considered even if they differ from what the older person wants. There may be an issue on general wards where the older patient is treated inadequately on the grounds of age, or staff members avoid the person with mental illness or cognitive impairment. The psychiatrist has a responsibility to advocate for the patient and family in the hospital setting, and perhaps more widely to ensure that the weaker members of society are treated fairly.

When there is an ethical problem, clarifying the issues through discussion may resolve the problem. The psychiatrist should gather information from all involved parties and educate them about the choices. The different courses of action and the seriousness or uncertainty of their outcomes need to be considered. Individuals place different weights on different principles. For example, the principle of autonomy may be more important to the patient, while the principle of non-maleficence matters most to the doctor. These differing weights of opinion need to be taken into account when considering options. Dialogue between parties may throw up alternatives that satisfy all, or compromises may have to be made.

Practical problems

Informed consent and competence

The requirement to gain informed consent to treatment and for other aspects of personal welfare and property matters is an acknowledgment of the importance placed on autonomy. However, a person who is not competent to make decisions cannot act autonomously.

All physicians should be able to evaluate a patient for the capacity to give informed consent, though not all feel comfortable doing so, especially if their training in this area has been inadequate. The liaison psychiatrist is called in if the assessment is difficult, if the primary physician feels mental illness is interfering with choice, or if the patient is making an apparently irrational decision (particularly if it conflicts with the physician's advice).

It is uncommon for treating doctors to request a competency assessment if the patient is going along passively with medical treatment, even if it is likely that the patient is incompetent. Some regard the non-refusal of treatment, such as taking and swallowing pills or putting an arm out for a blood test, as evidence of agreement to treatment. While this may seem inconsistent with our ideals of protecting the incapacitated person, it is unlikely that assessment and the appointment of a substitute decision-maker would make any difference to the management (Molloy *et al.* 1999, p. 208).

Defining capacity or competence

There is no uniform definition of competence or capacity, the words are used interchangeably in this chapter. Furthermore, definitions of 'competence' vary between jurisdictions (Molloy *et al.* 1999, p. 182).

It is worth noting that: 'Capacity deals with the process of decision-making, and does not depend on the actual choices made. Capable people are able to make rational decisions based on their values, goals, knowledge and understanding of the issues facing them. Apparently "inappropriate" choices, idiosyncrasy, or eccentricity, are not adequate reasons for declaring people incapable.' (Molloy *et al.* 1999, p.7)

English law uses the following concepts:

A person lacks capacity if some impairment or disturbance of mental function renders the person unable to make a decision whether to consent or to refuse treatment. That inability to make a decision will occur when:

(a) the patient is unable to comprehend and retain the information which is material to the decision, especially as to the likely consequences of having or not having the treatment in question;

(b) the patient is unable to use the information and weigh it in the balance as part of the process of arriving at the decision. (Lutteril 1997)

See Chapter 16 for a further discussion of legal aspects.

Assessing competence

While much has been written about assessing competence (Appelbaum and Grisso 1988; Molloy *et al.* 1999) no definitive rules exist on 'how to do it'.

It is important to clarify the meaning of a 'request for competency assessment' as 'competency for what?' The examiner should identify what specifically triggered the request before the patient is interviewed. Common issues include informed consent to, or refusal of, medical treatment; personal care decisions (usually relating to accommodation and the acceptance of support services); and property matters or planning for the future when the person may be unable to make decisions (such as appointing a power of attorney).

Competence may be partial, meaning a person could consent to one thing but not another. Although there are aspects universal to all competency assessments, the current issue needs to be the focus.

As part of the assessment, a full cognitive and mental state examination will be performed (see Chapter 5). However, the examiner should be aware that although there may be a mental disorder present, it will not necessarily impact on a person's ability to make a particular decision. For example, a person who delusionally believes that his family are evil and trying to do him out of his money may be competent to give informed consent to medical treatment but not to change his will.

There are special concerns in people suffering from dementia. Although we value the right to individual self-determination, we often find this is ignored in people who have dementia (Rosoff and Gottlieb 1987). Doctors sometimes presume incompetence, on the basis of a previous diagnosis of dementia or an abnormal cognitive test score, without properly examining the patient.

The issue may come down to one of whether the patient trusts the doctor making recommendations. In everyday life, people often have to make decisions beyond their level of competence. They rely on the advice of an expert whom they trust. If a competency assessment has been requested because of disagreement with the physician's recommendation, it may help if the psychiatrist acts as an intermediary between the two to clear up misunderstandings. Not infrequently, this resolves the issue without having to proceed with the assessment.

Decision-making ability will fluctuate depending on a variety of factors such as fatigue, mental disorder, pain, or unpleasant procedures. The examiner might need to return on another occasion when the patient's condition is better. Improving conditions for decision-making involves reducing emotional pressure and improving the patient's confidence by allowing him or her to make choices in areas where he or she already feels more confident (Oppenheimer 1999). Having supportive family present will be the norm in many ethnic groups and desirable for most people, as a family presence will generally increase the patient's feeling of safety.

The person should be informed at the outset of the reason for the assessment. Some people are annoyed that their competence is being questioned, or distressed by the intrusion into their affairs. However, explanation that the ultimate goal is protection of their interests, usually gains agreement. If the subject refuses evaluation and the issue is a life-threatening one, then the psychiatrist needs to obtain indirect evidence, i.e. history from others and observation of the patient's behaviour, to make an assessment. It may be necessary to lower the threshold at which a determination of probable incompetence is made.

The assessment

Molloy *et al.* (1999) write of the concept of a 'competency cell'. 'A competent person:

(1) understands the context of the decision;

(2) knows specific choices; and

(3) appreciates the consequences of the choices.' (Molloy *et al.* 1999, p.18).

In assessing capacity, this 'cell' adapts to the particular circumstance, whether it be informed consent to treatment, financial arrangements, or personal care options.

For example, the geriatric team may be concerned that a person can no longer manage to live independently and request assessment to determine the person's ability to decide about alternative arrangements. The context would include the person's understanding of possible risks at home and a realistic appreciation of their own handicaps and difficulties with self-care. The choices available may be home-help, living with a relative, or institutional care and the person should be aware of these and able to weigh their relative merits. The consequences of possible choices can then be queried: 'What might happen if you decide to go home/live with your daughter/go into care?'

To assess competence to give informed consent, the person must have available sufficient information to make a decision (the context). The examiner cannot assume that this is already the case. It can be useful for the attending doctor to discuss the pertinent information with the patient, in the presence of the assessor, possibly re-presenting it in different ways, simplifying, and clarifying to suit the patient. To test understanding, the person can be asked to paraphrase the information.

He or she needs to grasp that the information under discussion applies personally, that he or she has a choice, and what the main options are. Discussion about the choices and their consequences takes place and the patient should be able to reach a decision, which is reasonably consistent with the starting premises, or at least be able to identify the major factors in the decision and the importance assigned to them (Appelbaum and Grisso 1988).

Power of attorney

A power of attorney is a document signed by a person (the donor) to allow another person (the attorney) to make decisions, generally financial, on behalf of the donor. A durable or enduring power of attorney, covering welfare, financial issues, or both, remains valid even if the donor becomes incompetent. Legislation usually provides for the 'least restrictive alternative' so that the person yields independence only gradually as his or her condition deteriorates, i.e. retains as much autonomy as possible for as long as possible.

The liaison psychiatrist will occasionally be asked to assess capacity to appoint an attorney should a person decide while in hospital that this is a useful thing to do. For example, a man recovering from a cerebrovascular accident realizes he will no longer be able to manage his financial affairs and wishes to enable his daughter to act for him. The person should understand the context of the decision, that is, the powers of an enduring power of attorney, the reasons for considering it, the choice of who might act as attorney, what areas of life they should manage, and the likely consequences of appointing the chosen person.

A person is likely to remain competent to execute a power of attorney in the early stages of dementia, i.e. up to the point where there is decreased performance in demanding employment and social settings (Reisberg *et al.* 1987). However, the patient sometimes denies the diagnosis or prognosis of the illness and will not agree to execute the power of attorney. For example, an elderly man recently diagnosed with dementia understands the concept of power of attorney and agrees that it would be a good thing to have one, but does not think he needs one just yet.

The psychiatrist should ensure that the person signing the power of attorney is not being placed under undue influence, particularly where there are financial issues. This is sometimes extremely difficult to ascertain. The subject needs to be assessed alone, away from the person who may be coercive. Suspicion is raised if the person to be the attorney actively seeks to have the power of attorney signed, and if the donor is dependent on the potential attorney. Sometimes unscrupulous relatives seek to gain control of property when the older person is particularly vulnerable.

Case study 15.1

Mrs K., 87 years of age, suffering dementia and in hospital for treatment of a chest infection, was visited separately by five different family members who each requested that she give them power of attorney over her property. She thus signed the proffered forms five times before the nursing staff discovered what had happened. It was clear that she had no understanding of what she was doing.

Levels of competence

Various commentators have suggested the application of sliding scales for incompetence, based on the potential consequences of patients' decisions (Drane 1985; Schwarz and Blank 1986;). Buchanan and Brock (1989, p. 51–2) write:

> The standard of competence ought to vary in part with the expected harms or benefits to the patient of acting in accordance with the patient's choice ... just because a patient is competent to consent to a treatment, it does not follow that the patient is competent to refuse it, and vice versa. For example, consent to a low risk life-saving procedure ... should require only a minimal level of competence, but refusal of that same procedure ... should require the highest level of competence.

Critics of this approach think there should be an objective standard for competency, otherwise doctors will manipulate the result of assessment to get the answer they want. The consulting psychiatrist will sometimes feel pressured by the medical team to declare the patient incompetent so that the team can intervene as it believes is necessary (Katz et al. 1995). The alternative may be pressure to declare the patient competent so he or she can be discharged (Umapathy et al. 1999).

Result of a finding of incompetence

The conclusion that a person is incompetent does not end the consultation. It should also include an evaluation of the cause of the incapacity with recommendations for treatment, if possible. Treatment may restore competence for long enough to allow the person to make a decision. In many cases, if a person is found incompetent, medical staff accept a proxy decision by next-of-kin, and do not use formal legal procedures. However, a judicial decision may be requested if a risky procedure is contemplated or if there is consideration of a long-lasting curtailment of rights, for example involuntary placement in residential care. The possible outcomes of a judicial hearing will include, in most jurisdictions, a guardian being appointed or a specific order for ongoing management being made. If a guardian is appointed, that person is usually charged with encouraging the person under his or her care to make as many decisions as possible.

The reasons for deciding that the person lacks capacity should be clearly recorded, and a report written in the format appropriate to the local jurisdiction.

Ultimately the balance lies between the desire to protect patients from the consequences of bad decisions and the desire to protect their autonomy, i.e. between non-maleficence and autonomy.

End-of-life issues

Decisions about death and dying are made in all age groups and settings. The balance being considered may be between non-maleficence and autonomy (e.g. when withdrawing treatment at the patient's request), or between justice and beneficence (e.g. in the use of scarce resources in the hopelessly ill).

The psychiatrist may become involved if there is doubt about the patient's competence to make a choice for or against treatment because of cognitive impairment or psychiatric disorder. The request for psychiatric consultation may also arise if there is disagreement between staff, patient, or family as to the right course to follow for the dying person.

Truth-telling

The ethical issue in truth-telling is again a choice between non-maleficence and autonomy; the desire not to distress the dying person versus allowing that person enough information to make necessary decisions at this time.

Family or medical staff may believe that conveying information about a terminal condition will result in despair or depression. In some cultures, it is not thought proper or kind to inform the dying person, and that knowledge of the prognosis may speed death. Surveys in several countries (Harrison et al. 1997; Osuna et al. 1998), however, show that a high proportion of dying people want to know their prognosis. The proportion of patients wanting to know about their impending death is higher than the proportion of doctors or families who think the patient should not be informed. That is, most people with terminal conditions want to know about it, but doctors and families are more reluctant to disclose the information.

Families often think that imparting the diagnosis of dementia is likely to cause distress without serving any useful purpose, and may explicitly instruct that the patient is not to be told. The advent of cholinesterase inhibitors has changed this situation, and if informed consent for their use is to be obtained, the patient must know the diagnosis.

Failure to be truthful with the patient may cause him or her to feel isolated and the resulting distress can trigger a referral. The psychiatrist may also become involved at this stage, to assist in a complex family situation or to help resolve disagreements between staff about what to tell the patient.

Denial

The patient's denial of illness, even after being told the likely outcome, can complicate terminal management. Denial can impair competency, but knowledge about competency may not be particularly useful except on rare occasions when it seems necessary to override the patient's wishes. More often, it will be the psychiatrist's role to support the patient in coming to terms with the prognosis (as much as the patient chooses) so that he or she can benefit maximally from the available care. The psychiatrist also needs to assist family or staff in accepting the situation whether or not the person comes to terms with approaching death. Denial-like processes may aid coping strategies and may improve survival time (Cohen *et al.* 1997). The question is whether the denial processes should be confronted. Should patients be made to contemplate the grim realities of their future?

Case study 15.2

Mr G., a successful businessman with intractable heart failure, continued to pressure his physician to treat him vigorously. His doctor, upset by Mr G.'s demands in the face of his own therapeutic impotence referred him for psychiatric assessment. Mr G., a pushy man, used to 'making things happen', was aware of his diagnosis but had no intention of giving up without a fight—his usual way of facing challenges. Given the opportunity to acknowledge his frustration and to take back control over his life by returning home with a private nurse and having his daughter help run his business affairs, he became less demanding of those around him. He survived much longer than expected. The psychiatric team never directly addressed the issue of his terminal diagnosis.

Disagreements about treatment

Decisions about whether to treat a very old or seriously ill person are often difficult. An underlying agenda might be staff disagreement as to the worth of treatment, or the patient or family may be demanding treatment that the medical team thinks unjustified. However, the concern is usually that the person is turning down potentially life-prolonging treatment against the advice of the medical staff.

The psychiatrist's main role is to determine capacity for decision-making. Although treatment refusal reasonably triggers a capacity assessment, disagreement with the physician's opinion should not be taken as evidence of incompetence (Buchanan and Brock 1989). Appelbaum and Roth (1982) found that the reasons for the refusal of treatment could be grouped under the following headings: problems in communication, problems in trust, psychological and psychopathological factors, and hospital fatigue syndrome. Of 158 refusals, 62 were ascribed to psychological and psychopathological factors.

Psychiatric intervention may lead to resolution of the problem regardless of the patient's capacity (Steinberg 1997), or the psychiatrist may be able to help improve diminished capacity. The patient should be reassured that choosing to go against the physician's advice will not result in abandonment.

Depression and treatment refusal

The question of depression and passive suicide may arise. The treatment refused by the patient can be anything from major surgery to taking food and drink. The psychiatric role is to do a full examination and assessment of capacity. It can be hard to evaluate treatment refusal in depression, especially as the depressed person may be able to understand the medical facts in abstract but not apply them to his or her own life, and can give rational explanations for the choices made. It is difficult to distinguish realistic hopelessness from pathological hopelessness in the terminally ill patient.

Rather than superficially adhering to the ideal of patient autonomy, it is important to treat depression and other medical conditions before acceding to a wish to refuse treatment (Sullivan and Youngner 1994). Acceptance of life-sustaining treatment previously refused is associated with successful treatment of depression in the elderly (Ganzini *et al.* 1994; Hooper *et al.* 1996; Leeman 1999). Even in the palliative stages of care when the depression might be regarded as 'understandable', treatment can improve quality of life.

Refusal of food and fluids

Psychiatric assessment may be requested when an older person chooses to refuse food and fluids in a stated attempt to die. The issue is particularly difficult if there is no immediate cause for dying and the patient does not seem to have irremediable suffering. Nursing staff are often very distressed by this situation as they find it difficult to daily face a person who seems to be needlessly fading away, refusing their attempts at nourishment (Hamel *et al.* 1999).

If the person is competent to make an informed choice, the psychiatrist's role will be to validate this decision and to help the staff and family to accept it. This can put the psychiatrist in an uncomfortable role (Appelbaum and Roth 1982), but is less difficult on geriatric wards or in nursing homes where the staff are used to allowing death to occur without excessive intervention.

If there are adjustment issues the person would need an opportunity to ventilate these, although it is sometimes difficult to establish rapport with a person who has had to make such a desperate statement. Changes in the person's living arrangements or personal relationships may improve quality of life sufficiently for the person to decide to go on living. Removal of the person to a new situation may clarify diagnosis, reduce staff distress, or allow a patient to 'save face.'

Case study 15.3

After the death of a close male friend, Mrs B. (79 years of age), a widow living in institutional care, announced that life was not worth living and that she would starve herself to death. She had no life-threatening illnesses and no Axis I diagnosis. She was deemed competent. Enquiries indicated that she had previously responded dramatically to losses and a decision was made to allow her the time and opportunity to grieve.

Nevertheless, she continued to refuse food and fluids, causing great upset to the staff. The psychiatric team told her their concerns about the effect on the nurses and their own worries that they were missing a treatable psychiatric illness. She agreed to a short inpatient admission. Over the first few days she accepted parenteral rehydration and then spontaneously began to eat. She denied ever wishing to die and blamed physical illness for her anorexia. She was discharged home in good health and spirits, refusing psychiatric follow-up.

The situation is more difficult if the psychiatrist is involved late when the person is incapacitated by delirium from infection, dehydration, or electrolyte abnormalities. The issue is to decide, without access to the person, whether he or she is acting this way because of a treatable mental illness. Assessment requires discussion with family and friends, other clinical staff including the general practitioner, and review of notes. Advance directives should be read and the enduring power of attorney, if appointed, consulted. All this has to be done urgently and even then, if a decision is made to treat, it is often too late.

Advance directives (living wills)

Advance directives deal with future treatment decisions, which may need to be made when a person becomes incapacitated. They are widely recognized as directions for care when patients are unable to speak for themselves. In the US there is a requirement that federally funded nursing homes and hospitals inform newly admitted patients of their right to determine their future medical care (Janofsky and Rovner 1993; Kaufman 1998). The areas commonly addressed include treatment in the intensive-care unit, feeding, cardiopulmonary resuscitation, and, if relevant, blood transfusion. The directive may be 'instructional', that is giving explicit instructions (for example, stipulating various levels of care under specific conditions), or it may be a 'proxy' directive appointing a power of attorney for personal and healthcare decisions, or ideally both (Molloy *et al.* 1999, p. 132).

However, few elderly people have completed an advance directive or appointed an enduring power of attorney (Emanual *et al.* 1991; Janofsky and Rovner 1993). Cohen *et al.* (1997, p. 27) write about advance directives: 'it has been our impression that important and under-appreciated psycho-social barriers such as denial and avoidance commonly prevent people from formulating and expressing these wishes'. It is obviously helpful if there is prior consultation about life-prolonging treatments. However, patients may expect physicians to bring up the topic and physicians are reluctant to do so, as they fear unnecessarily alarming the patient or compromising their defence mechanisms (Kohn and Menon 1988).

The psychiatrist is unlikely to be involved in the writing of the advance directive, but may be required to assess the patient's capacity to do so.

Euthanasia

Active euthanasia (i.e. taking an action to deliberately shorten the life of an individual who is ill) has been decriminalized in The Netherlands and is now openly practised (Groenewoud *et al.* 1997; Jochemsen and Keown 1999). There have been attempts to legalize voluntary active euthanasia in many other countries, but these have so far been unsuccessful. Although active euthanasia and assisted suicide are illegal in most countries, they are thought nevertheless to be widely practised and accepted by many doctors (Kuhse *et al.* 1997; Meier *et al.* 1998). The ethics of active euthanasia continue to be widely debated in the medical and lay press. The principles involved are those of autonomy 'the patient's right to die' and non-maleficence, 'the sanctity of life'.

Passive euthanasia, i.e. the withholding or withdrawing of life-sustaining treatment, is accepted medical practice. As is the 'doctrine of double effect' in which treatment is given for relief of suffering in the knowledge that it may also speed up death, e.g. the giving of large doses of morphine for pain relief. In assisted suicide, the doctor provides the means (usually drugs) for the patient to end his or her life.

Although requests for active euthanasia or assisted suicide cannot legally be granted (outside The Netherlands), such a request should be taken seriously as a communication about the patient's experience of illness and quality of life.

Requests may represent several needs. They may be a 'cry for help' from someone whose suffering is too much. In The Netherlands, euthanasia was performed, according to medical practitioners' official reports, for 'intolerable suffering without prospect of improvement' in 74% of cases, 'to prevent loss of dignity' in 56%, and 'to prevent further suffering' in 47% (Jochemsen and Keown 1999). The request may be from a person who has difficulty in communicating needs, for example the farmer who asks to be 'put down' or a histrionic person who dramatically asks for help. Not infrequently, people misunderstand the term and are actually requesting that life-prolonging techniques not be used. However, it may be a genuine request for medical staff to speed up death for apparently rational reasons.

> Most patients in saying that they wish to die, are asking for assistance in living—for help in dealing with depression, anxiety about the future, grief, lack of control, dependence, physical suffering and spiritual despair. (Block and Billings 1995, p. 445).

The role of the psychiatric team is to assist in relieving pain and distress in whatever way possible to improve the care of the dying rather than to speed up death. This requires liaison with the treating team, and may involve the prescription of antidepressants or counselling. When depression is treated, requests for euthanasia remit in many elderly patients (Hooper *et al.* 1997).

Whenever public discussion of euthanasia becomes prominent, a few older people become fearful in hospital or refuse residential placement because they are afraid they will be involuntarily 'euthanased'. It is possible that non-voluntary euthanasia does indeed occur in The Netherlands (Jochemsen and Keown 1999), and perhaps in other countries. However, usually discussion of the local laws will relieve this anxiety. It may also be reassuring, at this point, to document the person's wishes regarding treatment at the end of life and to appoint a proxy.

There is ongoing discussion as to the rights of people with dementia with respect to euthanasia, either in the early stages of the illness while still competent or later, in response to an advance directive enacted at a predetermined stage of decline (Post 1997; Sheldon 1999). There are concerns that people with dementia may become the victims of involuntary euthanasia on the basis of a perceived 'loss of dignity' in their lives (Berghmans 1999).

There is understandable anxiety that if euthanasia becomes legal, older people may be pressured to request it. A former Governor of Colorado told an audience that elderly people 'have a duty to die and get out of the way' (Lamm 1984). Cicely Saunders of the British Hospice movement, noting a lack of healthcare resources and frequent negative attitudes towards elderly people, doubts that euthanasia would remain voluntary for long:

> Is there a society which would not exert pressure, however subtle, on the dependent to believe they are merely burdens with the responsibility to opt out or for exhausted care providers to beg or to act for their joint relief? (Saunders 1999, p. 195)

Confidentiality

The respect of confidentiality allows the patient to control his or her personal information and its dissemination and is an aspect of autonomy. The knowledge that the psychiatrist's consultation is private allows the honesty essential to gain an accurate understanding of the patient's condition.

However, confidentiality is not an absolute right. There will be times when parties not directly involved in the patient's treatment need to be informed, for example lawyers about the person's competency, or the court in mental health committal hearings. Generally, the need to breach confidentiality can be discussed with the person involved or the proxy, and only if there is a serious risk to the safety of the patient or others.

Patient confidentiality and the family

The liaison psychiatrist will often receive information from the family of a mentally ill person. This can put them in the difficult position of knowing more than the patient has disclosed. While total openness is a fine ideal, in reality families' fear damage to their relationship with the patient if that person knows how much has been told. It is important, therefore, to decide with the family how much information should be shared with the patient. At the same time one needs to be sure that the information provided is consistent with what is observed on the ward, and in one's own interactions with the person.

Advocacy

Balancing patient and family needs

A difficult problem that arises frequently is how to balance the needs and wishes of the family or caregiver against those of the older person. A common scenario is of the parent who expects her children to look after her, when the family would find this difficult. There are often unspoken underlying agendas, especially around property or complicated family dynamics.

Cultural expectations may be such that a particular family member, such as the oldest son or a daughter, is obliged to care for ageing parents. This may have been feasible in the family's native country, but immigration to Western countries means the usual supports are not available. Migration groups worldwide not only retain the customs of their country of birth but also from the era when they migrated, not realizing how much these customs may have changed over time. With the ageing of populations, especially in developing countries, the expected care may not be available in the home country either.

The psychiatrist may become involved in such issues when there are decisions to make about post-discharge accommodation, especially if there are strong emotions being expressed by the older person or family, if staff fear abuse, or there is a likelihood that the person is not competent to make a decision. It takes time to sort out these situations, and there is often pressure to move the patient on to 'free up the bed'. Nevertheless, the consultation needs to include discussion with the older person, the family separately, other caregivers in the community, and the patient's general practitioner. Sometimes a solution is negotiated that suits everyone, but often the wishes of the older person cannot be met. There is no point in sending the person back to a reluctant family, even with support. The situation will break down again and there is a risk of abuse or neglect.

Case study 15.4

Mr D., an 82-year-old man with early dementia, was admitted after a fall in which he sustained a minor injury. After assessment he was deemed safe enough to go home with community support. However, his three daughters strongly objected. He had previously turned away home help and demanded that they look after him. Mr D. had sexually abused all his daughters in their childhood. Despite (or because of) his previous treatment of them, the daughters were unable to withdraw and leave him to the care of formal support services. There was also a degree of animosity and competition between them, which Mr D exploited, by comparing how much each daughter did for him. The health of the daughters and their families were suffering. The crisis was an opportunity for them to be relieved of their burden. Mr D. reluctantly agreed to institutional care.

Advocacy on the medical ward

The liaison psychiatrist may be overtly or covertly placed in a position where he or she must advocate for the patient to achieve optimal treatment. Mental illness is frequently overlooked (McCartney and Palamateer 1985; Rapp *et al.* 1988; Ames and Tuckwell 1994) and general medical staff often feel unsure how to handle the person with a diagnosed mental disorder. A choice has to be made between the benefits of receiving treatment for the physical illness on the medical ward and transfer to a psychiatric ward, with its associated stigma and the possibility that physical care will be compromised. Whether or not the decision is made to leave the patient on the medical ward, the psychiatrist needs to educate staff and attempt to dispel myths about psychiatric illness. This can occur on a one-to-one basis or in a more formal manner. The psychiatrist will be seen as a role model and needs to show respect for each individual, recognizing cultural and cohort differences, and avoiding stereotyping and discrimination.

It may appear that the person is receiving too little, too much, or inappropriate medical care. Especially when resources are stretched, the mentally ill older person may be ignored or attempts made to discharge prematurely, despite the lack of optimal treatment for the illness. Requests may be made to admit a delirious patient to a psychiatric ward without adequate medical work-up. These situations can usually be resolved by discussion with the referrer.

Sometimes advice written after careful assessment is ignored by the treating team, much to the psychiatrist's annoyance. It is not be enough to say, 'well, I've done my bit . . .', and rationalize that the liaison psychiatrist is only there to advise. The geriatric psychiatrist needs to ensure that the best possible treatment is given. It is vital therefore to develop good communication and relationships with the referring teams (British Geriatric Society and the Royal College of Psychiatrists Joint Position statement 1992).

Institutional care

Some of the most difficult decisions in geriatric psychiatry practice are about placement in long-term care. There is no doubt that for many people, despite an initial reluctance, placement in long-term care is beneficial for both the older person and the family. As well as being relieved of the day-to-day worries about self-care, the resident has increased opportunities for social interaction and involvement in activities that would otherwise be unavailable. The person's quality of life should be better in residential care than he or she would have in any other setting (Wagner 1988, cited in Redfern 1997).

Quality of life, however, is mostly a subjective experience and it can be difficult for other people to decide what is best for a person.

Case study 15.5

Ms M., a cheerful, eccentric, 81-year-old lady, lived on her own in a flamboyantly decorated council flat in the central city. When visited, the floor was sticky with faeces and it was evident she had not cooked for a while. She was clearly dementing. She reluctantly accepted home help, but remained at some risk from 'street kids', whom she let into her flat where they probably stole things. She refused to even consider rest-home care and it was hard to imagine her fitting into institutional life.

She was admitted to hospital after being accosted and beaten. Ward staff and her niece were reluctant to let her go home again, although Ms M. had no memory of the event causing her hospitalization and no worries about her safety.

She was involuntarily placed in a secure facility. On follow-up she was well-nourished, taken for walks, and had done up her room to resemble her apartment. However, she was flat and irritable, had 'lost her spark'. Ms M. was 'safe', and the anxieties of family and health staff had been addressed, but it was unclear whether her quality of life had improved.

Elder abuse

Elder abuse is a recently recognized problem that affects 1–5% of the elderly population (Kurrle *et al.* 1997; Comijs *et al.* 1998). Abuse may be physical, psychological, sexual, or financial. Neglect by caregivers is also included, and some writers describe self-neglect. Most research has focused on abuse by family caregivers, but there is a growing awareness of abuse or neglect occurring in residential care (Pillemer and Moore 1989; Leetreweek 1994). Other more subtle forms of abuse associated with institutional stays include the use of restraint and excessive sedation (Collins 1993).

Physical or sexual abuse is most likely to be picked up by medical or nursing staff. Clues to abuse are: multiple traumas (including genital traumas), injuries that do not match the explanation given for them, postponed medical treatment, a reaction of fear or apprehension to the carer, and reluctance to investigation. Behaviour on the ward such as cringing or resistance to certain cares, for example toileting or bathing, may suggest abuse. Neglect is evident when the person arrives in the ward inadequately clothed and cold, with poor hygiene, and indications of non-compliance with essential treatment, perhaps without dentures, hearing aid, or glasses.

Patients rarely directly acknowledge abuse, especially as they are frequently dependent on the abuser. However, staff sometimes observe threats of abandonment by the carer, deference to the carer in decision-making, or excessive timidity or fearfulness. A family member may be reluctant to allow the older person privacy or demand to be present at interviews. The non-abusing family members who are concerned to see assets disappearing sometimes report financial abuse.

If the psychiatrist suspects elder abuse, management should be based on local protocols which may involve an 'adult protective service', 'elder abuse team', or experienced social workers. In some countries, reporting of elder abuse is mandatory (Capezuti *et al.* 1997). Where confidentiality is being broken, it is advisable to get the patient's permission. However, there are some situations, such as when the patient is incompetent and the next-of-kin is the abuser, when this may place the older person at more risk, for example of being abruptly removed from hospital. In many cases it will also be prudent to seek legal advice.

Elder abuse is a multifactorial problem and its management requires a team approach. After ensuring the person's safety, other interventions will depend on the situation. Counselling the older person and the family, increased social support, referral for treatment of the abuser, and protective legal interventions are all possible options.

The victim often suffers from a degree of cognitive impairment and may be unable to make decisions about future care. The liaison psychiatrist may be asked to assess competency about placement in a place of safety.

The psychiatrist must remember that not all institutional care can be regarded as safe.

Case study 15.6

Mr R., a poorly mobile but continent man with bipolar disorder, was cared for in a private hospital. On several visits he was found soaking wet and the visiting psychiatric team had to search for staff to change him. The psychiatric nurse discussed Mr R.'s need for regular toileting with the charge nurse, and with the manager when the problem persisted, but without avail. Mr R. was alert, competent, aware of his inadequate care, and the disagreement between private hospital and psychiatric staff. He was reluctant, however, to take the decision to move out. Eventually, the stress of the situation was too much and he developed a manic episode. He was admitted to the old age psychiatry ward where his mood quickly stabilized, his mobility and continence improved, and he was able to consider living elsewhere. As the psychiatric team were concerned that other patients were possibly also being neglected, they reported the incident to the monitoring agency.

The competent person who denies abuse or chooses to return to the abusive situation without intervention is difficult to deal with. As with other types of domestic abuse, all the health worker can do is to inform the person of the options available and await a later response. In such situations, autonomy overrules non-maleficence, although it is often difficult to decide whether to act more assertively and how much coercion of the older person is interfering with his or her decision-making. Issues such as the perceived risk to the person and their ability to obtain help if necessary need to be addressed.

Restraint

In the acute hospital setting the psychiatrist may be asked to review the need for physical restraint or sedation of someone whose behaviour, for example when delirious, is making care difficult. The use of restraint raises ethical issues such as the reduction of patient autonomy and the obtaining of informed consent (Evans *et al.* 1991), but it may appear necessary to prevent harm to the patient or others and to allow treatment. However, its deleterious effects on mental and physical health may outweigh benefits (Robbins *et al.* 1987; Donius and Rader 1994). Staff often resort to inappropriate management because they lack the expertise or numbers to deal with difficult behaviours, and the use of physical restraint remains relatively common worldwide (Karlson *et al.* 1996).

The liaison psychiatrist needs to weigh up the possible management options after examination of the patient and discussion with family, caregivers, and other treating staff. Sometimes it is possible to come up with a solution that avoids both physical restraint and excessive sedation. For example, a 'special' nurse or family member can supervise the person individually. Single rooms, the use of medication to reduce anxiety or hallucinations, or brief physical restraint for specific procedures are other options. Sometimes the patient can be moved to another ward more used to dealing with difficult behaviour, with the agreement that medical staff will still attend. Restraint of movement is a major assault on autonomy and not without negative consequences. Staff should be alerted to other less restrictive ways to prevent harm (Evans *et al.* 1991; Strumpf *et al.* 1992).

Rationing of healthcare on the basis of age

On the medical ward

Ageism and the stigmatization of mentally ill people may adversely affect decisions to provide medical or surgical treatment to those in need. If patients appear to be discriminated against on the basis of age or psychiatric condition, the liaison psychiatrist should discuss this with the treating doctor. With more information it may become clear that there are good clinical reasons for decisions which appeared discriminatory, and the psychiatrist can assist in explaining these to the patient and family. On the other hand, the psychiatrist may need to emphasize the anticipated improvements in quality of life or mental health to be obtained from some physical intervention. If care is being limited by the availability of resources this should be explained to the patient and family, who then have the option of looking elsewhere for care or, at least, complain.

Ongoing debates about funding certain treatments, e.g. the antidementia drugs, are driven by the need to distribute health resources justly. The elderly, often regarded as having reached their natural lifespan, are seen as having less call on available treatments, especially in the high technology areas. The older person may be less likely to undertake life-extending treatment, but this does not mean that life-extending treatments should be forcibly withheld from all persons once they have reached a certain age (Hunt 1993).

> Resource allocation based on age rather than need is ageism; a prejudice based on the presumptions that the elderly benefit little from healthcare intervention, are not in paid employment, are disproportionate consumers of benefits, and their life-expectancy is inevitably short. (Scharf *et al.* 1997, p. 9)

Various ethical guidelines state the requirement that doctors should advocate for their patients to ensure they have available the best possible health services (Royal College of Physicians 1994; Royal Australian and New Zealand College of Psychiatrists 1998). The Medical Council of New Zealand (1999) affirm that it is the doctor's responsibility 'to make clear to any patient to whom care of approved effectiveness is being denied by any funder or provider, that what is being provided is not optimal care, by generally agreed standards of medical practice.'

There is a role for the liaison psychiatrist in the general ward to encourage staff to step back from viewing their patient primarily as an 'old person', with the attendant stereotypic connotations, and to look more widely at other clinical and psychosocial aspects that should be taken into account when making decisions.

Older people with mental illness are often 'forgotten members of our society'. Theirs is not a well-organized constituency with a strong voice (Rosoff and Gottlieb 1987). Points to be considered in speaking for them include the recognition of universal human rights, a moral requirement to help the weak, and the acknowledgment of prior contribution even if the person is no longer economically productive (Siegler 1984). Older people with mental illness must rely on others not only to help them get along in life but also to design and implement the structures within which support can best be provided.

References

Ames, D. and Tuckwell, V. (1994). Psychiatric disorders among elderly patients in a general hospital. *Medical Journal of Australia*, **160**, 671–5.

Appelbaum, P. and Grisso, T. (1988). Assessing patients' capacities to consent to treatment. *New England Journal of Medicine*, **319**, 135–8.

Appelbaum, P.S. and Roth, L.H. (1982). Treatment refusal in medical hospitals. In *Report of the President's Commission for the study of ethical problems in medicine and biomedical and behavioural research*. Government Printing Office, Washington, DC.

Berghmans, R.L. (1999). Ethics of end-of-life decisions in cases of dementia: views of the Royal Dutch Medical Association with some critical comments. Alz*heimer Disease and Related Disorders*, **13**, 91–5.

Block, S. and Billings, J. (1995). Patient requests for euthanasia and assisted suicide in terminal illness: the role of the psychiatrist. *Psychosomatics*, **36**, 445–57.

British Geriatrics Society and the Royal College of Psychiatrists Standing Joint Committee. (1992). Revised Guidelines. *Psychiatric Bulletin*, **16**, 583–4.

Buchanan, A.E. and Brock, D.W. (1989). *Deciding for others: the ethics of surrogate decision-making*. Cambridge University Press, Cambridge.

Capezuti, E., Brush, B.L., and Lawson, W.T. (1997). Reporting elder mistreatment. *Journal of Gerontological Nursing*, **23**, 24–32.

Cohen, L.M., McCue, J.D., Germain, M., and Woods, A. (1997). Denying the dying, advance directives and dialysis discontinuation. *Psychosomatics*, **38**, 27–34.

Collins, J. (1993). *The resettlement game: policy and procrastination in the closure of mental handicap hospitals. Values into action report*. Joseph Rowntree Foundation, London.

Comijs, H.C., Pot, A.M., Swit, J.H., Bouter, L.M., and Jonker, C. (1998). Elder abuse in the community: prevalence and consequences. *Journal of the American Geriatrics Society*, **46**, 885–8.

Donius, M. and Rader, J. (1994). Use of siderails: rethinking of a standard practice. *Journal of Gerontological Nursing*, Nov, 23–7.

Drane, J.F. (1985). The many faces of competency. *Hastings Centre Report*, **14**, 17–21.

Emanuel, L.L., Barry, M.J., Stoeckle, J.D., and Ettleson, E.J. (1991). Advance directives for medical care: a case for greater use. *New England Journal of Medicine*, **324**(13), 889–95.

Evans, L.K., Strumpf, M.E., and Williams, C. (1991). Redefining a standard of care for frail older people. Alternatives to routine physical restraint. In *Advances in long term care*, Vol. 1 (ed. P. Katz, R. Kane, and M. Mezey), pp. 81–108. Springer, New York.

Ganzini, L., Lee, M., Heimtz, R., Bloom, J., and Fenn, D. (1994). The effect of depression treatment on elderly patient's preferences for life-sustaining treatment. *American Journal of Psychiatry*, **151**, 1631–6.

Groenewoud, J.H., van der Maas, P.J., van der Wal, G., Hengeveld, M.W., Tholen, A.J., Schudel, W.J., *et al.* (1997). Physician-assisted death in psychiatric practice in the Netherlands. *New England Journal of Medicine*, **336**, 1795–801.

Hamel, M.B., Teno, J.M., Goldman, L., Lynn, J., Davis, R.B., Galanos, A.N., *et al.* (1999). Patient age and decisions to withhold life-sustaining treatments from seriously ill, hospitalized adults. SUPPORT Investigators. Study to Understand Prognoses and Preferences for Outcomes and Risks of Treatment. *Annals of Internal Medicine*. **130**, 116–25.

Harrison, A., al-Saadi, A.M., al-Kaabi, M.R., al-Bedwawi, S.S., al-Kaabi, S.O., and al-Neaimi, S.B. (1997). Should doctors inform terminally ill patients? The opinions of nationals and doctors in the United Arab Republic. *Journal of Medical Ethics*, **23**, 101–2.

Hesse, K.A. (1993). Ethical issues and terminal management of the old old. *Abstracts of the meeting of The Boston Society for Gerontological Psychiatry Inc., 'Older Old People'*, Oct. 30th, 75–92.

Hooper, S.C., Vaughn, K.J., Tennant, C.C., and Perz, J.M. (1996). Major depression and refusal of life-sustaining medical treatment in the elderly. *Medical Journal of Australia*, **165**, 416–19.

Hooper, S.C., Vaughn, K.J., Tennant, C.C., and Perz, J.M. (1997). Preferences for voluntary euthanasia during major depression and following improvement in an elderly population. *Australian Journal on Ageing*, **16**, 3–7.

Hunt, R.W. (1993). A critique of using age to ration health care. *Journal of Medical Ethics*, **19**(1), 19–23.

Janofsky, J.S. and Rovner, B.W. (1993). Prevalence of advance directives and guardianship in nursing home patients. *Journal of Geriatric Psychiatry and Neurology*, **6**, 214–16.

Jochemsen, H. and Keown, J. (1999). Voluntary euthanasia under control? Further empirical evidence from the Netherlands. *Journal of Medical Ethics*, **25**, 16–21.

Karlson, S, Bucht, G., Eriksson, S., and Sandman, P. (1996). Physical restraints in geriatric care in Sweden: prevalence and patient characteristics. *Journal of the American Geriatrics Society*, **44**, 1348–54.

Katz, M., Abbey, S., Rydall, A., and Lowy, F. (1995). Psychiatric consultations for competency to refuse medical treatment. *Psychosomatics*, **36**, 33–4.

Kaufman, S.R. (1998). Intensive care, old age, and the problem of death in America. *The Gerontologist*, **38**, 715–25.

Kohn, M. and Menon, G. (1988). Life prolongation: views of elderly outpatients and health care professionals. *Journal of the American Geriatrics Society*, **36**, 840–4.

Kuhse, H., Singer, P., Baume, P., Clark, M., and Rickard, M. (1997). End of life decisions in Australian medical practice. *Medical Journal of Australia*, **199**, 191–6.

Kurrle, S.E., Sadler, P.M., Lockwood, K., and Cameron, I.D. (1997). Elder abuse: prevalence, intervention and outcomes in patients referred to four Aged Care Assessment Teams. *Medical Journal of Australia*, **166**, 119–22.

Lamm, R. (1984). *New York Times*, 28th Mar.

Leeman, C.P. (1999). Depression and the right to die. *General Hospital Psychiatry*, **21**, 112–15.

Leetreweek, G. (1994). Bedroom abuse: the hidden work in a nursing home. *Generations Review*, **4**, 2–4.

Lutteril, S. (1997). Assessing mental capacity for decisions about medical treatment. CME Bulletin, *Geriatric Medicine*, **1**,19.

McCartney, J. and Palamateer, L.L. (1985). Assessment of cognitive deficit in geriatric patients: a study of physician behaviour. *Journal of the American Geriatrics Society*, **33**, 467–71.

Medical Council of New Zealand. (1999). *Ethical guidelines for doctors' duties in an environment of competition or resource limitation*. Medical Council of New Zealand, Wellington.

Meier, D.E., Emmons, C., Wallenstein, S., Quill, T., Morrison, R., and Cassel, C. (1998). A national survey of physician assisted suicide and euthanasia in the United States. *New England Journal of Medicine*, **338**, 1193–201.

Molloy, D., Darzins, P., and Strang, D. (1999). *Capacity to decide* (1st edn). Newgrange Press, Troy, Ontario.

Oppenheimer, C. (1999). Ethics in old age psychiatry. In *Psychiatric ethics* (3rd edn) (ed. S. Bloch, P. Chodoff, and S.A. Green), p. 333, Oxford University Press, Oxford.

Osuna, E., Perez-Carceles, M., Esteban, M., and Luna, A. (1998). Right to information in the terminally ill patient. *Journal of Medical Ethics*, **24**, 106–9.

Pillemer, K. and Moore, D. (1989). Abuse of patients in nursing homes: findings from a survey of staff. *The Gerontologist*, **29**, 314–20.

Post, S. (1997). Physician-assisted suicide in Alzheimer's disease. *Journal of the American Geriatrics Society*, **45**, 647–51.

Rapp, S., Walsh, D., and Parisi, S. (1988). Detecting depression in elderly medical inpatients. *Journal of Consulting and Clinical Psychology*, **56**, 509–13.

Redfern, S. (1997). Supporting residents in long-stay settings. In *Mental health care for elderly people* (ed. I. Norman and S. Redfern), p. 499. Churchill Livingstone, Edinburgh.

Reisberg, B., Borenstein, J., Salob, S.P., Ferris, S.H., Franssen, E., and Georgotas, A. (1987). Behavioural symptoms in Alzheimer's disease: phenomenology and treatment. *Journal of Clinical Psychiatry*, **14**, Suppl. 9–15.

Robbins, L.J., Boyko, E., Lane, J., Cooper, D., and Jahnigen, D.W. (1987). Binding the elderly: a prospective study of the use of mechanical restraints in an acute care hospital. *Journal of the American Geriatrics Society*, **35**, 290–6.

Rosoff, A. and Gottlieb, G. (1987). Preserving personal autonomy for the elderly, competency, guardianship and Alzheimer's disease. *The Journal of Legal Medicine*, **8**, 1–47.

Royal Australian and New Zealand College of Psychiatrists. (1998). *The RANZCP Code of Ethics, Principle Ten*. RANZCP, Melbourne.

Royal College of Physicians. (1994). *Ensuring equity and quality of care for elderly people*. Royal College of Physicians, London.

Saunders, C. (1999). Medical ethics: dying in a technological age. In *The last dance: encountering death and dying* (5th edn) (ed. L.A. DeSpelder, A.L Strickland, and A. Lee), p. 203. Mayfield Publishing, Mountain View, California, USA.

Scharf, S., Flamer, H., and Christophidis, N. (1997). Age as a basis of health care rationing, arguments against agism. Guest Editorial. *New Ethicals*, March 1, 8–13.

Schwarz, H.I. and Blank, K. (1986). Shifting competency during hospitalization: a model for informed consent decisions. *Hospital and Community Psychiatry*, **37**, 1256–60.

Sheldon,T. (1999). Euthanasia endorsed in Dutch patient with dementia. *British Medical Journal*, **319**, 75.

Siegler, M. (1984). Should age be a criterion in health care? *Hastings Centre Report*, Oct. 24–27.

Steinberg, M. (1997). Psychiatry and bioethics, an exploration of the relationship. *Psychosomatics*, **38**, 313–20.

Strumpf, N.E., Evans, L.K., Wagner, J., and Patterson, J. (1992). Reducing physical restraints: developing an educational program. *Journal of Gerontological Nursing*, **18**, 21–7.

Sullivan, M. and Youngner, S. (1994). Depression, competence, and the right to refuse lifesaving medical treatment. *American Journal of Psychiatry*, **151**, 971–8.

Umapathy, C., Ramchandani, D., Lamdan, R., Kishel, L., and Schindler, B. (1999). Consultation evaluations on the consultation-liaison service: some overt and covert aspects. *Psychosomatics*, **40**, 28–33.

16 A legal perspective on issues in geriatric liaison psychiatry

Hanneke Bouchier

Summary

Obtaining the consent of patients with psychiatric disorders to medical or surgical treatment will often involve an assessment of competency to consent. In the absence of legal mental capacity, the attending medical practitioner should make enquiries about whether a substituted authority exists. This may include advanced directives, a living will, or the appointment of a welfare guardian by the patient. It may require an application to the Court for appointment of a welfare guardian or for the Court's authorization for the procedure. Alternatively, medical intervention may be justified because of necessity. This does not require an emergency. The circumstances and standards of care applicable is determined by the Bolam test. Where a patient in a medical or surgical ward requires possible psychiatric treatment, local mental health statutes will usually outline the processes for preliminary assessment and treatment of the patient, and these do not require the consent of the patient. The statutory provisions in mental health statutes restrict the all-important principle of autonomy and are for that reason interpreted narrowly by the Courts.

Introduction

Geriatric liaison psychiatry is concerned with the transfer of elderly patients from surgical or medical services to a psychiatric system of care, and vice versa. This patient group may be characterized by reduced mental capacity or no legal capacity. Thus, patients' further treatment, and transfer of their personal information between medical systems, raises specific legal issues that include consent to treatment, competency, absence of consent, treatment under statute, advanced directives, necessity, and privacy. These issues will be discussed in this chapter, noting that, generally, legal provisions will define the legal rights and obligations of both patient and medical practitioner.

This chapter will focus on the following areas:

1. Sources of law
2. Duty of care imposed by law
   • General duty to care
   • The doctor as fiduciary
   • Statutory duty of care
3. Consent
   • Form of consent
   • Some issues in competency
   • Consent via living wills (advanced directives)
4. Absence of consent
   • Third-party decision-making—welfare guardianship/enduring power of attorney
   • Statutory power to treat—Court appointment/authority
   • Necessity
5. Confidentiality

Sources of law

Law is a matter for each sovereign state, and unlike medicine, sovereign laws have no universal application. Nevertheless, there is considerable uniformity in the substantive principles in the Western world even where administrative processes differ.

Law arises from two sources—from statute, which is the written law issued by Parliament, or from common law, which is judge-made law through court cases. Common law principles may become 'codified', that is, reduced to a written form and in this way become statute law. However, the Courts continue to have a role in the interpretation of statutory provisions and thus the judgments of court cases provide an important source of law. For example, much of the law of negligence is still essentially in case law, and the standards of care continue to evolve as case law defines and refines the applicable criteria required to meet the duty of care.

However, statutes are a higher source of law than common law, and where common law becomes codified in statute, the statutory provisions will prevail in the event of conflict. Some common law is now replaced by statute. These may include legislative provisions for privacy, psychiatric treatment, advanced directives, and patient rights involving medical treatment. Countries, for example, New Zealand, with express human rights protection are likely to enshrine the fundamental principle of individual autonomy, which extends to the right to refuse medical even life-saving treatment (The New Zealand Bill of Rights Act 1990).[1]

Those involved with the medical care or treatment of geriatric psychiatric patients need to become familiar with the locally applicable laws and procedures. Medical practitioners need to be familiar with statutory provisions, which apply in the country and place where they work.

Duty of care imposed by law

General duty of care

When a doctor accepts responsibility for treatment of a patient, a general duty for the practitioner to use diligence, knowledge, skill and care in administering treatment applies. This duty is imposed by common law and medical ethics. There are circumstances in which the law imposes an additiional duty of care, discussed as follows.

The doctor as a fiduciary

The vulnerability of this patient group, and their dependence on caregivers, may give rise to circumstances that attract duties of a fiduciary nature. A fiduciary relationship is one in which the law imposes upon one person a paternalistic obligation of care towards another. In some circumstances, the common law, in its equity function, recognizes that certain relationships are characterized by the control by one party and the vulnerability of another. The most explicit fiduciary relationship exists between a trustee and a beneficiary. While North American Courts have been ready to characterize the doctor–patient relationship as fiduciary, other countries have been less willing to do so, preferring to recognize duties of care as those usually arising from the professional doctor–patient relationship. Nevertheless, even in the absence of a fiduciary relationship, the particular circumstances of a relationship may nevertheless incorporate some duties of a fiduciary kind. This is likely where particular vulnerability exists, such as with patients with a high degree of dependence such as the elderly or the psychiatrically impaired, and who require medical or psychiatric treatment but may be unable to arrange for their own care. This may give rise to a duty to be proactive in ensuring the patient obtains needed treatment, and to ensure that a lawful basis exists for such treatment.

Statutory duty of care

A duty of care can also be imposed by statute. This may arise where there is legislative recognition of the vulnerability of highly dependent persons and who are for that reason unable to provide the necessities of life for themselves. While such statutory provisions may be particularly relevant for the care of children, clearly any person with particular vulnerability, including the elderly, falls within their contemplation. Penal provisions may back this duty, so that a person's failure to provide basic care and safety for someone in their care may expose them to criminal sanction.

Consent

There are very few circumstances where a patient's consent is not required for medical treatment. They are broadly in areas of preliminary psychiatric assessment and compulsory treatment for mental disorder, and in some public health situations. In all other cases, the consent of the patient is required, or some other lawful basis for treatment must be present.

The significance of obtaining consent is twofold. It protects the health professional against any legal suit of assault or battery, since medical treatment may involve physical interventions, which would otherwise be unlawful and actionable. The second reason is clinical compliance by the patient. However, consent is not required where intervention is authorized by statute, and the medical practitioner can provide such medical treatment as falls within the statutory provisions, with legal immunity.

The three aspects to personal consent are competency, information, and freedom. Consent presupposes legal mental capacity, or competency. Any challenges to consent for general medical treatment involving psychiatric or cognitively impaired patients will usually be based on the patient's lack of competency. The kind and extent of information given to a patient may depend upon the capacity to understand.

Form of consent

Consent may be expressly given, or may be implied. Most health-provider institutions use consent forms. The advantage of such explicit consent is that the written form is evidence of both the fact of, and the nature of, the consent. Although consent, expressly given, need not be in a written form, the absence of such evidence can be disadvantageous if contest to these issues occurs subsequently.

Consent may also be implied from a person's conduct. This would most often occur when the patient allows an explained procedure without any expressed consent and without protest. When a person's mental status impairs autonomy, this kind of passive conduct can be mistaken for consent.

Some issues in competency

Competency is a prerequisite to a patient's legal capacity to personally consent to treatment. Health professionals can rely on the legal defence of 'consent' only if the patient is competent to grant consent. Ensuring that medical treatment is lawful must be of paramount concern to treating clinicians because consent is the only defence for potential allegations of assault, battery, or detention. Ultimately, the treating physician will be legally accountable for administering medical treatment, and where applicable, the health-provider organization will be vicariously liable.

The main approaches to measuring competency are: (1) status and (2) understanding.

Status

A common perception is that a person who has a mental disorder is precluded, by virtue of that status, from being able to give lawful consent to medical treatment. Professor Skegg has dismissed this view in his book *Law, ethics and medicine* (1984):

> The fact that a person is suffering from a mental disorder, as defined by the Mental Health Act 1983, does not of itself preclude that person from giving a legally effective consent. Whether the person is capable of doing so depends upon whether that person can understand and come to a decision upon what is involved. Most patients in mental hospitals are capable of giving a legally effective consent, including many who are compulsorily detained. (pp. 72, 73)

The basic principle is that the mentally disordered person is not, only by virtue of that status, legally incompetent to consent to treatment.

'Competency' is a not only a medical and psychiatric concept, but a social and legal issue as well, and one single test to establish competency is unlikely to be found. If an individual is not incompetent because of mental illness, then whether such a person is capable of consenting depends on their ability to understand what is involved in the treatment and their capacity to come to a decision (see Chapters 5 and 15).

Understanding

A patient, who is legally competent to consent to treatment, is equally competent to refuse treatment, however unreasonable such refusal might appear to be. However, refusal by the patient of reasonable treatment may be seen as 'evidence' of incompetence when the refusal disagrees with other views of what is reasonable and where the valence of the patient's refusal is against the risk:benefits ratio. It is important to discern the difference between the patient exercising autonomy, and inability to exercise autonomy; the patient's choice cannot, *per se*, be evidence of this.

The test for competency may vary from one context to another, so that an individual could be considered competent for one purpose but not for another. To satisfy any evaluation, tests must include reliability of application, be mutually comprehensible to the medical (and legal) fraternity, and be capable of providing a balance between preserving individual autonomy and providing necessary medical care. The test has more validity if it relies on manifest behaviour rather depending on inferred and unknown mental status.

There are a number of approaches to testing a patient's level of understanding for purposes of consenting to treatment. The following examples are based on observed practices:

1. In practical terms, there is a greater likelihood of presuming patient competency to consent where the patient's agreement to treatment aligns with the recommendation of the health professional. As there will usually be a bias on the part of doctors (and judges) in favour of providing beneficial treatment, a test of competency is applied that will permit the treatment to be given, irrespective of the patient's actual or potential understanding. However, there is a possible hazard in shortcutting the process where there is limited understanding because supposedly consent has been obtained. When the proposed treatment is invasive or has potential risks, the onus of establishing that the patient understood those risks may fall on the practitioner if there is an adverse outcome.

2. Measuring levels of competency—from low to high thresholds:

(a) The lowest-level test for competency is a reliance on the patient providing 'evidence for a choice'—through words (express) or behaviour (implied)— either for or against treatment. This test focuses on the choice made, not the quality of that choice. This can be illustrated by the depressed patient who, when interviewed and recommended for hospital admission, does not respond in any way. He neither agrees nor disagrees and does nothing even when he has the opportunity to walk away. As this test requires some evidence of a decision, the patient who proffers no preference at all may be considered incompetent. This is a low test of competency that does not assure the patient's understanding of the nature of what they consented to or refused.

(b) A slightly higher test is one that measures competency based upon the 'reasonableness' of the patient's decision. A measure of 'reasonableness' may be the congruency between the patient's decision and that of the reasonable person (or the doctor). However, by equating the patient's unreasonableness with incompetence, the promotion of social goals and individual health may be at the cost of patient autonomy. The failure to further investigate the issue means that there is an assumption of competence, which may not exist in fact.

(c) A higher test for competency is one based on 'rational reasons'. This looks to whether the reasons for the patient's decision are due to a mental illness. As with the above test, because of the medical profession's bias in favour of necessary treatment, congruence between the patient's decision and that of the medical professional is likely to avoid further enquiry as to competence. To illustrate, an elderly undernourished patient, who lives alone amidst the faeces of her cats, comes into hospital for treatment. Her thinking is fragmented and she appears delusional but is not hallucinating. She refuses a blood test because, 'You just want to spread my blood over the town'. Incompetence is assumed due to the irrationality of the decision. The doctor does not press for the blood sample then, but treatment is later given (and justified) on the grounds of necessity when the woman's blood pressure is found to be dangerously high.

(d) The highest test for competency is ascertaining the patient's ability to understand the risk and benefits of treatment. An irrational process or outcome is accepted, but the patient needs to demonstrate understanding even if the processing of information is different from that of the medical practitioner. Asking a series of relevant questions about the risk and benefits and about alternatives can test the level of understanding. For example, an elderly non-psychotic woman diagnosed as schizophrenic in remission may refuse amputation of her frostbitten toes. She understands the proposed treatment and the infection risk of no treatment, but is psychiatrically evaluated as having extreme denial. She declines treatment, insisting she wants to keep her toes on. Her decision is accepted. This test is probably the nearest to informed consent. Yet, this raises questions about how sophisticated the understanding should be for the patient to be considered competent.

The issue of competency in seeking consent needs careful attention where psychiatric patients require transfer to medical or surgical systems. The physician is liable not only for treatment given without lawful consent, but may also be liable for failing to provide treatment where refusal of consent is due to lack of competency of the patient. The issues are not always clear. As shall be discussed later, the legal basis for unauthorized medical intervention necessary for the patient's health or well-being is only prescribed when incompetency exists.

Consent via living wills/advanced directives

In the event that a person may suffer mental incapacity at some future time, he/she may make provision for their health and welfare by means of a document often called a 'living will'. Where, instead, a person appoints a proxy decision-maker by way of a power of attorney, this is not equivalent to the consent of the patient. This is discussed in more detail below. However, both these activities are 'advanced directives' since the patient makes prior arrangements for the making of health decisions at a future time.

A living will can be made only when a person is competent, and it becomes operative only when the circumstances contemplated by the document arise. A living will usually addresses future life-sustaining treatments in life-threatening situations, but may be drafted to include any healthcare situation in which people may anticipate an absence of capacity to make a decision at a future time. The controversy around their legal effectiveness and application is beyond the present discussion. However, when a living will is produced in circumstances where a life-sustaining decision must be made, any local legislation will determine the status and application of the specific document. In the absence of legislation, common law principles will apply. These have been discussed by the English Court of

Appeal in Re T (1992), which established four elements for a living will to be valid. They are:

1. The person is competent at the time the document is drawn up.
2. No undue influence is exerted on the person in creating the directive.
3. The directive must be made with informed consent.
4. The subsequent circumstances that arise must be those anticipated by the directive.

Discussion with relatives will often point to the existence of a living will. Where there is concern about the legal status of an advanced directive of this kind, medical practitioners should be cautious in complying with advance directives that are inconsistent with good medical practice, and should seek legal advice.

Verbal instructions may be given for medical treatment in future situations, but reliance on this alone would be hazardous by the treating doctor.

Absence of consent

Except where the proposed treatment is of a psychiatric nature (see below), the consent of the patient is always required. In the absence of personal consent, some other lawful basis for treatment is necessary.

A common view is that a spouse or a near relative can consent to medical treatment. However, the general rule is that no one can consent to medical treatment on behalf of an incompetent adult. Where competency cannot be established with any degree of confidence, another lawful basis for medical intervention is required. This may be via a lawfully appointed proxy decision-maker, being a welfare guardian appointed by the patient at an earlier date, or by a welfare guardian appointed through the Court under statutory provisions. Alternatively, authorization for specific treatment can be obtained from the Court on an *ad hoc* basis, noting that such authority is in fact a pronouncement on the lawfulness of the procedure, and not an order to treat. Alternatively, the existence of necessity can provide a lawful basis for medical treatment. These will be discussed in turn.

Third-party decision-making—welfare guardianship/enduring power of attorney

By personal appointment

A person may wish to appoint another person to make welfare decisions for them in the event they are unable to do so at a future time. An appointment made under a normal power of attorney cannot achieve this objective for two reasons. First, such appointment does not allow for health and personal welfare decisions to be made, as the power is essentially an agency for property affairs. Second, a power of attorney automatically ends when the appointer becomes mentally incapacitated, and that is the very time when the substituted decision-making would be required. To overcome these objections, some countries have passed statutes that allow for a power of attorney that becomes operative at the point of incapacity, and to provide for substituted consent in matters of health and welfare. This is another form of advanced directive. The relevant legislation sets out the requirements for such an appointment to be lawful. Medical practitioners can rely on the authority of appointees to administer medical treatment of the now incapacitated person. However, if consent is unreasonably withheld against the interests of the patient, the doctor should not rely on the appointee's refusal and should, instead, seek consent to the proposed treatment from the appropriate statutory body or Court.

Geriatric patients should be encouraged to appoint a welfare guardian whilst they are still competent, and treating physicians should enquire as to the existence of such appointment.

Statutory power to treat—Court appointment/authority

Many countries have some form of welfare statute that provides for the appointment by the Court of a welfare guardian for persons who are unable to make personal decisions for their own welfare. In the event of a person likely to remain incompetent for some time and needing medical treatment or other welfare decisions making, an application can be made to the Court for the appointment of a welfare guardian, if there is a statute providing for such appointment.

The Court's jurisdiction to make such an appointment will be based on evidence of incompetency. This is usually set at a lower threshold than that required to determine a mental disorder as defined by mental health statutes. The Court's jurisdiction to appoint a welfare guardian may arise if the patient lacks, wholly or partly, the capacity to understand the nature or consequences of decisions relevant to their personal welfare, or lacks the capacity to communicate such decisions. The statute will define the categories of possible applicants, which will usually include relatives, the doctor, or other health provider. There will be some legislative control over the proxy decision-making process.

Limitations set out in the relevant statute are likely to exclude power to consent to socially controversial treatments such as ECT, experimental surgery, or removal of tissue. The relevant legislation is also likely to prohibit refusal to consent to standard medical treatment or life-saving procedures. Doctors may safely provide treatment on the instructions of a Court-appointed welfare guardian acting within their statutory authority.

In the absence of a welfare guardian, when consent to one-off treatment is required, or when approval is required for a treatment outside the jurisdiction of a welfare guardian, authority to treat should be sought through the Court. This process avoids any potential challenges concerning lawful authorization for treatment.

Necessity

It is generally recognized that where a patient is unable to consent for any reason but requires medical treatment necessary to save his/her life or avoid serious harm, such treatment as is necessary for that purpose is legally justifiable, notwithstanding the absence of lawful consent. Legal justification usually contemplates the unconscious patient in a car accident and in the context of an emergency. However, the principle of justification based on necessity goes further and can apply to general medical treatment of incompetent people. The absence of a formal proxy or other means of obtaining lawful authorization presents a practical problem when incompetent people require medical treatment. The British House of Lords addressed this issue in Re F (1990) and concluded that the principle of necessity was not necessarily confined to emergencies. The principle is based on an agent, acting on behalf of a principal, when an intervention is justifiable because it is necessary. Pointing out that reliance on justification was available only in the absence of a lawfully appointed guardian or advance directives, the Law Lords applied this principle to the situation of an incompetent person in need of medical treatment.

In describing the circumstances of the application of the principle of necessity, Lord Goff in Re F (1990) stated:

> Another example ... is that of a mentally disordered person who is disabled from giving consent. I can see no good reason why the principle of necessity should not be applicable in his case as it is in the case of the victim of a stroke. Furthermore, in the case of a mentally disordered person, as in the case of a stroke victim, the permanent state of affairs calls for a wider range of care than may be requisite in an emergency, which arises from accidental injury. Where the state of affairs is permanent, or semi-permanent, action properly taken to preserve the life, health or well-being of the assisted person may well transcend and may extend to include such humdrum matters as routine medical or dental treatment, even simple care such as dressing and undressing and putting to bed.

He observed that in the circumstances of a temporarily unconscious or temporarily incompetent patient who requires life-saving surgery, the principle of justification is limited to essential treatment only, on the basis that the patient will be able to consent to additional treatment on gaining consciousness or resuming competency. However, this is not the case with the permanently mentally disabled:

> But where the state of affairs is permanent or semi-permanent, as be so in the case of a mentally disordered person, there is no point in waiting to obtain the patient's consent. The need to care for him is obvious; and the doctor must then act in the best interests of his patient, just as if he had received his patient's consent so to do.

Lord Goff determined that, where the doctor–patient relationship exists, the doctor might in fact have a duty to treat the patient.

He continued:

> I have said that the doctor has to act in the best interest of the assisted person. In the case of routine treatment of the mentally disordered person, there should be little difficulty in applying this principle. In the case of more serious treatment, I

recognise that its application may create problems for the medical profession; however, in making decisions about treatment, the doctor must act in accordance with a responsible and competent body of relevant professional opinion, on the principles set down in Bolam v Friern Hospital Management Committee [(1957)].

The 'Bolam test' accepts that a doctor would be acting in the best interest of his patient if 'a responsible and competent body of relevant professional opinion' would support the doctor's conduct. Some commentators have pointed out that while Bolam may be authoritative on the appropriateness of treatment, the issue of whether to treat at all is not necessarily confined to medical issues. While Lord Goff agrees that it is good practice to consult relatives and others concerned with the care of the patient, in practice differences may arise between the opinion of the treating physician and that of relatives. These differences may be about whether to treat at all, as well as the kind of treatment proposed. When confronted with opposing views from relatives, the physician may be reluctant to proceed to treat, despite medical evidence that supports treatment serving the patient's interest. In that case, the physician may wish to obtain the protection of a Court's authorization, whether the concern is over the decision to treat at all, or regarding the kind of treatment. In the case of the permanently incapacitated person, even if the Bolam test based on medical evidence appears to prevail, it is likely that a determination whether to treat at all will invoke a balancing of medical factors and issues of public interest.

Treatment authorized by statute

Treatment can be given, in proscribed circumstances, under statutory authority. Since most societies recognize that any kind of compulsory medical treatment significantly undermines the highly valued principle of autonomy, the circumstances of forced intervention are usually very narrowly and specifically defined. These will include treatment of the psychiatrically impaired person under the authority of Mental Health statutes. Medical practitioners relying on statutory provisions to assess and treat a patient against their will must take care to ensure strict compliance with the procedures set down in the statute. Furthermore, mental health laws cannot be used to justify medical treatment other than the treatment proposed by the statutes. Any detention and assessment pursuant to mental health provisions for treatments not related to psychiatric treatment, such as general medical or surgical procedures, are likely to be unlawful (*R* v. *Collins* [1998]).[2]

Confidentiality

The obligation to keep medical information confidential is universally recognized as one of the most fundamental duties owed by the doctor to the patient. This general right is recognized at common law. The collection and use of health information may be covered by statute.

For the purposes of the present chapter, the extent of lawful sharing of personal health information between medical systems for mentally impaired patients raises the question of the scope and the limits of the duty of confidentiality. There may be different views as to the basis of this duty. For example, it may be viewed in terms of the *status* of the relationship, so that the basis of this duty lies in the existence of the doctor–patient relationship and the patient's trust in the doctor not to reveal clinical information without permission. An alternative approach is based on *capacity*, so that the duty is premised on the ability of the patient to form a relationship of confidence with the doctor. Here, the duty does not arise where the patient is unable to form such a relationship. Whilst these views are usually explored in the context of the medical treatment of children, there are clear parallels for the permanently incompetent patient. The different approaches have significantly dissimilar legal implications, the first being against disclosure, where any exceptions must be justified, and the second favouring disclosure except where there is a good reason for not doing so. There are obvious problems that could arise for the mentally incompetent adult. The legal debate could be resolved by the law taking the view that the relationship between doctor and patient gives rise to some fiduciary duties, for example that the provision of medical care will impose a duty of confidentiality but allows disclosure of medical information to the extent necessary for the welfare of the patient.

When consent has been obtained more general legal principles allow disclosure or sharing of medical information to the extent necessary for treatment of the patient, especially when anticipated treatment involves a team of physicians, who may require a number of clinical investigations. The patient will be considered to have given consent to such sharing of information as is necessary to enable the treatments or investigations to take place. The treatment team, as a whole, has the obligation of confidentiality.

Some countries have codified the law in this area of general obligations of confidentiality with Privacy laws, which define both the obligation of confidence and the circumstances for lawful use and disclosure. When applied to medical situations, lawful disclosure provisions will usually involve situations of safety for the person or members of the public.

In conclusion

Obtaining the consent of psychiatric patients to medical or surgical treatment will often involve assessment of competency to consent. In the absence of legal mental capacity, the attending medical practitioner should make enquiries about whether a substituted authority exists. This may be an advanced directive, such as a living will or the appointment by the patient of a welfare guardian. It may require an application to the Court for appointment of a welfare guardian or for the Court's authorization for the procedure. Alternatively, medical intervention may be justified because of necessity. This does not require an emergency. The basis of the applicable circumstances and standards of care is the Bolam test.

Where a patient in a medical or surgical ward requires possible psychiatric treatment, local mental health statutes will usually outline the processes for preliminary assessment and treatment of the patient, and these do not require the consent of the patient. The statutory provisions in mental health statutes restrict the all-important principle of autonomy and are for that reason interpreted narrowly by the Courts.

References

Bolam v. *Friern Hospital Management Committee* [1957] 1 WLR 582.

R v. *Collins, ex parte* [1998] 3 All ER 673.

Re F (a mental patient: sterilisation) [1990] 2 AC 1.

Re T, [1992] 4 All ER 649.

Skegg, P.D.G. (1984). *Law, ethics and medicine: studies in medical law*. Clarendon Press, Oxford.

The New Zealand Bill of Rights Act (1990), s.11.

Notes

1. S.11 states, 'Everyone has the right to refuse to undergo any medical treatment'.
2. In *R* v. *Collins*, Ms Collins expressly refused a caesarean section against medical advice. Her decision raised concern over her mental state, which drove the hospital to detain her under the Mental Health Act 1983 and seek an *ex parte* order for surgery to be undertaken. The Court of Appeal set aside the High Court, and compensated Ms Collins in respect of that and the hospital's *ex parte* application for compulsory admission under the Mental Health Act 1983.

Glossary

Activities of daily living
Practical self-care activities such as toileting, bathing, feeding, transferring, walking. Instrumental activities of daily living include housework, telephoning, cooking, shopping, managing finances, and laundry.

ADARDS
Alzheimer and Related Disorders Society, is a lay organization of caregivers and professionals dedicated to the increased awareness of Alzheimer's disease and related dementias and to supporting caregivers of sufferers of the disease. Similar organizations exist in many countries and have a variety of names, e.g. Alzheimer's Association, Alzheimer Society, etc.

Advance directives/living wills
Advance directives deal with treatment decisions that may need to be made in the future if a person becomes incapacitated.

Affective disorders
Mental disorders that affect mood state. Examples are depressive illness, bipolar affective disorders.

Ageing
A progressive accumulation of changes over time, which causes the systems and structures of the organism to lose function, decline, and eventually die.

Ageism
A negative prejudice against older people on the grounds of chronological age.

Amnestic disorders
A group of disorders characterized by loss of memory in the absence of other cortical dysfunction.

Autonomy
People's right to make decisions for themselves.

Behavioural and psychological symptoms of dementia (BPSD)
The behavioural and psychological symptoms of dementia include: mood disorders, psychosis, wandering, inappropriate vocalization, aggression.

Behaviour therapy
Therapy targeted at specific behaviours in an attempt to extinguish unwanted behaviour and encourage desired behaviour.

Bibliotherapy
A therapy that involves giving the patient selected, educational reading matter in order to encourage self-help and psychological change.

Bioavailability
The physiological availability of a given amount of a drug, as distinct from its chemical potency; the proportion of the administered dose which is absorbed into the bloodstream.

Biopsychosocial model
Engels' holistic concept of perceiving a patient's problems by examining the impact and interplay of biological, psychological, and social processes.

Consultation liaison psychiatry
A branch of psychiatry in which a psychiatrist provides psychiatric consultations for patients admitted to non-psychiatric medical systems.

Carer or caregiver
A person who looks after or gives care to an elderly person, such as a nurse or family member.

Challenging incident
Behaviour that is considered to be a risk to the patient or others in the vicinity.

Cochrane review
A systematic review of similar randomized controlled trials or studies of a specified intervention; conducted according to the protocols of the Cochrane Collaboration, to establish where research results are consistent, eliminate bias, and reduce random error, in order to make meaningful, evidence-based decisions about the effects of healthcare.

Cognition
A generic term embracing the mental activities associated with thinking, learning, and memory. Any process whereby one acquires knowledge.

Cognitive appraisal

The mental process of assessment of an event from a personal perspective based on memory, learning, thinking, and emotion.

Cognitive–behavioural model

The idea that a person's thinking is structured into thoughts about the self, the world, and others. Emotions are dependent on thinking patterns and behaviour is the response to both.

Cognitive–behaviour therapy

A psychotherapy based on the cognitive–behavioural model

Comorbidity

The coexistence of more than one medical or psychiatric disorder in the same person.

Competency

The ability of a person to make rational decisions concerning personal affairs or welfare.

Counselling

A professional activity, whereby one person endeavours to help another to understand and to solve his or her adjustment problems. Counselling includes giving of advice, opinion, and guidance. Also see psychotherapy.

Countertransference

A psychoanalytical term, which refers to the analyst's transference (usually unconscious) toward the patient, of the therapist's emotional needs and feelings, to the detriment of the desired objective analyst–patient relationship.

Culture

A specific set of ideas, values, norms, expectations, and beliefs held by a group of people and constituting a shared basis for social action.

Diaschisis

A sudden inhibition of function produced by an acute focal disturbance in a portion of the brain at a distance from the original seat of injury, but anatomically connected with it through nerve fibre tracts.

Disability

Decreased functioning as a result of disease or illness.

Disease

An illness or sickness. An interruption, cessation, or disorder of body functions, systems, or organs. A morbid entity usually characterized by at least two of the following criteria: (1) recognized aetiological agent(s); (2) identifiable group of signs and symptoms; (3) consistent anatomical alterations.

Duty to care
An obligation, sanctioned by law, to provide care, attention, or medical treatment to those in need.

ECT
Electroconvulsive therapy used in the treatment of severe depressive illness.

Elder abuse
Physical, psychological, or financial harm committed against an older person.

Emergency room (ER)
A medical clinic dealing with accidents and emergencies. May be a facility of a hospital or a stand-alone clinic. Synonyms are Accident and Emergency, and Casualty.

Episodic memory
Memory for facts and personal 'episodes'.

Euthanasia
The intentional and consensual putting to death of a person with an incurable or painful disease.

Executive function
The functions of the frontal lobe of the brain

Fiduciary relationship
A relationship in which the law imposes upon one person a paternalistic obligation of care towards another.

Functional mental disorders
A mental disorder affecting social, occupational, or psychological functioning, for which a specific organic cause cannot be found. Examples are depressive disorders, anxiety, non-organic psychoses, and somatoform disorders.

Gerontology
The scientific study of the process and problems of ageing from a non-clinical perspective.

Geriatrics
The branch of medicine concerned with the medical problems and care of old people.

Gerontophobia
Fear of aged people, growing old, or the outward manifestations of ageing.

Gnosis
The perceptive faculty enabling a person to recognize the form and the nature of persons and things; the faculty of perceiving and recognizing.

Handicap
A physical, mental, or emotional condition that interferes with an individual's normal functioning. See also disability.

Illness
A subjective state of being, feeling, or perceiving oneself to be sick.

Impairment
Objective weakening, damage, or deterioration as a result of injury or disease.

Incidence
The number of new cases of a disease in a defined population over a specific period.

Legal jurisdiction
The mandate given by statute for a court to consider a question according to the law.

Legal necessity
An intervention considered justifiable, without informed consent, because it is considered necessary to health or life, when not to do so would result in serious harm to the individual.

Legal status (mental health)
Whether a patient is being treated by order of a Mental Health Act or not.

Life event
A significant event that poses emotional or physical change for the individual that can be perceived as problematic, harmful, stressful, or beneficial and productive.

Locus of control
The individual's personal sense of their ability to control events impinging upon them.

Memory clinic
A clinic, usually outpatient, that specializes in the assessment and management of people with disorders of memory.

Multidisciplinary team
A clinical team composed of several members from different disciplines (such as medical, nursing, occupational therapy, physical therapy, and psychology) who combine and share their expertise to effect holistic management plans.

Neuroimaging
Radiology of the central nervous system. Examples are: computed tomography (CT); magnetic resonance imaging (MRI); single-photon emission computed tomography (SPECT); and positron emission tomography (PET).

Normative transition
Changes that are expected according to the social norms for individuals at particular times in their lives, including events such as retirement, grandparenthood, etc.

Organic mental disorders (OMD)
Psychiatric syndromes that result from neuropathological, or physical disease.

Pain clinic
A clinic that specializes in the assessment and management of chronic pain disorders.

Pathological grief
Grief that persists and fails to resolve within the expected time, or otherwise presents with an atypical pattern of behaviour in response to a major loss.

Perseveration
The constant repetition of a meaningless word or phrase; or the uncontrollable repetition of a previously appropriate or correct response, even though the repeated response has since become inappropriate or incorrect.

'Pickwickian'
Refers to the characteristics illustrated by Mr Pickwick, the central character in Charles Dicken's Victorian novel *The Pickwick papers*, or to the social conditions that were common in nineteenth century England, and described in the novel.

Placement
Transfer of an elderly person to a residential facility such as a nursing home, residential hospital, or supervised hostel.

Polypharmacy
Prescription of multiple drugs in the same patient with the potential for drug–drug interactions and adverse effects

Power of attorney
The legal appointment of a person by another to act for the latter in decisions concerning their property or welfare if they become mentally incapacitated and unable to act for themselves.

Praxis
The performance of an action.

Prevalence
The number of cases of a disease existing in a given population at a specific time (period prevalence) or at a particular moment (point prevalence).

Primary-care physicians
General medical practitioners who are responsible for the initial assessment and treatment of people in a community. Variously known as family doctors, community physicians, general practitioners.

Psychopharmacology
Also known as neuropsychopharmacology. The use of drugs to treat mental and psychological disorders. The science of the relationship between drugs and behaviour.

Psychotherapy
The treatment of emotional, behavioural, personality, and psychiatric disorders based primarily upon verbal communication with the patient, in contrast to treatments utilizing chemical and physical measures.

Psychogeriatrics
Also known as the specialty of psychiatry of old age, geropsychiatry, or geriatric psychiatry.

Rehabilitation
Restoration, following disease, illness, or injury, of the ability to function in a normal or near-normal manner.

Restraint
An intervention to prevent an excited or violent patient from doing harm to himself or others. Restraint may involve the use of a physical restraint or sedative drugs.

Reversible dementia
Memory loss that recovers if the cause is identifiable and treatable.

Rumination
Periodic and repetitive reconsideration of the same subject.

Screening scales
Psychometric instruments that are designed to separate people or objects according to a fixed characteristic or property.

Semantic memory
Memory for the meaning and significance of language.

Social network
The type and extent of a person's social roles, contacts, and support mechanisms.

Stigma
Visible evidence of a disease. A mark of shame or discredit. A feeling of humiliation as a result of having an illness or disease.

Subcortical dementia
Dementia commencing in, or mainly affecting, the subcortex of the brain, beneath the cerebral cortex. Examples are Binswanger's disease, Parkinson's disease, Huntington's chorea, and subcortical vascular dementia.

Tardive dyskinesia
A movement disorder that occurs some weeks or months after taking certain psychotropic (generally antipsychotic) drugs, and which is characterized by abnormal movement of the face, lips, jaw, tongue, and sometimes the trunk and other extremities.

Transference
In psychoanalysis, transference is generally applied to the projection of feelings, thoughts, and wishes on to the analyst, who has come to represent some person from the patient's past. Displacement of affect or one idea from one person to another.

Triage
Medical screening of patients to determine their relative priority for treatment.

Wisdom
Ability to exercise good judgement about important but uncertain matters of life. The ability to understand human nature and the significance and context of events. Relativistic, flexible, and reflective thinking that focuses on the meaning of life and relationships.

Index